Primary Sclerosing Cholangitis

Lisa M. Forman
Editor

Primary Sclerosing Cholangitis

Current Understanding, Management, and Future Developments

Springer

Editor
Lisa M. Forman
Department of
Gastroenterology-Hepatology
University of Colorado
1635 Aurora Court, B-154
Aurora, CO 80045
USA

ISBN 978-3-319-40906-1 ISBN 978-3-319-40908-5 (eBook)
DOI 10.1007/978-3-319-40908-5

Library of Congress Control Number: 2016959029

Printed on acid-free paper

This Springer imprint is published by Springer Nature

Preface

Primary Sclerosing Cholangitis: Current Understanding, Management, and Future Developments grew out of a need I perceived within the fields of hepatology and liver transplantation. Primary sclerosing cholangitis (PSC) is a rare disease, with an incidence ranging from 0.04 to 1.30 per 1000,000 person years. Patients with PSC have variable presentations and there is significant variability in progression and prognosis. As a clinician, it has been frustrating that up until recently there has been little we could offer patients with PSC, other than liver transplantation, and little that we knew about its pathogenesis. In the liver community, much effort has been made into finding a cure for hepatitis C, a much more common chronic liver disease. With the development of successful antiviral therapies for hepatitis C, there has been a renewed interest into potential treatments of cholestatic diseases.

Indeed, it is an exciting time for PSC. Great work has been done to further clarify the role of genetics, immunology, and the microbiome with regard to the development and progression of PSC. Although liver transplantation remains the definitive treatment for advanced PSC, there are multiple new agents that are in clinical trials which will hopefully halt and even improve the fibrosis and subsequent complications associated with PSC. Endoscopic techniques have vastly improved over the past decade, and cholangiocarcinoma, a once universally fatal disease, can now be cured with liver transplantation.

In this book, recognized international experts in cholestatic diseases review the epidemiology, pathophysiology, current and future management of PSC, its variants, and associated complications. Up-to-date data regarding genetics, cholangiocyte biology, and immunology of PSC are presented. I hope that this publication will be of interest and utility to the medical and scientific community at large, with the ultimate goal of improving our understanding and treatment of this orphan disease.

Aurora, CO, USA Lisa M. Forman

Acknowledgments

I appreciate and gratefully acknowledge the dedicated, hardworking members of the Liver Team at the University of Colorado Denver: Gregory Everson, MD; James Burton, MD; Hugo Rosen, MD; Amanda Wieland, MD; Michael Kriss, MD; Igal Kam, MD; Thomas Bak, MD; Michael Wachs, MD; Trevor Nydam, MD; Kendra Conzen, MD; Catherine Ray, RN, BSN, MA; Maura McCourt, RN; Holley Reitz, RN; Kaitlyn Paus, RN; Catherine Behnke, RN; Mindy Stewart, RN; Lori McCoy, RN; Amy Huntsman, RN; Jaime Cisek, RN; Sarah Tise, PA; Lindsay Pratt, PA; Deidre Ellis, Administrator of the Transplant Center, Tracy Steinberg, RN, MS, CCTC; Lana Schoch, RN; Lauren Basham, RN; Amanda Kober, RN; Andrea Chester, RN, Kathleen Orban, RN, CCTC; Danica Farrington, RN; Jenny Sanderson, LCSW; John Scheid, LSW; and finally, my research team-Jennifer DeSanto, RN; Halley Isberg, BA; and Allison Pabisch BS. I am lucky to work with such a dedicated group of people who are committed to the care and management of patients with liver disease.

Special thanks to Ricky Safer and her wonderful advocacy group, PSC Partners Seeking a Cure. Most importantly, I wish to acknowledge all my patients with PSC and their families whose stories have inspired me, who have put their trust in me, and who have challenged me to become a better physician.

Finally, this book would not have been possible without the efforts of the authors – I appreciate their enthusiasm, critical thinking, and willingness to participate in this project.

Contents

Contributors

Christopher L. Bowlus, MD Division of Gastroenterology and Hepatology, University of California Davis, Sacramento, CA, USA

James R. Burton Jr. University of Colorado Hospital, Anschutz Outpatient Pavilion, Aurora, CO, USA

Tamsin Cargill, MBBS, BSc(Hons) Translational Gastroenterology Unit, John Radcliffe Hospital, Oxford, UK

Nuffield Department of Medicine, University of Oxford, Oxford, UK

Roger W. Chapman, MD, FRCP, FAASLD Nuffield Department of Medicine, University of Oxford, Oxford, UK

Nuffield Department of Medicine, Translational Gastroenterology Unit, Level 5, John Radcliffe Hospital, Oxford, UK

Kendra Conzen, MD Division of Transplant Surgery, Department of Surgery, University of Colorado School of Medicine, Aurora, CO, USA

Emma L. Culver, MBChB, BSc(Hons), MRCP, PhD Translational Gastroenterology Unit, John Radcliffe Hospital, Oxford, UK

Nuffield Department of Medicine, University of Oxford, Oxford, UK

Albert J. Czaja, MD Division of Gastroenterology and Hepatology, Mayo Clinic College of Medicine, Rochester, MN, USA

Janette D. Durham, MD Division of Interventional Radiology, University of Colorado School of Medicine, Aurora, CO, USA

Blair Fennimore, MD Assistant Professor of Medicine, Division of Gastroenterology and Hepatology, University of Colorado School of Medicine, 12700 E. 19th Ave. MS B-146, Aurora, CO 80045, USA

Mark E. Gerich, MD Assistant Professor of Medicine, Division of Gastroenterology and Hepatology, University of Colorado School of Medicine, 12700 E. 19th Ave. MS B-146, Aurora, CO 80045, USA

Hazem T. Hammad, MD Section of Interventional Endoscopy, Division of Gastroenterology and Hepatology, University of Colorado Anschutz Medical Campus, Aurora, CO, USA

Gideon M. Hirschfield Centre for Liver Research, NIHR Birmingham Liver Biomedical Research Unit, University of Birmingham, Birmingham, UK

Bing Q. Huang Division of Gastroenterology and Hepatology, Mayo Clinic Center for Signaling in Gastroenterology, Mayo Clinic, Rochester, MN, USA

Thor Johnson, MD Division of Interventional Radiology, University of Colorado School of Medicine, Aurora, CO, USA

Tom Hemming Karlsen Norwegian PSC Research Center, Division of Cancer Medicine, Surgery and Transplantation, Department of Transplantation Medicine, Oslo University Hospital Rikshospitalet, Oslo, Norway

Section of Gastroenterology, Division of Cancer Medicine, Surgery and Transplantation, Department of Transplantation Medicine, Oslo University Hospital Rikshospitalet, Oslo, Norway

Institute of Clinical Medicine, Faculty of Medicine, University of Oslo, Oslo, Norway

Research Institute of Internal Medicine, Division of Cancer Medicine, Surgery and Transplantation, Oslo University Hospital, Oslo, Norway

Craig Lammert, MD Division of Gastroenterology and Hepatology, Indiana University School of Medicine, Indianapolis, IN, USA

Nicholas LaRusso Division of Gastroenterology and Hepatology, Mayo Clinic Center for Signaling in Gastroenterology, Mayo Clinic, Rochester, MN, USA

Keith D. Lindor, MD College of Health Solutions, Arizona State University, Phoenix, AZ, USA

Lorena Loarca Division of Gastroenterology and Hepatology, Mayo Clinic Center for Signaling in Gastroenterology, Mayo Clinic, Rochester, MN, USA

Cara L. Mack, MD Section of Pediatric Gastroenterology, Hepatology and Nutrition, Children's Hospital Colorado, University of Colorado School of Medicine, Aurora, CO, USA

Dania Molla-Hosseini, MD Section of Pediatric Gastroenterology, Hepatology and Nutrition, Children's Hospital Colorado, University of Colorado School of Medicine, Aurora, CO, USA

Leslie Morton Division of Gastroenterology and Hepatology, Mayo Clinic Center for Signaling in Gastroenterology, Mayo Clinic, Rochester, MN, USA

Larissa Muething University of Colorado Hospital, Anschutz Outpatient Pavilion, Aurora, CO, USA

Trevor L. Nydam, MD Division of Transplant Surgery, Department of Surgery, University of Colorado School of Medicine, Aurora, CO, USA

Steven O'Hara Division of Gastroenterology and Hepatology, Mayo Clinic Center for Signaling in Gastroenterology, Mayo Clinic, Rochester, MN, USA

María José Lorenzo Pisarello Division of Gastroenterology and Hepatology, Mayo Clinic Center for Signaling in Gastroenterology, Mayo Clinic, Rochester, MN, USA

Emilie H. Regner, MD Assistant Professor of Medicine, Division of Gastroenterology and Hepatology, University of Colorado School of Medicine, 12700 E. 19th Ave. MS B-146, Aurora, CO 80045, USA

Paul D. Russ, MD, FACR Department of Radiology, University of Colorado Hospital, University of Colorado Denver, Anschutz Medical Campus, Aurora, CO, USA

Raj J. Shah, MD, FASGE, AGAF Section of Interventional Endoscopy, Division of Gastroenterology and Hepatology, University of Colorado Anschutz Medical Campus, Aurora, CO, USA

Patrick Splinter Division of Gastroenterology and Hepatology, Mayo Clinic Center for Signaling in Gastroenterology, Mayo Clinic, Rochester, MN, USA

Mark G. Swain, MD, MSc, FRCPC, FAASLD Cal Wenzel Family Foundation Chair in Hepatology, Professor of Medicine, Head, Division of Gastroenterology and Hepatology, University of Calgary, Section Head, Section of Gastroenterology and Hepatology, Calgary Zone, Alberta Health Services, TRW Building, 3280 Hospital Dr., NW, Calgary, Alberta, Canada T2N 4N1

James H. Tabibian, MD, PhD Division of Gastroenterology, University of Pennsylvania, Philadelphia, PA, USA

Center for Endoscopic Education, Innovation, and Training, University of Pennsylvania, Philadelphia, PA, USA

James F. Trotter, MD Director, Hepatology, Baylor University Medical Center, 3410 Worth Street #860, Dallas, TX 75246, USA

John M. Vierling, MD, FACP, FAASLD Division of Abdominal Transplantation, Department of Medicine and Surgery, Baylor College of Medicine, Baylor-St. Luke's Medical Center, Houston, TX, USA

Raj Vuppalanchi, MD Division of Gastroenterology and Hepatology, Indiana University School of Medicine, Indianapolis, IN, USA

Epidemiology and Natural History of Primary Sclerosing Cholangitis

1

Christopher L. Bowlus

Introduction

Primary sclerosing cholangitis (PSC) is a rare, heterogeneous, idiopathic, inflammatory disorder of the bile ducts resulting in strictures of the intrahepatic and/or extrahepatic bile ducts. The classic form of PSC, which accounts for the majority of PSC cases, as originally described has several characteristic features in addition to the classic cholangiographic features of strictures in the large and medium-sized bile ducts. The so-called large duct PSC occurs predominantly in men (male-to-female ratio, 3:2), is coexistent with IBD in 60–80 % of cases, and typically presents with cholestasis. The IBD typically is a pancolitis with frequent ileitis and rectal sparing. A small group of PSC patients present with clinical and histologic features compatible with PSC, except for the lack of typical cholangiographic findings and have been defined as small duct PSC [1]. IgG4-related sclerosing cholangitis, often found in association with autoimmune pancreatitis as one of many diseases associated with elevated IgG4 serum levels and tissue infiltration of IgG4 plasma cell, represents a separate disease entity and should be distinguished from PSC.

C.L. Bowlus, MD
Division of Gastroenterology and Hepatology, University of California Davis, 4150 V Street, PSSB 3500, Sacramento, CA 95817, USA
e-mail: clbowlus@ucdavis.edu

Although the great majority of PSC patients have inflammatory bowel disease (IBD), only ~5 % of IBD patients will develop PSC, the underlying causes of this association remaining poorly understood. PSC affects all age groups and has been described in a variety of ethnic and racial groups but is best characterized in populations of Northern European descent. The natural history of PSC is variable in terms of liver disease progression with numerous possible clinical outcomes. In addition to progression to portal hypertension, cirrhosis, and its complications, PSC patients may also suffer from bacterial cholangitis, cholangiocarcinoma, gallbladder cancer, and colorectal adenocarcinoma. Increasing collaboration has led to an improved understanding of the epidemiology of PSC, the heterogeneity of its presentation, and its natural history.

Diagnosis

According to the American Association for the Study of Liver Disease (AASLD) practice guidelines, the diagnosis PSC can be made in "patients with a cholestatic biochemical profile, when cholangiography (e.g., magnetic resonance cholangiography [MRC], endoscopic retrograde cholangiography [ERC], percutaneous transhepatic cholangiography) shows characteristic bile duct changes with multifocal strictures and segmental dilatations, and secondary causes of sclerosing cholangitis have been excluded" [2].

L.M. Forman (ed.), *Primary Sclerosing Cholangitis*, DOI 10.1007/978-3-319-40908-5_1

The AASLD guidelines also consider patients with clinical, biochemical, and histological features compatible with PSC but have a normal cholangiogram, to be classified as small duct PSC. However, these criteria are problematic for number of reasons.

First, not all patients with PSC demonstrate cholestatic liver test yet otherwise fulfill these criteria. Second, interpretation of cholangiograms can be difficult to quantify and limited by technical and interobserver variability. Although MRCP remains the initial diagnostic imaging tool of choice with a sensitivity 86 % and specificity 94 % of for the diagnosis of PSC [3, 4], a negative MRCP does not obviate the need for ERCP as MRCP lacks sensitivity in early PSC and can lack specificity in cirrhosis [5]. Third, the classic "onion-skinning" of concentric fibrosis is found in only a minority of PSC cases and is not specific to PSC. Finally, excluding secondary causes of sclerosing cholangitis can be difficult, particularly in patients without IBD who may have undergone cholecystectomy during an evaluation of cholestasis. In light of these limitations, there has yet to be a set of objective criteria upon which a case definition can be established. In fact, the defining features of the PSC cholangiogram may represent numerous different pathways leading to the same clinical disease. As we better understand the various clinical phenotypes, immunologic abnormalities, and genetic basis of PSC, the development of a more rigorous diagnostic framework may arise.

Signs and Symptoms

The typical symptoms of PSC include right upper quadrant abdominal discomfort and fatigue. Pruritus can occur but is typically episodic, coinciding with biliary obstruction. Signs and symptoms of bacterial cholangitis, including fever and right upper quadrant pain with or without jaundice, may also occur sporadically. Weight loss may also be reported at presentation. Although the majority patients have a concomitant IBD, it is frequently quiescent. Therefore, a colonoscopy is mandatory at PSC diagnosis in all patients. This should also include intubation of the terminal ileum to rule out ileitis.

Diagnostic Evaluation

As noted above, the diagnosis of PSC is typically entertained in the setting of cholestatic biochemical abnormalities. However, the diagnosis should also be considered in the setting of advanced liver disease of unknown etiology, particularly in individuals with IBD. Although no serologic markers have sufficient accuracy in diagnosing PSC, they are helpful in establishing the certainty in difficult cases. Serum IgG levels are elevated 1.5 times the upper limit of normal in approximately 60 % of PSC patients, and IgG4 levels can be found to be elevated in approximately 10 % of patients. The latter is of particular importance along with imaging and histology in order to exclude the diagnosis of IgG4-sclerosing cholangitis. In addition, a number of autoantibodies can be found with high prevalence. Notably, the atypical perinuclear anti-neutrophil cytoplasmic antibody (pANCA) is present in up to 80 % PSC patients but is also commonly found in patient with autoimmune hepatitis. Antinuclear antibody and anti-smooth muscle antibody are also frequently present, but alone should not be considered diagnostic of overlap with autoimmune hepatitis. The importance of liver biopsy and the diagnostic evaluation of PSC have decreased over time. Given that this is a disease of the medium and large-sized bile ducts that may be regionally affected, liver biopsy frequently does not reflect the disease or its severity. Nevertheless, liver biopsy remains an important diagnostic tool when there is a disproportionate elevation of serum aminotransferase levels to rule out overlap with autoimmune hepatitis or when the cholangiogram is normal and small duct PSC is suspected.

Epidemiology

The incidence and prevalence of PSC appears to be highest in North America and Northern Europe where it has been most extensively studied, and estimates of approximately incidence and prevalence rates of 1–1.5 cases per 100,000 person-years and 6–16 cases per 100,000 inhabitants, respectively, have been reported [6–8]. However, there are several limitations to our understanding of PSC epidemiology, and current data may underestimate the true prevalence of PSC. Notably, prior to the widespread use of MR cholangiography, diagnosis relied upon liver biopsy or invasive cholangiographic methods such as endoscopic retrograde cholangiography (ERC) to diagnose PSC. For a disease with no proven therapy, many clinicians may have decided not to pursue the diagnosis of PSC in patients with IBD and abnormal liver tests. In addition, liver biochemistries may not be particularly sensitive to identify PSC among IBD patients. Without routine imaging of the biliary tree, the true prevalence of PSC cannot be known. Lack of awareness of PSC may lead to underdiagnosis as well. PSC is a rare disease and not well appreciated by general practitioners who may not entertain the diagnosis.

In addition to underdiagnosis, other structural limitations have prevented an accurate estimate of PSC prevalence and incidence. Specifically, most studies derive data from limited populations from specialized centers in specific geographic areas and are not truly population based. In addition, the lack of an International Classification of Diseases, 9th Revision, Clinical Modification (ICD-9) code defining PSC has hampered true population-based estimates of PSC from administrative data. ICD-10 does little to rectify this issue but there is movement to change this for ICD-11.

Prevalence and Incidence Rates

Early studies of cohorts estimated that the incidence of PSC in North America and Northern Europe was approximately 0.9–1.3 cases per 100,000 person-years (Table 1.1) [6, 9, 10]. Subsequent population-based studies have estimated similar incidence rates [8, 11], while several other studies have placed the estimates at approximately 0.4–0.5 cases per 100,000 [12–14]. Importantly, two of these studies have demonstrated increasing incidence over time suggesting either an increasing incidence of disease or increasing rate of detection [8, 12].

Data on the prevalence of PSC in other parts of the world are limited. From questionnaire data from Spain and Japan, the estimated prevalence rates were 0.22 and 0.95 cases per 1000,000 inhabitants, respectively [15, 16]. PSC appears to be rare in native Alaskans [17], but PSC dispro-

Table 1.1 Estimates of incidence and prevalence of primary sclerosing cholangitis

Region	Study period	Number of cases	Incidence[a]	Prevalence[b]	Reference
Northern Europe					
Norway	1986–1995	17	1.3	8.5	[9]
Sweden	1992–2005	199	1.22	16.2	[8]
Netherlands	2000–2007	519	0.5	6.0	[12]
UK	1984–2003	46	0.91	12.7	[10]
UK	1987–2002	149	0.41	3.85	[13]
North America					
Rochester, MN	1976–2000	22	0.9	13.6	[6]
California	2000–2006	169	0.41	4.15	[14]
Calgary, Canada	2000–2005	49	0.92	NA	[11]
Spain	1984–1988	43	0.07	0.22	[15]
Japan	2007	415	NA	0.95	[16]

NA not available
[a]Per 100,000 person-years
[b]Per 100,000 inhabitants

portionately accounts for African-Americans listed for liver transplantation suggesting that they have a prevalence similar to whites [18].

Demographics

The demographic characteristics of patients with PSC have been similar regardless of the cohort being described. PSC disproportionately affects men with approximately two-thirds of patients with PSC being male. The age of diagnosis of PSC ranges from children to the elderly, but the median age of diagnosis is typically in the fourth decade [6–8, 12]. Notably, the peak incidence in men is younger than women. Approximately 10 % of cases are in children. The association between PSC and IBD has been consistently reported; however, earlier data suggested that approximately 80 % of patients with PSC had concomitant IBD. In contrast, more recent data estimate this value to be in the range of 65–70 %, with women having a lower prevalence of IBD compared to men with PSC [6–8, 12]. Across all series, nearly 80 % of PSC patients with IBD have ulcerative colitis, while fewer than 20 % have Crohn's disease [6–8, 12].

Natural History

Understanding the natural history of PSC is complicated by a multitude of challenges, most notably an unknowable onset of disease (Fig. 1.1). There is likely to be a preclinical period between the onset of disease and the abnormal cholangiographic findings, which represent established fibrosis. In addition, delay in diagnosis is common resulting in an artificially shortened time from diagnosis to clinical outcome. Further, there are several clinically important outcomes, such as cholangiocarcinoma and colorectal cancer, which are unrelated to liver disease severity. Finally, as with the epidemiology of PSC, changes in technology and increased awareness of the disease have likely lead to the diagnosis of less severe cases. Overall, this might lead to the erroneous conclusion that PSC is becoming more common but less severe.

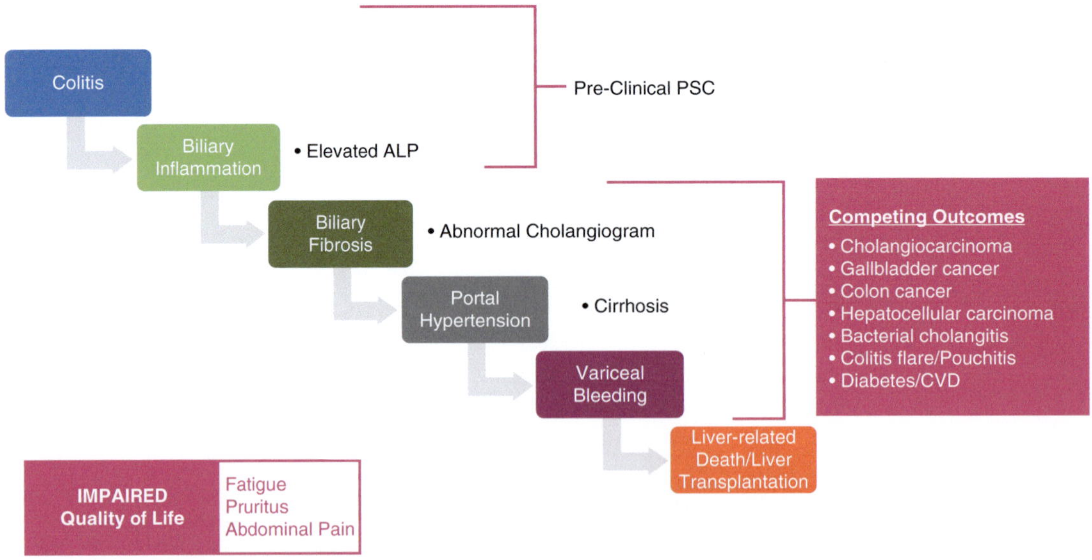

Fig. 1.1 The natural history of primary sclerosing cholangitis (PSC). Prior to the diagnosis of PSC, there is a preclinical stage, which likely involves colitis leading to biliary inflammation. Not until biliary fibrosis is present can the diagnosis of PSC be made by an abnormal cholangiogram. Subsequently, there is a progression of biliary fibrosis leading to portal hypertension, cirrhosis, and its complications. In addition, there are competing risk unrelated to the progression of the liver fibrosis

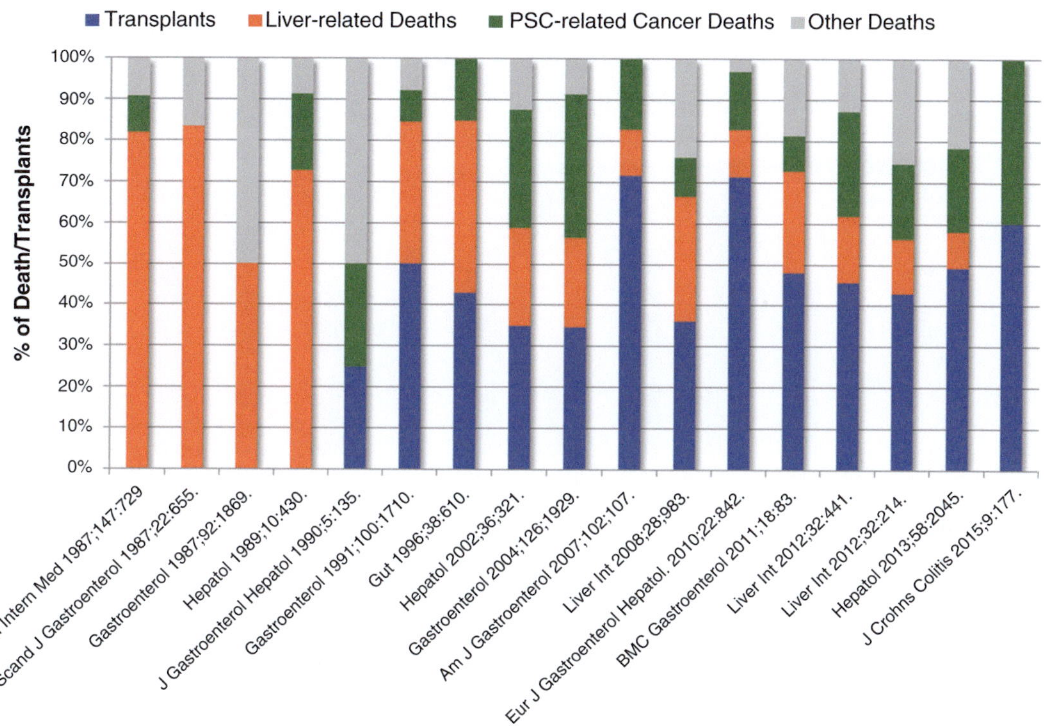

Fig. 1.2 Distribution of outcomes of death and liver transplantation among patients with PSC. In early studies, the majority of deaths were related to liver failure. Increasingly, the primary outcome has become liver transplantation with a smaller percentage dying from liver failure. A variable, but minor, percentage developed PSC-related cancers or die from unrelated causes [12, 19, 48–55]

Most commonly, PSC progresses similar to other chronic liver diseases with liver fibrosis leading to portal hypertension and its associated complications. In early studies, liver-related deaths accounted for approximately 70–80 % of mortality (Fig. 1.2). More recent studies suggest little change with clinical end points of liver transplantation and liver-related deaths still accounting for similar proportion of outcomes. Cancers related to PSC, including cholangiocarcinoma, gallbladder cancer, and colorectal cancer, make up 10–20 % of death in PSC. Like other biliary forms of liver disease, portal hypertension tends to be presinusoidal with esophageal varices developing early in the course of disease. In addition to cirrhosis, biliary strictures can lead to bacterial cholangitis and jaundice. Risks of malignancy are also increased. This includes not only a risk of cholangiocarcinoma and gallbladder cancer but also an increased risk of colorectal cancer in those patients with concomitant IBD.

The estimated median time from diagnosis of PSC to either death or liver transplantation based upon early studies ranged from 9 to 18 years (Fig. 1.3) [19–21]. However, these studies were from tertiary care and liver transplant centers with the potential for significant referral bias. This was illustrated by a study of all PSC patients treated at 44 hospitals in a large geographically defined area in the Netherlands comprising over 8 million people. In this population-based study, the estimated median survival from diagnosis of PSC until liver transplantation or PSC-related death was 21.3 years in the entire cohort compared to only 13.2 years for patients receiving care at a transplant center [12].

Risk Prediction in PSC

Predicting outcomes from PSC is important not only for individual patients but also for clinical

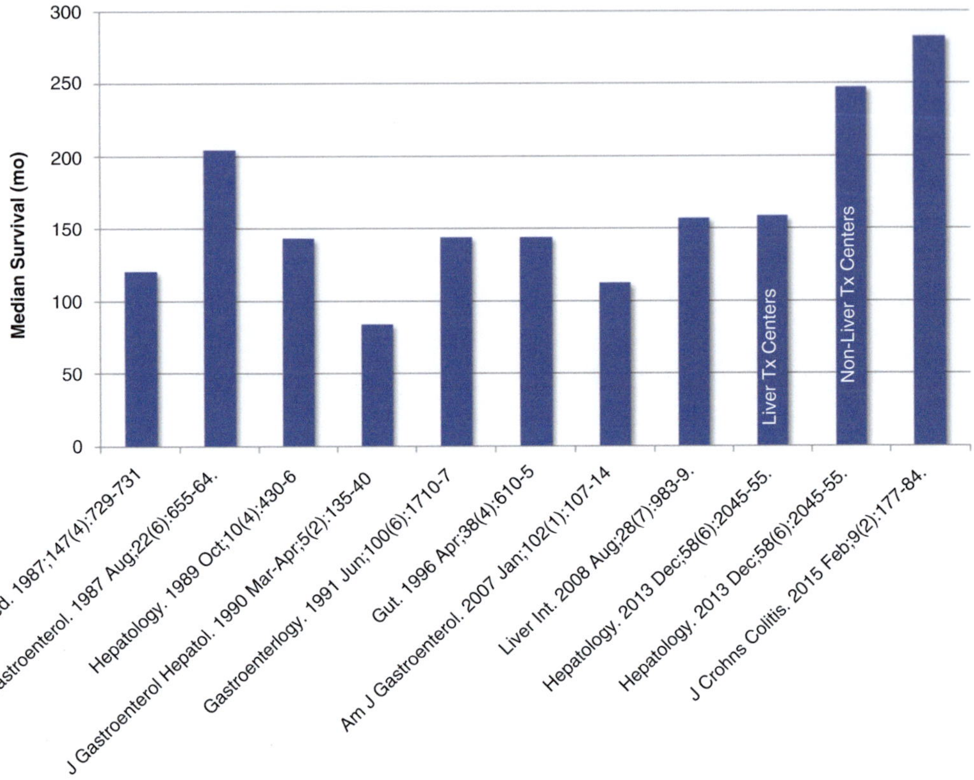

Fig. 1.3 The median transplant-free survival across multiple studies [12, 19, 48–55]

trial design and decisions on liver transplantation. Although the model of end-stage liver disease (MELD) score is used universally for predicting outcomes in patients with cirrhosis regardless of etiology, it is worth noting that the MELD score has not been studied in PSC patients with cirrhosis. Because cholestasis occurs relatively early in PSC compared to hepatocellular-based causes of cirrhosis, commonly used models for cirrhosis such as the Child-Turcotte-Pugh (CTP) classification and the MELD score may not adequately predict outcomes in PSC. In contrast, several risk models have been developed over time to prognosticate and predict outcomes in patients with PSC regardless of cirrhosis status. These models have incorporated different combinations of clinical, histological, and/or laboratory parameters (Table 1.2). As expected, bilirubin and markers of portal hypertension are common to all of the PSC models described. However, it is quite informative that only one model carried alkaline phosphatase into the final predictive model given recent findings that suggest normalization of alkaline phosphatase portends good long-term transplant-free survival.

The Mayo risk score, which unlike some other models, does not include histological criteria requiring a liver biopsy, is the only validated model, and remains the most commonly used [22]. It was developed and validated to prognosticate outcomes in patients with all stages of disease and is based purely on objective clinical and laboratory criteria. The revised Mayo risk score includes serum bilirubin, albumin, aspartate aminotransferase, age, and history of variceal bleeding. In derivation and validation cohorts, this score estimated survival up to 4 years after calculation [23].

Limitation of the Mayo risk score and other models include the lack of long-term predictions of outcome and lack of responsiveness to intervention making them less attractive as end points

Table 1.2 Prognostic models of survival in primary sclerosing cholangitis [19, 23, 52, 53, 56]

	King's (n=126)	Hannover (n=273)	Sweden[a] (n=305)	Europe[b] (n=330)	Revised Mayo (n=405;124)
Demographics					
Age	⊗	⊗	⊗	⊗	⊗
Laboratory/pathology					
Alkaline phosphatase	⊗				
Aspartate aminotransferase (AST)					⊗
Total bilirubin		⊗[c]	⊗	⊗	⊗
Albumin		⊗		⊗	⊗
Biopsy stage	⊗		⊗		
Clinical findings					
Hepatomegaly	⊗	⊗			
Splenomegaly	⊗	⊗			
Clinical events					
Variceal bleeding					⊗

[a]Cases with variceal bleeding (4 % of total) excluded
[b]Time-dependent model
[c]Persistently elevated bilirubin

in clinical trials. Noninvasive fibrosis markers, including measures of liver stiffness by transient elastography and serum markers of fibrosis, are currently being evaluated. In a prospective study of patients with PSC, liver stiffness measurement (LSM) using vibration-controlled transient elastography (VCTE) was accurate at differentiating PSC patients into those with minimal to no fibrosis versus those with severe fibrosis and cirrhosis [24]. VCTE was superior to other noninvasive markers of fibrosis in patients with PSC, notably the FIB-4 score and the Mayo risk score. Furthermore, among 142 patients monitored with VCTE for an average of 3.9 ± 2.1 years, LSM demonstrated a slow progression in those patients with minimal fibrosis (F0 or F1) but an exponential increase in stiffness over time once patients reached a fibrosis stage of F2 or greater. Once patients reached an F4 stage of fibrosis (cirrhosis), the median time from compensated to decompensated cirrhosis was 3.6 years, with a significantly increased risk of liver-related complications in patients with either a greater amount of baseline fibrosis or a more rapid increase in their LSM [24].

The Enhanced Liver Fibrosis (ELF) score combines three serum markers: tissue inhibitor of metalloproteinases-1 (TIMP-1), hyaluronic acid (HA), and intact N-terminal propeptide of type III procollagen (PIIINP) and has also been studied in PSC patients [25]. Importantly, the ELF score was significantly great in PSC compared to ulcerative colitis patients without PSC, and ulcerative colitis disease activity did not appear to affect the ELF score. However, the ELF score did distinguish between mild and severe PSC disease defined by clinical outcome of transplantation or death with an area under the receiver-operator curve (AUROC) of 0.81. Additionally, in multivariable survival models, the ELF score was significantly associated with transplant-free survival, independent from the Mayo risk score. The ELF risk score correlated with VCTE in separate assessments, which highlights the applicability of either of these noninvasive measures of fibrosis as a means to prognosticate outcomes of patients with PSC [25].

Clinical Phenotypes

In addition to risk models and noninvasive markers, a variety of clinical features have been associated with differences in natural history and clinical outcomes. The classic form of PSC, which accounts for the majority of PSC cases, as originally described has several characteristic features in addition to the classic cholangiographic features of strictures in the large and medium-sized bile ducts. Namely, large duct PSC occurs predominantly in men (male-to-female ratio, 3:2), is coexistent with IBD in 60–80 % of cases, and typically presents with cholestasis. The IBD typically is a pancolitis with frequent ileitis and rectal sparing. In addition, the IBD is commonly mild and asymptomatic. The association between PSC and IBD appears to be greater in Northern latitudes, although, even there, the frequency of non-IBD PSC is increasing.

Dominant bile duct strictures, defined as strictures with a diameter of less than 1.5 mm of the common bile duct or less than 1.0 mm of a hepatic duct within 2 cm of the bifurcation, develop in approximately half of PSC patients and are associated with poor outcomes even with endoscopic management [26, 27]. This decreased survival has been suggested to be due to the increased prevalence of cholangiocarcinoma. In contrast, small duct PSC, which comprises approximately 10 % of PSC cases, rarely progresses to large duct PSC and has a favorable outcome [1].

The impact of IBD, both in terms of its absence or type, on the natural history of PSC has increasingly been recognized. PSC in the absence of IBD tends to be equally distributed among men and women, is diagnosed at an older age [28], and may have a better prognosis [29]. The presence of Crohn's disease has also been associated with a better prognosis in recent studies [30, 31]. However, differentiating between ulcerative colitis and Crohn's disease is often difficult given that fistulizing or fibrostenotic Crohn's disease is rare in PSC. Studies of PSC in non-Caucasians are limited, but African-Americans listed for liver transplantation with PSC are younger and with greater MELD scores compared to whites with PSC [18].

Overlap between PSC and autoimmune hepatitis remains a controversial issue, especially regarding diagnostic criteria. The prevalence of this overlap has been reported to be between 1 and 53.8 % reflecting the lack of agreed-upon criteria. Case reports and clinical experience suggest two types of presentation. One in which there is coexisting features of both diseases; the other in which a typical case of autoimmune hepatitis transforms into a cholestatic variant. Interestingly, 10 % or more of patients with autoimmune hepatitis will have cholangiographic features consistent with PSC [32, 33]. Overlap with autoimmune hepatitis also appears to be more frequent in pediatric cases of PSC as discussed in Chaps. 4 and 6.

Recently, the rate of inflammatory bowel disease among African-Americans has been increasing with distinct clinical and genetic features. Not surprisingly, PSC has also been demonstrated to be prevalent in African-Americans. Genetically, there is still a strong HLA association with HLA-B8. In addition, among African-Americans listed for liver transplantation with the diagnosis of PSC, the male predominance is less pronounced, the frequency of the inflammatory valve disease is less, but the patients are listed at a younger age and with a greater MELD score suggesting a more aggressive disease [14, 18].

In addition to demographic and clinical features, laboratory markers may have prognostic value in distinguishing patients with PSC into groups with elevated IgG4 and normal serum alkaline phosphatase. Contrasting results on the impact of elevated serum IgG4 and disease course have been reported with the first study suggesting that an elevated IgG4 levels was associated with a shorter time from disease presentation to liver transplantation, while a second report was unable to replicate this finding[34, 35]. More consistent has been the finding that reduction and/or normalization in serum alkaline phosphatase levels is associated with longer survival times, irrespective of treatment leading to this normalization [36–39].

Complications

Malignancy in PSC

Patients with PSC are not only at risk for progressive liver fibrosis and liver failure but also are at significantly increased risks of three cancers:

cholangiocarcinoma, colorectal adenocarcinoma, and gallbladder carcinoma. Importantly, unlike the risk of hepatocellular carcinoma in chronic viral hepatitis, the risks of these cancers in PSC are not related to disease stage. In fact, aside from a greater incidence of cholangiocarcinoma in the first year following diagnosis, the annual incidence rates of these cancers appear to be constant. Details regarding hepatobiliary and colorectal malignancies are addressed in Chaps. 2 and 3, respectively.

Nonmalignant Outcomes of PSC

In addition to the progression to end-stage liver disease and malignant complications, there are several important nonmalignant outcomes related to PSC. These include the development of the dominant stricture, which as noted above is associated with a lower rate of survival, bacterial cholangitis, and hepatic osteodystrophy.

Dominant Stricture

Dominant strictures occur with a cumulative frequency of 36 to 57 % of patients with PSC. The presence of a dominant stricture is of particular concern for cholangiocarcinoma and should be evaluated by brush cytology and/or biopsy [45]. In the short term, management of dominant structures involves endoscopic evaluation and treatment. However, whether there is benefit to regular dilation in the absence of symptoms or worsening cholestasis has not been adequately studied.

Bacterial Cholangitis

The prevalence, incidence, and natural history a bacterial cholangitis and PSC have been rarely studied, primarily because the diagnosis is a clinical one. Patients with PSC frequently have abdominal pain and often report transient episodes of fever, which may resolve spontaneously. Among patients with PSC listed for liver transplantation, 48 % were reported to have developed bacterial cholangitis while awaiting transplantation [46]. Interestingly, there was no increase in wait-list removal for death or deterioration associated with bacterial cholangitis.

Hepatic Osteodystrophy

Osteopenic bone disease is frequent in patients with cirrhosis from any cause and has been well studied in patients with primary biliary cholangitis (PBC). Although PSC affects primarily younger men who are at very low risk of low bone mineral density, approximately 15 % of PSC patients have osteoporosis defined by a T-score less than −2.5 [47]. The presence of age ≥54 years or older, body mass index ≤24 kg/m^2, and inflammatory bowel disease for ≥19 years all correlated with osteoporosis.

Conclusion

PSC is a rare inflammatory disease of the bile ducts that is often associated with inflammatory bowel. It is unique among autoinflammatory diseases in its strong male predominance. The disease frequently progresses over decades to biliary cirrhosis and liver failure but may also result in malignancies of the bile ducts, gallbladder, and colon. These latter outcomes that are unrelated to disease stage make the development of prognostic models and surrogate markers problematic. In addition, the rarity of PSC and its heterogeneity requires international collaboration and cooperation to fully understand and classify the subphenotypes, which may lead to a better understanding of the underlying pathophysiology as well as more accurate predictive models.

References

1. Bjornsson E, Olsson R, Bergquist A, Lindgren S, Braden B, Chapman RW, et al. The natural history of small-duct primary sclerosing cholangitis. Gastroenterology. 2008;134(4):975–80.
2. Chapman R, Fevery J, Kalloo A, Nagorney DM, Boberg KM, Shneider B, et al. Diagnosis and management of primary sclerosing cholangitis. Hepatology (Baltimore, Md). 2010;51(2):660–78.
3. Dave M, Elmunzer BJ, Dwamena BA, Higgins PD. Primary sclerosing cholangitis: meta-analysis of diagnostic performance of MR cholangiopancreatography. Radiology. 2010;256(2):387–96.
4. Hekimoglu K, Ustundag Y, Dusak A, Erdem Z, Karademir B, Aydemir S, et al. MRCP vs. ERCP in the evaluation of biliary pathologies: review of current literature. J Dig Dis. 2008;9(3):162–9.

5. Weber C, Kuhlencordt R, Grotelueschen R, Wedegaertner U, Ang TL, Adam G, et al. Magnetic resonance cholangiopancreatography in the diagnosis of primary sclerosing cholangitis. Endoscopy. 2008;40(9):739–45.
6. Bambha K, Kim WR, Talwalkar J, Torgerson H, Benson JT, Therneau TM, et al. Incidence, clinical spectrum, and outcomes of primary sclerosing cholangitis in a United States community. Gastroenterology. 2003;125(5):1364–9.
7. Eaton JE, Talwalkar JA, Lazaridis KN, Gores GJ, Lindor KD. Pathogenesis of primary sclerosing cholangitis and advances in diagnosis and management. Gastroenterology. 2013;145(3):521–36.
8. Lindkvist B, Benito de Valle M, Gullberg B, Bjornsson E. Incidence and prevalence of primary sclerosing cholangitis in a defined adult population in Sweden. Hepatology (Baltimore, Md). 2010;52(2):571–7.
9. Boberg KM, Aadland E, Jahnsen J, Raknerud N, Stiris M, Bell H. Incidence and prevalence of primary biliary cirrhosis, primary sclerosing cholangitis, and autoimmune hepatitis in a Norwegian population. Scand J Gastroenterol. 1998;33(1):99–103.
10. Kingham JG, Kochar N, Gravenor MB. Incidence, clinical patterns, and outcomes of primary sclerosing cholangitis in South Wales, United Kingdom. Gastroenterology. 2004;126(7):1929–30.
11. Kaplan GG, Laupland KB, Butzner D, Urbanski SJ, Lee SS. The burden of large and small duct primary sclerosing cholangitis in adults and children: a population-based analysis. Am J Gastroenterol. 2007;102(5):1042–9.
12. Boonstra K, Weersma RK, van Erpecum KJ, Rauws EA, Spanier BW, Poen AC, et al. Population-based epidemiology, malignancy risk, and outcome of primary sclerosing cholangitis. Hepatology (Baltimore, Md). 2013;58(6):2045–55.
13. Card TR, Solaymani-Dodaran M, West J. Incidence and mortality of primary sclerosing cholangitis in the UK: a population-based cohort study. J Hepatol. 2008;48(6):939–44.
14. Toy E, Balasubramanian S, Selmi C, Li CS, Bowlus CL. The prevalence, incidence and natural history of primary sclerosing cholangitis in an ethnically diverse population. BMC Gastroenterol. 2011;11:83.
15. Escorsell A, Pares A, Rodes J, Solis-Herruzo JA, Miras M, de la Morena E. Epidemiology of primary sclerosing cholangitis in Spain. Spanish Association for the Study of the Liver. J Hepatol. 1994;21(5):787–91.
16. Tanaka A, Takikawa H. Geoepidemiology of primary sclerosing cholangitis: a critical review. J Autoimmun. 2013;46:35–40.
17. Hurlburt KJ, McMahon BJ, Deubner H, Hsu-Trawinski B, Williams JL, Kowdley KV. Prevalence of autoimmune liver disease in Alaska Natives. Am J Gastroenterol. 2002;97(9):2402–7.
18. Bowlus CL, Li CS, Karlsen TH, Lie BA, Selmi C. Primary sclerosing cholangitis in genetically diverse populations listed for liver transplantation: unique clinical and human leukocyte antigen associations. Liver Transpl. 2010;16(11):1324–30.
19. Broome U, Olsson R, Loof L, Bodemar G, Hultcrantz R, Danielsson A, et al. Natural history and prognostic factors in 305 Swedish patients with primary sclerosing cholangitis. Gut. 1996;38(4):610–5.
20. Ponsioen CY, Vrouenraets SM, Prawirodirdjo W, Rajaram R, Rauws EA, Mulder CJ, et al. Natural history of primary sclerosing cholangitis and prognostic value of cholangiography in a Dutch population. Gut. 2002;51(4):562–6.
21. Angulo P, Maor-Kendler Y, Lindor KD. Small-duct primary sclerosing cholangitis: a long-term follow-up study. Hepatology (Baltimore, Md). 2002;35(6): 1494–500.
22. Kim WR, Poterucha JJ, Wiesner RH, LaRusso NF, Lindor KD, Petz J, et al. The relative role of the Child-Pugh classification and the Mayo natural history model in the assessment of survival in patients with primary sclerosing cholangitis. Hepatology (Baltimore, Md). 1999;29(6):1643–8.
23. Kim WR, Therneau TM, Wiesner RH, Poterucha JJ, Benson JT, Malinchoc M, et al. A revised natural history model for primary sclerosing cholangitis. Mayo Clinic Proc Mayo Clinic. 2000;75(7):688–94.
24. Corpechot C, Gaouar F, El Naggar A, Kemgang A, Wendum D, Poupon R, et al. Baseline values and changes in liver stiffness measured by transient elastography are associated with severity of fibrosis and outcomes of patients with primary sclerosing cholangitis. Gastroenterology. 2014;146(4):970–9; quiz e15–6.
25. Vesterhus M, Hov JR, Holm A, Schrumpf E, Nygard S, Godang K, et al. Enhanced liver fibrosis score predicts transplant-free survival in primary sclerosing cholangitis. Md).: Hepatology (Baltimore; 2015.
26. Bjornsson E, Lindqvist-Ottosson J, Asztely M, Olsson R. Dominant strictures in patients with primary sclerosing cholangitis. Am J Gastroenterol. 2004;99(3):502–8.
27. Rudolph G, Gotthardt D, Kloters-Plachky P, Kulaksiz H, Rost D, Stiehl A. Influence of dominant bile duct stenoses and biliary infections on outcome in primary sclerosing cholangitis. J Hepatol. 2009;51(1):149–55.
28. Eaton JE, Juran BD, Atkinson EJ, Schlicht EM, Xie X, de Andrade M, et al. A comprehensive assessment of environmental exposures among 1000 North American patients with primary sclerosing cholangitis, with and without inflammatory bowel disease. Aliment Pharmacol Ther. 2015;41(10):980–90.
29. Ngu JH, Gearry RB, Wright AJ, Stedman CA. Inflammatory bowel disease is associated with poor outcomes of patients with primary sclerosing cholangitis. Clin Gastroenterol Hepatol Off Clin Pract J Am Gastroenterol Assoc. 2011;9(12):1092–7; quiz e135.
30. Halliday JS, Djordjevic J, Lust M, Culver EL, Braden B, Travis SP, et al. A unique clinical phenotype of primary sclerosing cholangitis associated with Crohn's disease. J Crohns Colitis. 2012;6(2):174–81.
31. Fevery J, Van Steenbergen W, Van Pelt J, Laleman W, Hoffman I, Geboes K, et al. Patients with large-duct primary sclerosing cholangitis and Crohn's disease have a better outcome than those with ulcerative colitis, or without IBD. Aliment Pharmacol Ther. 2016;43(5):612–20.

32. Abdalian R, Dhar P, Jhaveri K, Haider M, Guindi M, Heathcote EJ. Prevalence of sclerosing cholangitis in adults with autoimmune hepatitis: evaluating the role of routine magnetic resonance imaging. Hepatology. 2008;47(3):949–57.
33. Lewin M, Vilgrain V, Ozenne V, Lemoine M, Wendum D, Paradis V, et al. Prevalence of sclerosing cholangitis in adults with autoimmune hepatitis: a prospective magnetic resonance imaging and histological study. Hepatology. 2009;50(2):528–37.
34. Mendes FD, Jorgensen R, Keach J, Katzmann JA, Smyrk T, Donlinger J, et al. Elevated serum IgG4 concentration in patients with primary sclerosing cholangitis. Am J Gastroenterol. 2006;101(9): 2070–5.
35. Benito de Valle M, Muller T, Bjornsson E, Otten M, Volkmann M, Guckelberger O, et al. The impact of elevated serum IgG4 levels in patients with primary sclerosing cholangitis. Digest Liver Dis Off J Ital Soc Gastroenterol Ital Assoc Study Liver. 2014;46(10): 903–8.
36. Stanich PP, Bjornsson E, Gossard AA, Enders F, Jorgensen R, Lindor KD. Alkaline phosphatase normalization is associated with better prognosis in primary sclerosing cholangitis. Digest Liver Dis Off J Ital Soc Gastroenterol Ital Assoc Study Liver. 2011;43(4):309–13.
37. Lindstrom L, Hultcrantz R, Boberg KM, Friis-Liby I, Bergquist A. Association between reduced levels of alkaline phosphatase and survival times of patients with primary sclerosing cholangitis. Clin Gastroenterol Hepatol Off Clin Pract J Am Gastroenterol Assoc. 2013;11(7):841–6.
38. Talwalkar JA, Chapman RW. The resurgence of serum alkaline phosphatase as a surrogate biomarker for prognosis in primary sclerosing cholangitis. Clin Gastroenterol Hepatol Off Clin Pract J Am Gastroenterol Assoc. 2013;11(7):847–9.
39. Hilscher M, Enders FB, Carey EJ, Lindor KD, Tabibian JH. Alkaline phosphatase normalization is a biomarker of improved survival in primary sclerosing cholangitis. Ann Hepatol. 2016;15(2):246–53.
40. Rustagi T, Dasanu CA. Risk factors for gallbladder cancer and cholangiocarcinoma: similarities, differences and updates. J Gastrointest Cancer. 2012;43(2): 137–47.
41. Claessen MM, Vleggaar FP, Tytgat KM, Siersema PD, van Buuren HR. High lifetime risk of cancer in primary sclerosing cholangitis. J Hepatol. 2009;50(1): 158–64.
42. Fevery J, Henckaerts L, Van Oirbeek R, Vermeire S, Rutgeerts P, Nevens F, et al. Malignancies and mortality in 200 patients with primary sclerosering cholangitis: a long-term single-centre study. Liver Int. 2012; 32(2):214–22.
43. Thackeray EW, Charatcharoenwitthaya P, Elfaki D, Sinakos E, Lindor KD. Colon neoplasms develop early in the course of inflammatory bowel disease and primary sclerosing cholangitis. Clin Gastroenterol Hepatol Off Clin Pract J Am Gastroenterol Assoc. 2011;9(1):52–6.
44. Ananthakrishnan AN, Cagan A, Gainer VS, Cheng SC, Cai T, Szolovits P, et al. Mortality and extraintestinal cancers in patients with primary sclerosing cholangitis and inflammatory bowel disease. J Crohns Colitis. 2014;8(9):956–63.
45. Bowlus CL, Olson KA, Gershwin ME. Evaluation of indeterminate biliary strictures. Nat Rev Gastroenterol Hepatol. 2016;13(1):28–37.
46. Goldberg DS, Camp A, Martinez-Camacho A, Forman L, Fortune B, Reddy KR. Risk of waitlist mortality in patients with primary sclerosing cholangitis and bacterial cholangitis. Liver Transpl. 2013;19(3):250–8.
47. Angulo P, Grandison GA, Fong DG, Keach JC, Lindor KD, Bjornsson E, et al. Bone disease in patients with primary sclerosing cholangitis. Gastroenterology. 2011;140(1):180–8.
48. Lebovics E, Palmer M, Woo J, Schaffner F. Outcome of primary sclerosing cholangitis. Analysis of long-term observation of 38 patients. Arch Intern Med. 1987;147(4):729–31.
49. Aadland E, Schrumpf E, Fausa O, Elgjo K, Heilo A, Aakhus T, et al. Primary sclerosing cholangitis: a long-term follow-up study. Scand J Gastroenterol. 1987;22(6):655–64.
50. Wiesner RH, Grambsch PM, Dickson ER, Ludwig J, MacCarty RL, Hunter EB, et al. Primary sclerosing cholangitis: natural history, prognostic factors and survival analysis. Hepatology (Baltimore, Md). 1989;10(4):430–6.
51. Jeffrey GP, Reed WD, Laurence BH, Shilkin KB. Primary sclerosing cholangitis: clinical and immunopathological review of 21 cases. J Gastroenterol Hepatol. 1990;5(2):135–40.
52. Farrant JM, Hayllar KM, Wilkinson ML, Karani J, Portmann BC, Westaby D, et al. Natural history and prognostic variables in primary sclerosing cholangitis. Gastroenterology. 1991;100(6):1710–7.
53. Tischendorf JJ, Hecker H, Kruger M, Manns MP, Meier PN. Characterization, outcome, and prognosis in 273 patients with primary sclerosing cholangitis: a single center study. Am J Gastroenterol. 2007;102(1): 107–14.
54. Tanaka A, Takamori Y, Toda G, Ohnishi S, Takikawa H. Outcome and prognostic factors of 391 Japanese patients with primary sclerosing cholangitis. Liver Int. 2008;28(7):983–9.
55. Yanai H, Matalon S, Rosenblatt A, Awadie H, Berdichevski T, Snir Y, et al. Prognosis of primary sclerosing cholangitis in Israel is independent of coexisting inflammatory Bowel disease. J Crohns Colitis. 2015;9(2):177–84.
56. Boberg KM, Rocca G, Egeland T, Bergquist A, Broome U, Caballeria L, et al. Time-dependent Cox regression model is superior in prediction of prognosis in primary sclerosing cholangitis. Hepatology (Baltimore, Md). 2002;35(3):652–7.

Malignancy and Primary Sclerosing Cholangitis: Cholangiocarcinoma, Hepatocellular Carcinoma, and Gallbladder Carcinoma

2

Larissa Muething and James R. Burton Jr.

Technical Terms and Abbreviations

AASLD	American Association for the Study of Liver Diseases
AFP	Alpha-fetoprotein
AJCC	American Joint Committee on Cancer
BCLC	Barcelona Clinic Liver Cancer
CCA	Cholangiocarcinoma
CLIP	Cancer of the Liver Italian Program
CT	Computerized tomography
CTP	Child-Turcotte-Pugh
DDLT	Deceased donor liver transplantation
ERCP	Endoscopic retrograde cholangiopancreatography
EUS	Endoscopic ultrasound
FISH	Fluorescence in situ hybridization
FNA	Fine needle aspiration
GBC	Gallbladder carcinoma
HCC	Hepatocellular carcinoma
LDLT	Living donor liver transplantation
MELD	Model for end-stage liver disease
MRCP	Magnetic resonance cholangiopancreatography
MRI	Magnetic resonance imaging
NCCN	National Comprehensive Cancer Network
OLT	Orthotopic liver transplantation
PDT	Photodynamic therapy
PIVKA II	Prothrombin induced by vitamin K absence II
PSC	Primary sclerosing cholangitis
RFA	Radiofrequency ablation
TACE	Transarterial chemoembolization
TNM	Tumor, node, metastasis
UCSF	University of California, San Francisco
UNOS	United Network for Organ Sharing
US	Ultrasound
Y-90	Yttrium-90

L. Muething (✉) • J.R. Burton Jr.
University of Colorado Hospital,
Anschutz Outpatient Pavilion, 7th Floor,
Transplant Center, 1635 Aurora Court, B154,
Aurora, CO 80045, USA
e-mail: James.Burton@UCDenver.edu

Cholangiocarcinoma

Introduction

Cholangiocarcinoma (CCA) is a common and devastating malignancy associated with primary sclerosing cholangitis (PSC). Cholangiocarcinoma is classified into intrahepatic CCA and extrahepatic CCA. Intrahepatic cholangiocarcinomas are located within the hepatic parenchyma. The anatomic boundary between intrahepatic CCAs and extrahepatic CCAs are the second-order bile ducts. Extrahepatic CCA is further differentiated into perihilar tumors, also known as Klatskin tumors, and distal tumors. The cystic ducts serve

L.M. Forman (ed.), *Primary Sclerosing Cholangitis*, DOI 10.1007/978-3-319-40908-5_2

as the anatomic boundary between perihilar and distal tumors. The location of CCA affects both the management and prognosis. The majority of CCAs associated with PSC are perihilar. Overall CCA has a poor prognosis in PSC.

Epidemiology

Individuals with PSC are at significantly higher risk for developing CCA. Bergquist et al. found that in a Swedish cohort, the incidence of hepatobiliary malignancy was 161 times higher in individuals with PSC compared to the general population [5]. The incidence of CCA in PSC reported in the literature varies widely but is most frequently reported to be in the range 7–14 % in population-based studies [5, 12, 38]. A higher incidence is reported in transplant studies with 10–36 % of incidental diagnoses of CCA at the time of transplant for PSC [1, 27, 34, 49, 52]. Up to 50 % of cases of cholangiocarcinoma are diagnosed within the first year of PSC diagnosis [10]. The exact reason is not known; however, we suspect that this may be due in part that the symptoms associated with malignancy prompt the diagnosis of PSC. After the first year, the annual incidence is 0.5–1.5 % [5, 15, 19, 29].

Pathogenesis

CCA arises from the bile duct epithelial cells (cholangiocytes) (Fig. 2.1) [16]. Chronic inflammation in the biliary tract, as is found in PSC, predisposes individuals to the development of CCA. Conversion from normal to malignant bile epithelium likely involves an accumulation of successive genetic mutations, similar to colorectal carcinoma. The oncogenesis in PSC, however, is not as well understood. The mechanism of chronic inflammation leading to somatic mutations is thought to be in part facilitated by inducible nitric oxide synthase (iNOS). Studies have found iNOS expression in PSC cholangiocytes, and formation of iNOS is thought to cause oxidative DNA damage and inactivation of the DNA repair process [35]. Mutations in several genes involved in cell growth and tumor suppression have been identified in the oncogenesis of PSC-associated CCA. Overexpression of the *p53* tumor suppressor gene has been identified in up to 93 % of PSC-associated CCA; other genes include *p16*, *EGFR*, *and Her2/neu* [64]. In addition polymorphisms in *NKG2D*, an activating receptor on the surface of T lymphocytes and natural killer cells, have been found to be associated with increased risk of cholangiocarcinoma in PSC [64]. Identifying additional molecular targets is an area of avid research in PSC-associated CCA with the ultimate goal of developing new targeted therapies.

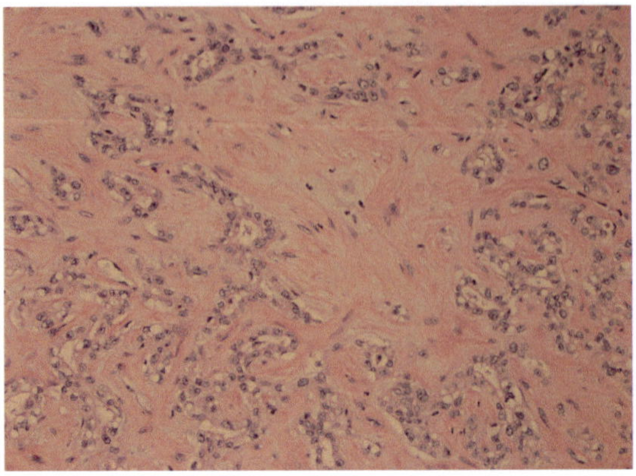

Fig. 2.1 Cholangiocarcinoma is represented by infiltrative glands with morphologic atypia with nuclear hyperchromasia and distinct nucleoli with surrounding desmoplastic tissue (200×; Courtesy of Dr. Jeffery Kaplan)

Risk Factors

There are several risk factors associated with an increased risk of CCA (both intrahepatic and extrahepatic) in the general population including parasitic infections [62] and biliary tract disorders. In PSC, specifically, several risk factors have also been linked to an increased risk of developing PSC. High alcohol consumption has been found to be associated with a higher risk of CCA. Chalasani et al. found alcohol consumption had an odds ratio of 2.95 (95 % CI 1.04–8.3) for developing CCA [17]. A case control study of 20 patients found smoking to be higher in PSC patients with CCA ($p < 0.0004$) [6]. However, subsequent studies have failed to replicate this correlation [15, 17]. Predictors of developing CCA in individuals with PSC include degree of serum bilirubin elevation, variceal bleeding, Mayo score >4, the presence of chronic ulcerative colitis with colorectal cancer or dysplasia, and the duration of inflammatory bowel disease [10]. Interestingly, the duration of PSC has not been found to be associated with a higher risk of CCA in contrast to the higher risk of colonic dysplasia associated with duration of ulcerative colitis. None of these risk factors or predictors have proven to be clinically useful in targeting a population to screen for CCA, however.

Screening

Currently the American Association for the Study of Liver Disease does not have published guidelines for routine screening for CCA in patients with PSC due to lack of highly sensitive and cost-effective diagnostic testing. The American College of Gastroenterology recommends considering screening with ultrasound or MRI and serial CA 19-9 every 6–12 months [43]. While consensus guidelines have not yet been established, most providers do screen for CCA in patients with PSC with routine liver chemistries every 3–6 months and annual MRI/MRCP and CA 19-9. Based on the results of these studies as well as clinical information, those with suspicion for CCA often undergo ERCP to assess for a dominant stricture where biliary tract brushings for cytology and fluorescent in situ hybridization (FISH) are typically performed [63].

Diagnosis

Overview

Diagnosis of CCA can be challenging. A dominant stricture in a patient with PSC is a stenosis with a diameter of ≤1.5 mm in the common bile duct or ≤1 mm in the hepatic ducts [9]. It is often difficult to distinguish a benign dominant stricture from PSC from a malignant stricture; thus, one should have a high index of suspicion for CCA when a patient develops evidence of biliary obstruction (jaundice, cholestasis, pruritus, cholangitis), unexplained weight loss, or abdominal pain. A multidisciplinary approach is often needed to diagnose CCA including laboratory studies, cross-sectional imaging, cholangioscopy, and pathology.

Imaging

A variety of imaging modalities are used in the diagnosis of CCA including ultrasound (US), computerized tomography (CT), and magnetic resonance imaging (MRI) with concurrent magnetic resonance cholangiopancreatography (MRCP) (see Chap. 13). The positive predictive value is nearly 100 % if a characteristic lesion is found on US, CT, or MRI (Table 2.1). Characteristic lesions, however, are not commonly seen, especially in early-stage CCA. The overall positive predictive value for US, CT, and MRI are 48 %, 38 %, and 40 %, respectively [19].

CA 19-9

The most commonly used laboratory test besides routine liver enzymes to detect CCA is CA 19-9. CA 19-9 is an antibody that binds to the tumor surface marker Sialyl-Lewis A. CA 19-9 is found to be elevated (normal typically up to 35 U/ml) in multiple other diseases and bile duct conditions including ascending cholangitis, hepatocellular carcinoma, alcoholic liver disease, primary biliary cirrhosis, chronic viral hepatitis, autoimmune hepatitis, and pancreatitis. Levy et al. found that in PSC, a CA 19-9 of ≥129 U/mL had a sensitiv-

Table 2.1 Characteristic appearance of cholangiocarcinoma on various imaging modalities

Imaging modality	Appearance of characteristic lesion
Ultrasound	Well-defined mass with echogenicity different from that of the liver
CT	Well-defined mass with hypoattenuating enhancement relative to the liver on portovenous phase and hyperattenuating on delayed phase imaging
MRI	Well-defined mass hypointese on T1-weighted imaging and hyperintense on T2-weighted imaging

ity of 79 %, a specificity of 98 %, and a positive predictive value of 79 % for CCA [40]. A change in CA 19-9 of ≥63.2 U/mL had a sensitivity of 90 %, specificity of 98 %, and a positive predictive value of 42 %.

Biliary Brushing

Endoscopic retrograde cholangiopancreatography (ERCP) is often used in patients with PSC to further investigate and characterize biliary strictures and to manage biliary obstruction with balloon dilation and stenting. Tissue sampling of dominant strictures is often achieved through bile duct brushings for cytology. Routine biliary cytology alone has been found to be highly specific (95–100 %) but to have lower sensitivity (36–83 %) [42]. The broad range in sensitivity cited in literature is due to the definition of a positive cytology results. Studies that defined a positive finding as both high-grade and low-grade dysplasia had a higher sensitivity than those that only defined high-grade dysplasia as a positive result.

Fluorescence In Situ Hybridization

Fluorescence in situ hybridization (FISH) can be used in addition to cytology to increase sensitivity for malignancy. Fluorescence in situ hybridization uses fluorescently labeled DNA probes to detect chromosomal aneuploidy (losses or gains of chromosomes). Abnormalities are characterized as trisomy, tetrasomy, and polysomy of chromosomes 3 and/or 7. Trisomy refers to ≥10 cells with three copies of chromosome 3 and 7, tetrasomy refers to ≥10 cells with four copies of all probes, and polysomy refers to ≥5 cells with ≥3 signals in two or more of the four probes [3]. Trisomy and tetrasomy of chromosomes 3 and 7 have low specificity for PSC as these findings are frequently found in biliary tree inflammation without malignancy. In contrast, polysomy has a specificity of 88 % for CCA [3]. It is difficult to interpret positive FISH polysomy in the setting of negative cytology. Patients with positive polysomy on serial brushings are significantly more likely to be diagnosed with cholangiocarcinoma than those with subsequent nonpolysomy results [4]. The presence of both polysomy and CA 19-9 ≥ 129 U/mL was a significant predictor for developing CCA (hazard ratio of 20.4 (95 % CI 7.94–52.63)) for polysomy and CA 19-9 ≥ 129 U/mL versus nonpolysomy and CA 19-9 < 129 U/mL [4]. If a patient with PSC is found to have negative cytology and polysomy, they should be followed up closely with repeat ERCP and biliary brushings for cytology and FISH especially if there is a non-resolving dominant stricture and/or elevated CA 19-9. Compared with other prognostic features, multifocal (multiple areas of the biliary tree) polysomy carries the highest risk for cholangiocarcinoma compared to unifocal polysomy HR 82.4 (95 % CI 24.5–277.3) vs. 13.27 (95 % CI 3.32–53.1), respectively, on univariate analysis [24]. Multifocality remains a stronger predictor of CCA even when adjusting for CA 19-9, cytology, and prior abnormal FISH. Patients with unifocal polysomy with suspicious cytology remain at increased risk. If serial polysomy is detected in a malignant appearing stricture, even in the setting of negative cytology, liver transplantation should be considered. Figure 2.2 summarizes the approach to managing a dominant stricture in patients with PSC.

Cholangioscopy with Biopsy

Cholangioscopy allows for direct visualization of the biliary tree and theoretically improves sampling as it allows for directed bile duct biopsies. Visual characteristics suspicious for malignancy are exophytic lesions, ulcerations, papillary mucosal projections, dilated tortuous vessels, and raised lesions [20, 60]. A meta-analysis showed that cholangioscopy with targeted biopsies of dominant strictures was able to detect CCA with a sensitivity and specificity of 66.2 % and 97 %, respectively [37].

Endoscopic Ultrasound

Endoscopic ultrasound (EUS) with fine needle aspiration (FNA) of a biliary stricture has also been used for additional tissue sampling in the setting of indeterminate biliary brushings and FISH. However, this method carries a risk of tract seeding and peritoneal metastasis and should be avoided, especially in patients potentially eligible for liver transplantation. In one study, 83 % of individuals who underwent a transperitoneal or trans-

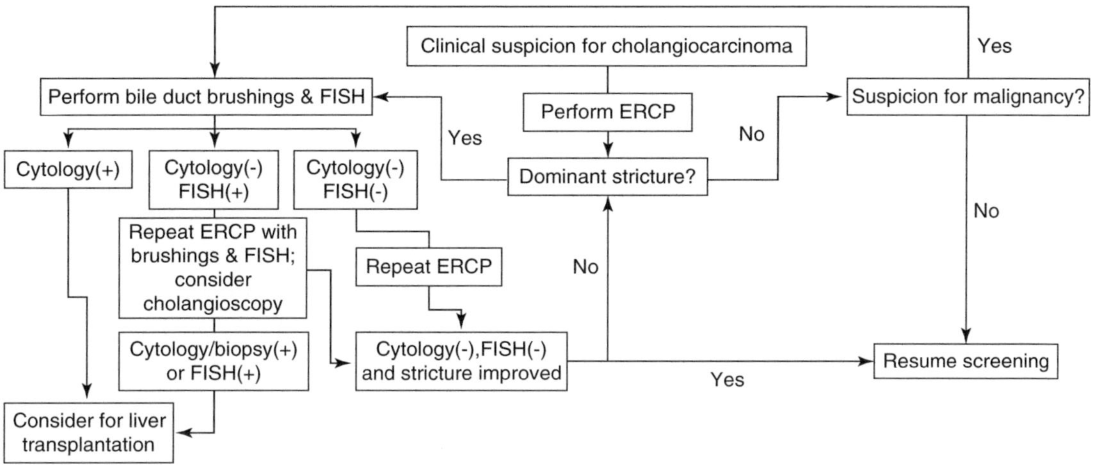

Fig. 2.2 Evaluation of the primary sclerosing cholangitis patient with clinical suspicion for cholangiocarcinoma. A dominant stricture in a patient with PSC is a stenosis with a diameter of ≤1.5 mm in the common bile duct or ≤1 mm in the hepatic ducts. Positive cytology and biopsy refers to that which is diagnostic for cholangiocarcinoma, and positive fluorescence in situ hybridization (FISH) refers to the presence of polysomy (*ERCP* endoscopic retrograde cholangiopancreatography)

luminal biopsy of biliary strictures had peritoneal metastasis compared to 8 % peritoneal metastasis in those who did not undergo biopsy [32]. EUS with FNA may be useful to sample lymph nodes to evaluate for metastatic disease in those being considered for liver transplantation and is often done prior to exploratory laparotomy.

Management

The mainstay of treatment for CCA is surgery. The only potential curative therapies include either liver resection or liver transplant. Patients with PSC are often not candidates for surgical resection due to the presence of diffuse bile duct disease and/or the presence of advanced hepatic fibrosis or cirrhosis. Patients with distal common bile duct tumors may be amenable to surgical resection if advanced liver disease is not present.

Surgical Resection

Surgical resection is an option for localized lesions with otherwise normal hepatic parenchyma. Contraindications to surgical resection of hilar CCA include bilateral tumor extension involving the left and right secondary biliary radicles, unilobar involvement with encasement of contralateral portal vein or hepatic artery, bilateral vascular involvement, distant metastases, underlying liver disease (advanced fibrosis or cirrhosis), future liver remnant <25–30 % with no or poor response to portal vein occlusion, and severe comorbidities [33, 55]. Due to the diffuse nature of PSC and risk for advanced hepatic fibrosis, PSC patients with CCA are often not candidates for resection.

Liver Transplantation

Most patients with PSC and the diagnosis of hilar CCA will need to be considered for liver transplantation (LT) as means for a definitive cure. Liver transplantation is not generally considered a treatment for intrahepatic or distal bile duct tumors. The management of the latter is a Whipple procedure which in a patient with severe end-stage liver disease may require concurrent liver transplantation. Historically, LT for CCA has been associated with very poor outcomes. In 2000, The Mayo Clinic developed a protocol for both patient selection and treatment of patients with CCA undergoing LT [23]. Patients fulfilling the so-called Mayo criteria showed superior outcomes with LT compared to historical controls. One study found a median survival of 3.3 years after LT prior to the publication of the Mayo results in

May 2000 compared to a median survival of 7.8 years for LTs done after May 2000 [58].

The Mayo protocol employs neoadjuvant therapy followed by LT as a definitive therapy for patients with hilar CCA. The criteria include patients with biliary duct obstruction and cytologically proven CCA or a mass lesion seen on cross-sectional imaging with biliary obstruction (Table 2.2). The protocol utilizes external and intraductal radiation therapy followed by chemotherapy (capecitabine) until the patient undergoes LT. All patients undergo exploratory surgery prior to LT to exclude extrahepatic disease, either after completing radiation or just prior to transplant. Using this protocol, Rea et al. found that LT with neoadjuvant chemoradiation had significantly improved 5-year survival when compared to conventional resection (82 % vs. 21 %) and had fewer recurrences (12 % versus 27 %) [56]. Overall survival of patients with PSC is approximately 70 % at 5 years. This approach has been externally validated at centers outside Mayo having nearly identical outcomes (65 % 5-year survival) [21]. Currently the United Network for Organ Sharing allows model for end-stage liver disease (MELD) exception points for patients meeting the criteria outlined in the Mayo protocol.

Table 2.2 Criteria for managing cholangiocarcinoma with liver transplantation

Eligible candidates for evaluation:
1. Unresectable hilar cholangiocarcinoma or cholangiocarcinoma in setting of primary sclerosing cholangitis
2. No clinical evidence of metastases
Diagnosis:
1. Intraluminal brush cytology or biopsy positive for cholangiocarcinoma
2. In case of negative cytology, malignant appearing stricture with at least one of the following:
(a) CA 19-9 > 100 ng/ml
(b) Biliary polysomy by FISH
Exclusion criteria:
Medical and psychosocial conditions that preclude transplantation
Prior abdominal radiation preventing further radiation or other malignancy within 5 years
Prior attempted resection with violation of tumor plane or attempt at transperitoneal biopsy of tumor
The presence of mass lesion >3 cm radial margin (longitudinal margin not a contraindication). Vascular encasement, the presence of poorly defined hilar enhancement, and length of hilar stricture not considered exclusion criteria
Intrahepatic metastases
Evidence of extrahepatic disease – includes regional lymph node involvement
Intrahepatic cholangiocarcinoma (tumor originating from second branch (segmental branch) or the proximal branch of bile duct – further classified into hilar type and peripheral type) or gallbladder involvement

Contributing to the excellent outcomes of this protocol are the strict selection criteria. Predictors of pre-LT dropout include CA 19-9 ≥ 500 U/mL, mass lesion ≥3 cm, malignant brushing or biopsy, and biological lab MELD score ≥20. Predictors of post-LT recurrence include elevated CA 19-9, portal vein encasement, and residual tumor on explant [22]. Finally, it is important to note that this protocol does not require the diagnosis of CCA but includes the presence of polysomy alone or elevation in CA 19-9 > 100 with a concurrent malignant appearing dominant stricture. It is possible that excellent outcomes with this protocol are further explained by the fact that patients simply did not have cancer. This is supported by the external validation of this protocol at 12 large volume transplant centers which found that patients without residual CCA on explant did better and had a significantly lower chance of recurrence than those with residual tumor tissue on explant [22]. It is impossible to determine whether these individuals never had CCA to begin with or that their CCA was effectively treated with neoadjuvant chemoradiation.

Palliative Therapies

For patients with unresectable cancers and those who are ineligible for LT, there are a variety of palliative therapies. Multiple locoregional therapies, including transarterial chemoembolization (TACE), radiofrequency ablation (RFA), and transarterial hepatic yttrium-90 (Y-90) can be utilized for debulking and biliary decompression. Systemic chemotherapy with gemcitabine and cisplatin are used in those with unresectable or metastatic disease. Biliary stenting (endoscopic and percutaneous) is utilized for palliation of obstructive jaundice. Photodynamic therapy (PDT) has recently emerged as an endoscopic palliative treatment modality. Kahaleh et al. found that ERCP with PDT decreased mortality in patients with unresectable cholangiocarcinoma compared to ERCP alone (56% vs. 82% at 12 months, respectively) [36].

Hepatocellular Carcinoma

Introduction

Hepatocellular carcinoma (HCC) is a primary malignancy of hepatocytes. It most commonly develops in the setting of cirrhosis, though can occur without cirrhosis in patients with chronic hepatitis B virus infection and hemochromatosis. In the setting of PSC, HCC is almost always seen in the setting of cirrhosis. Hepatocellular carcinoma is a leading cause of cancer in the world, largely contributed to chronic hepatitis B virus infection. Each year HCC is diagnosed in more than half a million people worldwide and 20,000 people in the United States [28].

Epidemiology

There is limited data on the incidence of HCC in PSC, but studies suggest that the cumulative incidence is lower than what is described for other etiologies of cirrhosis. One review of 134 patients with PSC undergoing LT found a prevalence of 2% [31]. In another study with 119 patients with cirrhosis secondary to PSC, none were diagnosed with HCC over a median follow-up of 7 years [69].

Pathogenesis

Not a lot is known about the specific mechanism of HCC development in PSC, but the pathogenesis is likely similar to other etiologies of cirrhosis. Chronic inflammation in PSC leads to hepatocyte necrosis and regeneration. The repetitive necrosis and regeneration leads to the development of benign hyperplastic nodules. Genomic instability and mutations in key oncogenes and tumor suppression genes then lead to the development of dysplastic polyps and ultimately HCC (Fig. 2.3). The exact oncogenesis of HCC is not as well understood as that of other malignant processes; however, several key events have been identified. Important genetic events include inactivation of tumor suppressor *p53*, mutations in β-catenin, overexpression of ErbB receptor family members, and overexpression of the MET receptor [26]. *p53*, in particular, plays a critical role in destabilizing the HCC genome [30]. Specific genomic alterations that have been shown to frequently be present in HCC include chromosomal gains in 1q, 6p, 8q, 11q, and 17q and chromosomal loses in 1p, 4q, 8p, 13q, and 17p [26]. Future studies in this area include utilizing genomic characteristics to help stage and predict recurrence as well as developing targeted therapies.

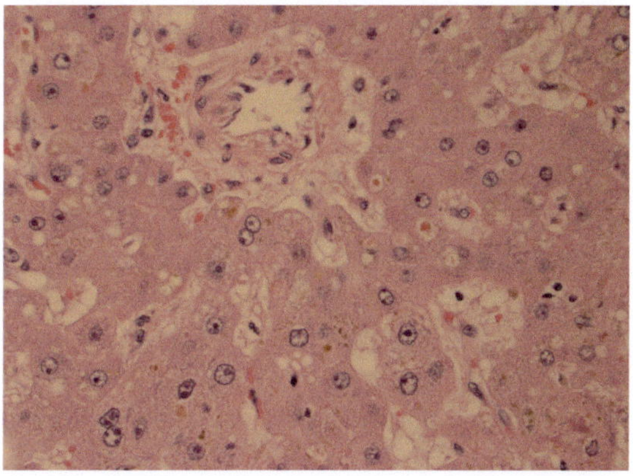

Fig. 2.3 Hepatocellular carcinoma resembles normal hepatocytes with more than 2–3 cell-thick hepatocellular plates or cords, nuclear atypia as evident by enlarged nuclei (high N/C ratio) with prominent nucleoli, and the absence of portal tracks. Bile production is pathognomonic for hepatocyte differentiation and aids in differentiating metastatic neoplasms and intrahepatic cholangiocarcinomas (400×; Courtesy of Dr. Jeffery Kaplan)

Risk Factors

The most significant risk factor for PSC-associated HCC is cirrhosis. The stage of cirrhosis and activity of liver disease influences the risk of HCC. Child-Pugh class B/C cirrhosis carries at three- to eightfold increased risk of HCC compared to Child-Pugh class A [28]. One should have a high suspicion for HCC in patients with previously compensated cirrhosis who develop decompensated disease with ascites, jaundice, variceal bleeding, or encephalopathy. Ongoing inflammation in the liver also increases the risk of HCC as evidenced by an increased risk of HCC observed in patients with persistently elevated ALT levels compared to those with normal levels [28]. Additional independent risk factors associated with HCC in cirrhotic patients are age >55 and male sex, which each carry a two- to fourfold increased risk [25, 28].

Screening

Despite the lower risk of HCC in PSC compared to other etiologies of cirrhosis, screening for HCC is important to perform in all patients who have cirrhosis or advanced fibrosis regardless of the etiology of liver disease. Screening tests fall into two categories, serological and radiological. Alpha-fetoprotein (AFP) has been the most extensively studied. Alpha-fetoprotein can be elevated in both chronic liver disease and HCC; however, an AFP >500 ng/mL (normal is 10–20 ng/mL) is considered diagnostic for HCC [8]. While previously recommended as a screening test for HCC, given its low sensitivity of only about 60 %, AASLD no longer recommends utilizing AFP to screen patients for HCC. Other serological tests such as prothrombin induced by vitamin K absence II (PIVKA II), descarboxyprothrombin, and AFP-L3 have not performed significantly better. Guidelines by AASLD currently recommend screening with ultrasonography (US) every 6 months [13]. Nodules detected on US that are >1 cm in diameter should be further evaluated with contrasted computed tomography (CT) or magnetic resonance imaging (MRI). Nodules < 1 cm should be followed with US every 3 months. If no growth is detected over 2 years, regular surveillance can be resumed. As a screening test, US has been reported to have sensitivity between 65 and 80 % and specificity >90 % [11]. While US is the recommended imaging modality for HCC screening in cirrhosis, CT and MRI should be considered in patients with PSC given concurrent need for CCA screening for which US is not adequate.

Diagnosis

Imaging

Diagnosis of HCC is primarily radiographic. The diagnosis of HCC on cross-sectional imaging requires CT or MRI with three phases: arterial, venous, and delayed. Hepatocellular carcinomas are typically supplied by the hepatic arterial system and not the portal venous system; therefore, characteristic lesions are hyperintense compared to the background liver parenchyma in the arterial phase and hypointense in the venous phase. Another diagnostic feature of HCC is pseudoencapsulation. The presence of these characteristic findings is considered diagnostic of HCC and does not require liver biopsy. Rarely, HCCs can be hypovascular, and such characteristic findings are not present. In such cases biopsy may need to be pursed.

Biopsy

Percutaneous biopsy of liver nodules suspicious for HCC should only be performed in lesions that were nondiagnostic with cross-sectional imaging. Biopsy carries the risk of bleeding and malignant seeding of the biopsy tract. A meta-analysis found the incidence of needle tract tumor seeding to be 2.7 % [62]. When biopsy is performed, per AALSD guidelines, lesions should be evaluated by expert pathologists. Staining for tumor markers including CD34, CK7, glypican 3, Hsp60, and glutamine synthetase can help characterize lesions that are not clearly HCC on biopsy. If biopsy is negative, lesions should be followed every 3–6 months until they disappear, enlarge, or display diagnostic characteristics of HCC. If the lesions enlarge but imaging remains atypical, repeat biopsy should be pursued.

Staging

There is no universal staging system for HCC. The four most commonly used are the Barcelona Clinic Liver Cancer (BCLC) staging system; the tumor, node, metastasis (TNM) staging system; the Okuda system; and the Cancer of the Liver Italian Program (CLIP) score. The BCLC staging system has four stages based on the extent of primary lesion, degree of invasion, symptoms, and performance status [46]. The American Joint Committee on Cancer (AJCC) TNM staging system is based on the number and size of primary tumors, the presence of regional lymph node metastasis, the distance metastasis, and the fibrosis score [2]. The Okuda staging system classifies individuals into three stages based on the presence of four criteria: tumor size >50 % of the area of the liver, the presence of ascites, albumin <3 mg/dL, and bilirubin >3 mg/dL [52]. The CLIP is a prognostic scoring system based on tumor morphology, AFP levels, the presence or absence of portal vein thrombosis, and the severity of cirrhosis. A score from 0 to 6 is calculated based on subscores from variables. For scores 0, 1, 2, 3, and 4–6, median survival was 36, 22, 9, 7, and 3 months, respectively [47]. Regardless of which stage of disease is utilized, in clinical practice the main determinate of management is whether a patient is a candidate for surgical resection or OLT.

Management

The management of HCC depends largely on the size and number of tumors, the presence of macrovascular invasion, and the presence of cirrhosis and portal hypertension.

Surgical Resection

Resection is the treatment of choice for solitary HCCs in individuals without cirrhosis or those with compensated cirrhosis (Child-Pugh class A). Patient with multifocal HCC and/or Child-Pugh class B/C, evidence of portal hypertension (transhepatic pressure gradient >10 mmHg or platelets <100,000/μL and splenomegaly), or elevated bilirubin are at high risk for surgical resection and require consideration for LT. Patients with PSC who develop HCC are not likely to be surgical candidates due to chronic biliary disease, and therefore management is focused on LT and locoregional therapy.

Liver Transplantation and the Milan Criteria

Liver transplantation is the mainstay of treatment for HCC in PSC as it is the only potentially curative therapy. Mazzaferro et al. demonstrated that LT in patients with a single tumor ≤5 cm or 2–3 separate lesions, all ≤3 cm with no evidence of macrovascular invasion or extrahepatic disease resulted in a 5-year survival of 75 %, similar to the survival rate of non-HCC patients undergoing OLT [50]. This so-called Milan criteria are the most widely used criteria for determining eligibility for LT. Patients fulfilling these criteria are eligible for automatic MELD exception points as long as the tumor remains within Milan criteria. Depending on when a patient may be transplanted which currently depends on regional donor availability and whether living donor liver transplantation is considered, locoregional therapy with TACE or RFA is often performed to keep patients within the Milan criteria while awaiting LT. Table 2.3 summarizes the diagnostic criteria of HCC eligible for standard MELD exceptions on the transplant list. Currently patients fulfilling the Milan criteria are granted a MELD exception of 28 points 6 months after the initial upgrade request. Once to 28 points, a MELD score equivalent to a 10 % mortality risk is added every 3 months to a maximum of 34 points (i.e., initially 28, then 29, then 31, then 33, and finally 34). The 6-month delay in receiving MELD exception points was recently included in the allocation of livers for HCC to allow time to assess tumor biology at transplant centers that do transplants at low MELD scores (<25). The cap of 34 points was so patients with HCC do not participate in regional sharing of donor livers which is the case for MELD scores ≥35 (see Chap. 15).

Expanded Criteria

There have been several studies that have looked at expanding the criteria for transplanting HCC

Table 2.3 Organ procurement and transplantation network diagnosis, classification and reporting of hepatocellular carcinoma, and eligibility for MELD exceptions

OPTN Class 5B nodules
T2 lesion(s)
1 lesion ≥2 cm and ≤5 cm
2–3 lesions ≥1 cm and ≤3 cm
And
Increased contrast enhancement on late arterial imaging
And
One of the following:
1. Washout on portal venous/delayed phases
2. Late capsule or pseudocapsule enhancement
3. Growth by >50 % on CT or MRI <6 months apart
4. Biopsy
OPTN Class 5A nodules
Single nodule, ≥1 cm and <2 cm (T1 lesion) with increased contrast enhancement on late arterial images
And
Both of the following:
1. Washout during portal venous/delayed phases
2. Peripheral rim enhancement on delayed phase
Or
Biopsy
Eligible for automatic MELD exception
Two 5A lesions
One 5A and one 5B
One 5B (≤5 cm)
Two 5B (both <3 cm)
Not eligible for automatic MELD exception
One 5A lesion

beyond the Milan criteria. The University of California, San Francisco (UCSF), has demonstrated equivalent outcome compared to Milan criteria by expanding criteria to a single tumor ≤6.5 cm, maximum of three total tumors with none >4.5 cm, and cumulative tumor size <8 cm [66]. The 5-year survival of these so-called UCSF criteria was 72.4 % similar to that of the Milan criteria, suggesting the Milan criteria may be too strict [67]. AASLD guidelines, however, state there is inadequate evidence to support LT outside of the Milan criteria [13]. UCSF has also shown good outcomes with transplant for patients outside Milan criteria who are downstaged to within the Milan criteria with locoregional therapy and remain within Milan criteria for a minimum of 3 months. Results of this protocol showed similar outcomes to the Milan criteria with 5-year posttransplant survival of 77.8 % in the downstaging group versus 81 % in the Milan group ($p=0.69$) [67]. Patients fulfilling either of these expanded criteria do not receive automatic MELD exception points as is the case with those fulfilling Milan criteria, but rather must appeal to the regional review board on a case-by-case basis.

Living Donor Transplantation

Given the long wait times for deceased donor liver transplantation (DDLT) in many areas of the United States and the associated risk of HCC progression to point of exceeding criteria for LT, many transplant centers offer the option of living donor liver transplantation (LDLT). In one retrospective study of LDLT versus DDLT, overall 5-year survival was similar in the two cohorts: 73 % in the LDLT cohort and 71 % in the DDLT cohort [7]. Dropout rates were significantly lower in the LDLT cohort (0 % versus 18 %), and waiting time to LT was significantly shorter (2.6 versus 7.9 months) [7]. Given the potential risk to a living donor, LDLTs in general should only be performed in candidates who meet standard criteria for LT.

Non-curative Treatment

The goals of therapy for patients who are not candidates for surgical resection or LT are aimed at both extending life expectancy and symptomatic management.

Locoregional Therapy

The main goal of locoregional therapy is to reduce tumor burden and extend survival. Overall there are no consensus guidelines, and choice of modality is often based on institutional preferences. Transarterial chemoembolization is the most commonly employed locoregional therapy. This therapy utilizes HCC's dependence on the arterial blood supply by inducing acute arterial obstruction leading to ischemic tumor necrosis in addition to the local effects of chemotherapy administration. It is contraindicated in patients with portal vein tumor thrombus as well as those with Child-Pugh class C cirrhosis due to increased risk of liver failure and death. Survival is improved compared to conservative management. In a randomized control trial, TACE was found to have a 2-year survival of 63 % compared to 27 % in the conservative management group [46]. An issue specific to patients with PSC is TACE cannot be done after in the setting of biliary obstruction or after sphincterotomy due to biliary infectious complications and liver abscess.

Radiofrequency ablation utilizes a needle electrode to deliver high-frequency alternating current from the tip of the electrode to the surrounding tissues which results in increased temperature and subsequent necrosis [51]. It is most often selected for tumors ≤5 cm in diameter as the rate for complete necrosis decreases with larger lesions [45].

Radioembolization using intra-arterial injection of yttrium-90 is another regional therapy utilized to induce tumor necrosis as well as provide local radiotherapy. However, similar to TACE, radioembolization also cannot be used in the setting of prior sphincterotomy and biliary obstruction. Percutaneous ethanol injection is also utilized: 95 % ethanol is injected directly into tumor to induce necrosis and tissue ischemia.

Systemic Chemotherapy

Overall systemic chemotherapy is of limited utility in HCC as it is a relatively chemotherapy-refractory tumor, and patients often do not tolerate chemotherapy due to underlying liver dysfunction associated with HCC. Newer molecularly targeted agents have shown some promise for unresectable, metastatic HCC. The agent with the most data is sorafenib which is a multikinase inhibitor which inhibits tumor angiogenesis through the vascular endothelial growth factor receptor and platelet-derived growth factor receptor as well as directly inhibiting tumor cell proliferation and survival [44]. The SHARP trial, which compared sorafenib to placebo, showed a significant difference in overall survival (10.7 versus 7.9 months; $p<0.05$) in patients who were CTP-A and not candidates for surgical resection [48].

Gallbladder Carcinoma

Introduction

Gallbladder carcinoma (GBC) is an adenocarcinoma arising from the epithelial lining of the gallbladder. Just as chronic inflammation in the biliary tract leads to an increased risk of CCA, patients with PSC are also at an increased risk for gallbladder dysplasia and carcinoma due to chronic inflammation and stasis within the gallbladder.

Epidemiology

In the general population, GBC is a relatively rare disease. Patients with PSC, however, have greater than a tenfold increased risk of GBC compared to the general population. The prevalence of gallbladder carcinoma in patients with PSC is reported to be 3.5–7 % compared to 0.35 % in the general population [14, 57].

Risk Factors

Risk factors for GBC in general are chronic infection with salmonella and gallbladder stones. While there is an increased risk of gallbladder stones in PSC alone, PSC appears to be an independent risk factor for GBC.

Pathogenesis

Not much is known about the pathogenesis of PSC-associated GBC, but the underlying mechanism is likely related to chronic inflammation. The gallbladder epithelium is continuous with the extrahepatic bile duct system, and 25 % of individuals with PSC have been found to have cholecystitis, the majority of which is not associated with gallbladder stones [57]. It has been proposed that there is a metaplasia-dysplasia-carcinoma sequence in PSC-associated GBC [41]. Gallbladder dysplasia, carcinoma in situ, and invasive carcinoma have been shown to have high rates of *p53* mutation; in contrast gallbladder adenomas tend to lack *p53* mutations and have K-*ras* mutations, which are less likely to be found in GBC [41].

Screening

The AASLD recommends annual screening for gallbladder polyps with ultrasound [18]. Whether CT and MRI/MRCP typically used to screen for CCA is adequate to screen for GBC is unclear. In the general population, gallbladder polyps <1 cm are often nonmalignant and can be followed with serial imaging. In PSC, however, even small polyps detected on US are often malignant, and therefore all PSC patients with gallbladder polyps should be considered for cholecystectomy [39].

Diagnosis

The diagnosis of GBC is a histologic one. Most diagnoses of GBC in the general population are detected incidentally during cholecystectomy. Laboratory analysis is of limited utility especially in PSC where patients will have aberrations in serum bilirubin, alkaline phosphatase, and CA 19-9 due to their chronic biliary disease. Suspicious US findings include a mass occupying or replacing the gallbladder lumen, focal or diffuse asymmetric wall thickening, and gallbladder polyps [65]. MRI/MRCP is utilized to further differentiate between benign gallbladder lesions and malignant ones and is also useful in the preoperative staging of GBC [59, 68].

Treatment

Surgical Management

As with CCA and HCC, surgical management is the only potentially curative treatment. Therapy for GBC is largely based on TNM staging. Cholecystectomy alone is sufficient for early tumors which are confined to the mucosa (Tis) or lamina propria (T1a). A radical cholecystectomy with resection of the liver bed is recommended for T1b and T2 lesions [70]. T3 and T4 lesions often involve significant invasion of adjacent organs and surgical resection carries substantial morbidity and mortality. This is especially true in PSC given preexisting hepatic disease. Due to the relative rarity of GBC, there are no large randomized trials to evaluate the role of adjuvant radiation and chemotherapy. 5-Fluorouracil (5-FU)-based chemotherapy regimens are often combined with radiation as adjuvant therapy in ≥T2 disease.

Advanced Stage

For unresectable T3 and T4 lesions, debulking and palliative therapies are similar to those utilized in CCA. For locoregionally advanced and unresectable lesions, external beam radiation with concurrent 5-FU-based chemotherapy is used to attempt to decrease tumor size. For distal metastases, the National Comprehensive Cancer Network (NCCN) recommends gemcitabine and/or a platinum or fluoropyrimidine-based regimen [54]. Percutaneous or endoscopic stenting is also utilized to relieve obstructive jaundice.

Prognosis

The overall prognosis of GBC is poor and declines rapidly with more advanced stages. The 5-year survival of stages I, II, III, and IV in the general population was 54 %, 32 %, 9–10 %, and 2–3 %, respectively [53].

Conclusion

Individuals with PSC are at increased risk for hepatobiliary malignancies which is a significant cause of morbidity and mortality. Surgical resection or liver transplantation in highly selected cases is usually the only curative therapy. Resection is amenable typically in early-stage carcinomas, necessitating early diagnosis in a surveillance program for cholangiocarcinoma, hepatocellular carcinoma, and gallbladder carcinoma. Cholangiocarcinoma is the most common hepatobiliary malignancy associated with PSC and is a common reason for liver transplantation in such patients. Diagnosis of CCA in PSC is challenging due to the difficulty distinguishing benign from malignant biliary strictures. PSC-associated HCC is rare and only arises in cirrhosis. Diagnosis and management is similar to HCC associated with other etiologies of cirrhosis. Gallbladder carcinoma is the less common and less researched hepatobiliary carcinoma associated with PSC; however, it is associated with significant mortality as it is often detected in later stages. More research in the diagnosis and targeted therapies could significantly improve the mortality of PSC-associated hepatobiliary malignancies.

References

1. Abu-elmagd KM, Malinchoc M, Dickson ER, et al. Efficacy of hepatic transplantation in patients with primary sclerosing cholangitis. Surg Gynecol Obstet. 1993;177(4):335–44.
2. AJCC Cancer Staging Manual. 6th ed. New York: Springer; 2002.
3. Bangarulingam SY, Bjornsson E, Enders F, Barr Fritcher EG, Gores G, Halling KC, Lindor KD. Long-term outcomes of positive fluorescence in situ hybridization tests in primary sclerosing cholangitis. Hepatology. 2010;51:174–80.
4. Barr Fritcher EG, Kipp BR, Voss JS, et al. Primary sclerosing cholangitis patients with serial polysomy fluorescence in situ hybridization results are at increased risk of cholangiocarcinoma. Am J Gastroenterol. 2011;106(11):2023–8.
5. Bergquist A, Ekbom A, Olsson R, et al. Hepatic and extrahepatic malignancies in primary sclerosing cholangitis. J Hepatol. 2002;36(3):321–7.
6. Bergquist A, Glaumann H, Persson B, Broomé U. Risk factors and clinical presentation of hepatobiliary carcinoma in patients with primary sclerosing cholangitis: a case–control study. Hepatology. 1998;27(2):311–6.
7. Bhangui P, Vibert E, Majno P, et al. Intention-to-treat analysis of liver transplantation for hepatocellular carcinoma: living versus deceased donor transplantation. Hepatology. 2011;53(5):1570–9.
8. Bialecki ES, Di Bisceglie AM. Diagnosis of hepatocellular carcinoma. HPB (Oxford). 2005;7(1):26–34.
9. Björnsson E, Olsson R. Dominant strictures in patients with primary sclerosing cholangitis-revisited. Am J Gastroenterol. 2004;99(11):2281.
10. Boberg KM, Lind GE. Primary sclerosing cholangitis and malignancy. Best Pract Res Clin Gastroenterol. 2011;25(6):753–64.
11. Bolondi L, Sofia S, Siringo SE, et al. Surveillance programme of cirrhotic patients for early diagnosis and treatment of hepatocellular carcinoma; a cost effectiveness analysis. Gut. 2001;48:251–9.
12. Broome U, Olsson R, Loof L, et al. Natural history and prognostic factors in 305 Swedish patients with primary sclerosing cholangitis. Gut. 1996;38:610–5.
13. Bruix J, Sherman M. Management of hepatocellular carcinoma: an update. Hepatology. 2010;53(3):1020–2.
14. Buckles D, Lindor K, et al. In primary sclerosing cholangitis, gallbladder polyps are frequently malignant. Am J Gastroenterol. 2002;97:5.
15. Burak K, Angulo P, Pasha TM, Egan K, Petz J, Lindor KD. Incidence and risk factors for cholangiocarcinoma in primary sclerosing cholangitis. Am J Gastroenterol. 2004;99:523–6.
16. Cardinale V, et al. Multiple Cells of origin in cholangiocarcinoma underlie biological, epidemiological and clinical heterogeneity. World J Gastrointest Oncol. 2012;4:94–102.
17. Chalasani N, Baluyut A, Ismail A, et al. Cholangiocarcinoma in patients with primary sclerosing cholangitis: a multicenter case–control study. Hepatology. 2000;31(1):7–11.
18. Chapman R, Fevery J, Kalloo A, Nagorney DM, Boberg KM, Shneider B, Gores GJ. Diagnosis and management of primary sclerosing cholangitis. Hepatology. 2010;51:660–78.
19. Charatcharoenwitthaya P, Enders FB, Halling KC, Lindor KD. Utility of serum tumor markers, imaging, and biliary cytology for detecting cholangiocarcinoma in primary sclerosing cholangitis. Hepatology. 2008;48:1106–17.
20. Chen YK, Pleskow DK. SpyGlass single-operator peroral cholangiopancreatoscopy system for the diagnosis and therapy of bile-duct disorders: a clinical feasibility study (with video). Gastrointest Endosc. 2007;65(6):832–41.
21. Darwish Murad S, Kim WR, Harnois DM, et al. Efficacy of neoadjuvant chemoradiation, followed by liver transplantation, for perihilar cholangiocarcinoma at 12 US centers. Gastroenterology. 2012;143(1):88–98.e3.
22. Darwish Murad S, Kim WR, Therneau T, et al. Predictors of pretransplant dropout and posttransplant recurrence in patients with perihilar cholangiocarcinoma. Hepatology. 2012;56(3):972–81.
23. De Vreede I, Steers JL, Burch PA, et al. Prolonged disease-free survival after orthotopic liver transplantation plus adjuvant chemoirradiation for cholangiocarcinoma. Liver Transpl. 2000;6:309–16.
24. Eaton JE, Barr Fritcher EG, Gores CJ, et al. Biliary multifocal chromosomal polysomy and cholangiocarcinoma in primary sclerosing cholangitis. Am J Gastroenterol. 2015;110:299–309.
25. El-serag HB. Hepatocellular carcinoma. N Engl J Med. 2011;365(12):1118–27.
26. Farazi PA, Depinho RA. Hepatocellular carcinoma pathogenesis: from genes to environment. Nat Rev Cancer. 2006;6(9):674–87.
27. Farrant JM, Hayllar KM, Wilkinson ML, et al. Natural history and prognostic variables in primary sclerosing cholangitis. Gastroenterology. 1991;100(6):1710–7.
28. Fattovich G, Stroffolini T, Zagni I, Donato F. Hepatocellular carcinoma in cirrhosis: incidence and

risk factors. Gastroenterology. 2004;127(5 Suppl 1): S35–50.
29. Fevery J, Verslype C, Lai G, Aerts R, Van Steenbergen W. Incidence, diagnosis, and therapy of cholangiocarcinoma in patients with primary sclerosing cholangitis. Dig Dis Sci. 2007;52:3123–35.
30. Gollin SM. Mechanisms leading to chromosomal instability. Semin Cancer Biol. 2005;15(1):33–42.
31. Harnois DM, Gores GJ, Ludwig J, Steers JL, Larusso NF, Wiesner RH. Are patients with cirrhotic stage primary sclerosing cholangitis at risk for the development of hepatocellular cancer? J Hepatol. 1997;27(3): 512–6.
32. Heimbach JK, Sanchez W, Rosen CB, Gores GJ. Trans-peritoneal fine needle aspiration biopsy of hilar cholangiocarcinoma is associated with disease dissemination. HPB Off J Int Hepato Pancreato Biliary Assoc. 2011;13(5):356–60. doi:10.1111/j.1477-2574.2011.00298.
33. Hong JC, Jones CM, Duffy JP, et al. Comparative analysis of resection and liver transplantation for intrahepatic and hilar cholangiocarcinoma: a 24-year experience in a single center. Arch Surg. 2011;146(6):683–9. Kozarek RA. Single-operator cholangioscopes in the diagnosis of cholangiocarcinoma: seeing is believing. Is belief enough to allow treatment? Gastrointest Endosc. 2015;82(4):615–7.
34. Ismail T, Angrisani L, Powell JE, et al. Primary sclerosing cholangitis: surgical options, prognostic variables and outcome. Br J Surg. 1991;78(5):564–7.
35. Jaiswal M, Larusso NF, Burgart LJ, Gores GJ. Inflammatory cytokines induce DNA damage and inhibit DNA repair in cholangiocarcinoma cells by a nitric oxide-dependent mechanism. Cancer Res. 2000;60(1):184–90.
36. Kahaleh M, Mishra R, Shami VM, et al. Unresectable cholangiocarcinoma: comparison of survival in biliary stenting alone versus stenting with photodynamic therapy. Clin Gastroenterol Hepatol. 2008;6(3):290–7.
37. Kozarek RA. Single-operator cholangioscopes in the diagnosis of cholangiocarcinoma: seeing is believing. Is belief enough to allow treatment? Gastrointest Endosc. 2015;82(4):615–7.
38. Kronfeld D, Ekbon A, Ihre T. Survival and risk of CCA in patient with primary sclerosing cholangitis. Scand J Gastroenterol. 1997;32:1042–5.
39. Leung UC, Wong PY, et al. Gallbladder polyps in sclerosing cholangitis: does the 1-cm rule apply? ANZ J Surg. 2001;77(5):355–7.
40. Levy C, Lymp J, Angulo P, Gores GJ, Larusso N, Lindor KD. The value of serum CA 19–9 in predicting cholangiocarcinomas in patients with primary sclerosing cholangitis. Dig Dis Sci. 2005;50(9):1734–40.
41. Lewis JT, Talwalkar JA, Rosen CB, Smyrk TC, Abraham SC. Prevalence and risk factors for gallbladder neoplasia in patients with primary sclerosing cholangitis: evidence for a metaplasia-dysplasia-carcinoma sequence. Am J Surg Pathol. 2007;31(6):907–13.
42. Linderg B, Arneio U, Bergquist A, et al. Diagnosis of biliary strictures in conjunction with endoscopic retrograde cholangiopancreatography, with special reference to patients with primary sclerosing cholangitis. Endoscopy. 2002;34:909–16.
43. Lindor KD, Kowdley KV, Harrison ME. ACG clinical guideline: primary sclerosing cholangitis. Am J Gastroenterol. 2015;110:646–59.
44. Liu L, Cao Y, Chen C, et al. Sorafenib blocks the RAF/MEK/ERK pathway, inhibits tumor angiogenesis, and induces tumor cell apoptosis in hepatocellular carcinoma model PLC/PRF/5. Cancer Res. 2006; 66(24):11851–8.
45. Livraghi T, Goldberg SN, Lazzaroni S, et al. Hepatocellular carcinoma: radio-frequency ablation of medium and large lesions. Radiology. 2000;214(3): 761–8.
46. Llovet JM, Brú C, Bruix J. Prognosis of hepatocellular carcinoma: the BCLC staging classification. Semin Liver Dis. 1999;19(3):329–38. Llovet JM, Bruix J. Prospective validation of the Cancer of the Liver Italian Program (CLIP) score: a new prognostic system for patients with cirrhosis and hepatocellular carcinoma. Hepatology. 2000;32(3): 679–80.
47. Llovet JM, Real MI, Montaña X, et al. Arterial embolisation or chemoembolisation versus symptomatic treatment in patients with unresectable hepatocellular carcinoma: a randomised controlled trial. Lancet. 2002;359(9319):1734–9.
48. Llovet JM, Ricci S, Mazzaferro V, et al. Sorafenib in advanced hepatocellular carcinoma. N Engl J Med. 2008;359(4):378–90.
49. Marsh JW, Iwatsuki S, Makowka L, et al. Orthotopic liver transplantation for primary sclerosing cholangitis. Ann Surg. 1988;207(1):21–5.
50. Mazzaferro V, Regalia E, Doci R, Andreola S, Pulvirenti A, Bozzetti F, Montalto F, Ammatuna M, Morabito A, Gennari L. Liver transplantation for the treatment of small hepatocellular carcinoma in patients with cirrhosis. N Engl J Med. 1996; 334(11):693.
51. Mcgahan JP, Brock JM, Tesluk H, Gu WZ, Schneider P, Browning PD. Hepatic ablation with use of radio-frequency electrocautery in the animal model. J Vasc Interv Radiol. 1992;3(2):291–7.
52. Okuda K, Ohtuiki T, Obata H, et al. Cancer. 1985;56:918.
53. Nashan B, Schlitt HJ, Tusch G, et al. Biliary malignancies in primary sclerosing cholangitis: timing for liver transplantation. Hepatology. 1996;23(5):1105–11.
54. www.nccn.org/professionals/physicians/f_guidelines.asp.
55. Petrowsky H, Hong JC. Current surgical management of hilar and intrahepatic cholangiocarcinoma: the role of resection and orthotopic liver transplantation. Transplant Proc. 2009;41(10):4023–35.
56. Rea DJ, Heimbach JK, Rosen CB, et al. Liver transplantation with neoadjuvant chemoradiation is more effective than resection for hilar cholangiocarcinoma. Ann Surg. 2005;242(3):451–8.

57. Said K, Glaumann H, Bergquist A. Gallbladder disease in patients with primary sclerosing cholangitis. J Hepatol. 2008;48(4):598–605.
58. Salgia RJ, Singal AG, Fu S, Pelletier S, Marrero JA. Improved post-transplant survival in the United States for patients with cholangiocarcinoma after 2000. Dig Dis Sci. 2014;59(5):1048–54.
59. Schwartz LH, Black J, Fong Y, et al. Gallbladder carcinoma: findings at MR imaging with MR cholangiopancreatography. J Comput Assist Tomogr. 2002; 26(3):405–10.
60. Shah RJ, Langer DA, Antillon MR, Chen YK. Cholangioscopy and cholangioscopic forceps biopsy in patients with indeterminate pancreaticobiliary pathology. Clin Gastroenterol Hepatol. 2006;4(2):219–25.
61. Shin H-R, Oh J-K, Masuyer E, Curado M-P, Bouvard V, Fang Y-Y, Wiangnon S, Sripa B, Hong S-T. Epidemiology of cholangiocarcinoma: an update focusing on risk factors. Cancer Sci. 2010;101:579–85.
62. Silva MA, Hegab B, Hypde C, Guo B, Buckels JA, Mirza DF. Needle track seeding following biopsy of liver lesions in the diagnosis of hepatocellular cancer: a systematic review and meta-analysis. Gut. 2008;57(11):159.
63. Sumera R, Eaton JE, Gores GJ. Primary sclerosing cholangitis as a premalignant biliary tract disease: surveillance and management. Clin Gastroenterol Hepatol. 2015;13(12):2152–65.
64. Timmer MR, Beuers U, Fockens P, et al. Genetic and epigenetic abnormalities in primary sclerosing cholangitis-associated cholangiocarcinoma. Inflamm Bowel Dis. 2013;19(8):1789–97.
65. Vijayakumar A, Vijayakumar A, Patil V, Mallikarjuna MN, Shivaswamy BS. Early diagnosis of gallbladder carcinoma: an algorithm approach. ISRN Radiol. 2013;2013:239424.
66. Yao FY, Ferrell L, Bass NM, et al. Liver transplantation for hepatocellular carcinoma: expansion of the tumor size limits does not adversely impact survival. Hepatology. 2001;33(6):1394–403.
67. Yao FY, Mehta N, Flemming J, et al. Downstaging of hepatocellular cancer before liver transplant: long-term outcome compared to tumors within Milan criteria. Hepatology. 2015;61(6):1968–77.
68. Yoshimitsu K, Honda H, Kaneko K, et al. Dynamic MRI of the gallbladder lesions: differentiation of benign from malignant. J Magn Reson Imaging. 1997;7(4):696–701.
69. Zenouzi R, Weismüller TJ, Hübener P, et al. Low risk of hepatocellular carcinoma in patients with primary sclerosing cholangitis with cirrhosis. Clin Gastroenterol Hepatol. 2014;12(10):1733–8.
70. Zhu A, Theodore H, et al. Current management of gallbladder carcinoma. Oncologist. 2010;15(2):168–81.

Primary Sclerosing Cholangitis-Associated Inflammatory Bowel Disease

3

Blair Fennimore, Emilie H. Regner, and Mark E. Gerich

Epidemiology of PSC-Associated IBD (PSC-IBD)

Approximately 60–80 % of PSC cases in North American and Western European populations are associated with IBD; generally, over two-thirds of the IBD cases are diagnosed as ulcerative colitis (UC) [1, 2]. It has been suggested that the prevalence of IBD among PSC patients of non-Caucasian background may be lower. For instance, IBD prevalence rates of 20–34 % have been reported in studies of Asian PSC patients; however, these studies were either very small or relied on provider surveys without rigorous methods of IBD case ascertainment [3–6].

The diagnosis of IBD precedes that of PSC in the majority of patients with concomitant PSC and IBD. Indeed, the diagnosis of PSC may be made many years after the diagnosis of IBD and can even occur after proctocolectomy [7–15]. The prevalence of PSC in population-based studies of UC patients ranges from 2 to 8 %. Among patients with Crohn's disease (CD), the prevalence of PSC approaches 1 %, and it appears to occur much less frequently among patients with CD that is isolated to the small bowel [1, 15–17]. It has been reported that no statistically significant differences were seen in the prevalence of PSC among African-American, Hispanic, and non-Hispanic white patients with IBD enrolled in the National Institute of Diabetes and Digestive and Kidney Diseases (NIDDK) Inflammatory Bowel Disease Genetics Consortium (IBDGC) repository; however, only 20 patients with PSC were in this study [18].

Pathophysiology of PSC-IBD

Although a variety of hypothesis-generating associations have been identified between PSC and IBD, the specific underlying pathophysiology has yet to be elucidated. The strong heritability of disease coupled with identification of multiple shared genetic risk loci between PSC and IBD suggests a significant genetic contribution. Familial occurrence of PSC has been well documented [19]. PSC also confers greater than a threefold increased risk of UC among first-degree relatives [20]. This risk exists even in the absence of concomitant IBD in the proband, strongly suggesting a shared genetic susceptibility between the diseases [20].

Interestingly, although a variety of HLA- and non-HLA-associated risk loci have been described for both PSC and UC [21–23], specific HLA haplotypes [24] and major IBD-associated genes such as CARD15 and MDR1 [25] do not appear to be shared between the two. While overlap involving various non-HLA-associated risk

B. Fennimore, MD (✉)• E.H. Regner, MD
M.E. Gerich, MD
Assistant Professor of Medicine, Division of Gastroenterology and Hepatology, University of Colorado School of Medicine, 12700 E. 19th Ave. MS B-146, Aurora, CO 80045, USA
e-mail: blair.fennimore@ucdenver.edu; emilie.regner@ucdenver.edu; mark.gerich@ucdenver.edu

L.M. Forman (ed.), *Primary Sclerosing Cholangitis*, DOI 10.1007/978-3-319-40908-5_3

loci does support a shared genetic susceptibility, the discrepancy between HLA haplotypes supports the assertion that PSC-IBD is a distinct clinical and genetic phenotype [26–28].

Beyond the significant role of genetics in PSC-IBD, there have been multiple other theories attempting to explain the pathophysiologic connection between PSC and IBD. One such theory involves specific anti-neutrophil autoantibodies termed atypical perinuclear-staining anti-neutrophil cytoplasmic antibodies (pANCA) which can be detected in ~80 % of patients with both PSC and UC [29]. The finding that atypical pANCA react with the autoantigen β-tubulin isotype 5 (TBB5) as well as its highly conserved evolutionary bacterial precursor, protein FtsZ [30], supports a possible role for molecular mimicry in which an abnormal immune response to intestinal microorganisms results in loss of tolerance to self-antigens and autoimmunity in genetically susceptible individuals [31].

Translocation of bacterial antigens into the portal circulation as a result of intestinal inflammation and barrier disruption has also been implicated in the pathogenesis of PSC-IBD [32]. Prior endoscopic retrograde cholangiopancreatography (ERCP) appears to be an important confounding factor, however, since the majority of ERCP-naïve PSC patients have been found to have negative bile cultures [33]. This theory also fails to explain the development of PSC either preceding or in the absence of IBD and its associated intestinal barrier dysfunction.

The most promising theory linking hepatic and intestinal inflammation involves aberrant lymphocyte trafficking of gut-specific T cells to the liver. PSC is characterized by a massive infiltration of mononuclear cells with a predominance of CD8+ T cells in the periportal regions [34]. Uniquely, up to 20 % of the lymphocytic liver infiltrate in PSC is comprised of gut-specific T cells that have both α4β7 integrin and chemokine receptor 9 (CCR9) on their cell surface [35]. The α4β7 integrin and CCR9 on circulating T cells bind the intestine-specific adhesion molecule mucosal vascular addressin cell adhesion molecule 1 (MAdCAM-1) and chemokine ligand CCL25, respectively. MAdCAM-1 and CCL25 are responsible for facilitating recruitment of α4β7+/CCR9+ gut-homing lymphocytes to sites of mucosal injury, are significantly upregulated within the intestine in active IBD, and are typically expressed exclusively in the intestinal endothelium [36, 37]. Aberrant hepatic endothelial expression of MAdCAM-1 and CCL25 in PSC-IBD results in recruitment of gut-specific α4β7+/CCR9+ lymphocytes to the liver, indicating a direct interplay between intestinal and hepatic inflammation [35, 38].

IBD Phenotype in PSC-IBD Patients

The clinical features of PSC-IBD appear to be distinct from those of IBD in the absence of PSC. Nearly all studies of PSC-IBD phenotype have reported a higher prevalence of extensive colitis in PSC-IBD patients than IBD controls [39]. Notably, although the colitis in PSC-IBD tends to be extensive, it is often mild and may be present only histologically [40]. Right-sided predominant colitis with relative rectal sparing and backwash ileitis are commonly described features of PSC-IBD [12, 41–43]. Rectal sparing and/or the presence of backwash ileitis may prompt a diagnosis of Crohn's disease or indeterminate colitis in patients with PSC-associated IBD; however, other more definitive characteristics of Crohn's disease such as perianal involvement, transmural inflammation, skip lesions, strictures, or isolated small bowel disease are generally lacking [12, 42, 44, 45]. Patients with PSC-IBD appear to have a more quiescent clinical course in terms of their IBD, with less frequent need for immunosuppression or hospitalization [46–48].

Colorectal Cancer Risk, Prevention, and Management in PSC-IBD Patients

Multiple studies have shown an increased risk of colorectal cancer (CRC) in patients with UC and Crohn's colitis, although the risk appears to be declining over time [49–51]. The magnitude of relative risk depends upon a variety of factors including anatomical disease extent, duration,

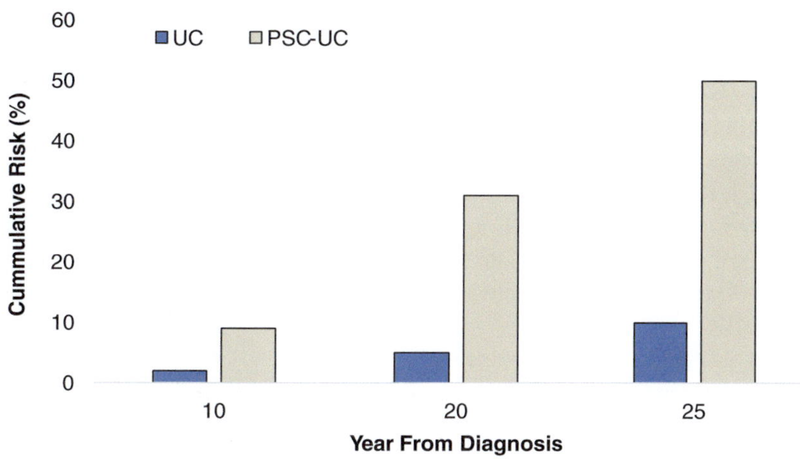

Fig. 3.1 Absolute cumulative risk for colorectal dysplasia or cancer over time among patients with UC and those with PSC-UC [1]

severity, and family history of CRC [52]. More extensive colonic disease confers the greatest risk; pancolitis is associated with a 15-fold increased risk of CRC as compared to a threefold or twofold increased risk with left-sided colitis and proctitis, respectively [53]. Likewise, CRC risk rises with increasing disease duration with an estimated incidence rate of 0.91, 4.07, and 4.55 per 1000 patient-years after 10, 20, and 30 years of disease, respectively [51].

The risk of CRC in PSC patients without concomitant IBD is low, with an estimated 2 % risk after 20 years of disease [39, 54]. Conversely, PSC is an independent risk factor for CRC in patients with a coexisting diagnosis of UC (PSC-UC), conferring a four- to fivefold increased risk above the already elevated CRC risk in isolated UC [55] (Fig. 3.1). Data regarding the risk of CRC among PSC patients with a coexisting diagnosis of CD (PSC-CD) is conflicting and limited by the low prevalence of CD diagnoses among PSC patients [39, 44, 56]. Ultimately, the risk for CRC in PSC-CD is likely comparable to PSC-UC after accounting for disease distribution and extent. Among patients with PSC-IBD, the diagnosis of CRC appears to occur at a younger age and closer to the time of IBD diagnosis than among patients with isolated IBD [39]. The mechanisms underlying the increased risk of CRC in PSC-IBD remain unknown. Altered colonic bile salt exposure has been postulated as a cause as has the delay in IBD diagnosis among PSC patients with subclinical colitis [57]. While colonic neoplasia among patients with UC alone typically presents in the rectosigmoid colon, neoplasia in PSC-IBD presents more commonly in the proximal colon [12, 39, 58].

Given the apparent increased incidence of colorectal neoplasia in PSC-IBD patients, a variety of medications have been evaluated as chemoprevention agents. Two recent meta-analyses with similar study inclusions have suggested a possible decrease in CRC risk associated with low- to medium-dose ursodeoxycholic acid (UDCA) [59, 60]. Hansen et al. reported a nonsignificant trend toward benefit with an RR of 0.64 (95 % CI 0.38–1.07, $p=0.09$) for CRC with UDCA dosed less than 25 mg/kg/day [59]. Conversely, Singh et al. found a statistically significant benefit with an OR of 0.18 (95 % CI 0.06–0.52) for CRC with UDCA dosed between 8 and 15 mg/kg/day [60]. Neither analysis demonstrated any benefit with higher-dose UDCA; however, definitions of high-dose UDCA differed. While low-dose UDCA may be associated with reduced CRC risk among PSC-IBD patients, there remains a lack of certainty that is reflected in the discordant recommendations from the American Gastroenterology Association (AGA) and American Association for the Study of Liver Diseases (AASLD) for and against the use of UDCA as CRC chemoprevention, respectively [2, 61].

Despite discrepant results among available observational studies, a 2010 AGA technical review favored the use of aminosalicylates (5-ASA) for chemoprevention in colitis-associated

CRC [62]. Thiopurines have been variably associated with a protective effect in reducing colitis-associated CRC; however, their risk profile limits their appeal as chemoprevention agents when not necessary for the treatment of colitis [63–67]. Results to date regarding the chemopreventative benefit of anti-TNF agents are limited and conflicting [68, 69]. Folate supplementation does not appear to protect against CRC in patients with IBD.

Patients with PSC-IBD are recommended to undergo rigorous surveillance colonoscopy to identify and manage colonic neoplasia as early as possible. Given the higher incidence of subclinical or mildly symptomatic colitis among PSC patients, current guidelines recommend a full colonoscopy with random segmental biopsies at the time of PSC diagnosis to assess for coexistent IBD. Patients with PSC-IBD should undergo serial colonoscopy for dysplasia surveillance every 1–2 years starting at the time of IBD diagnosis according to the AASLD; several other society guidelines recommend annual colonoscopic surveillance [2, 61, 70, 71]. There are no current guidelines regarding additional colonoscopic surveillance in PSC patients without concomitant IBD at initial colonoscopy.

Current surveillance colonoscopy guidelines for IBD patients recommend both targeted biopsies of visible lesions and extensive segmental biopsies with four-quadrant biopsies every 10 cm [70, 72, 73]. It should be noted, however, that guidelines for dysplasia surveillance and management differ among societies and are evolving as endoscopic imaging techniques improve the detection of dysplasia [70, 74]. Although the merits of continued surveillance versus colectomy for low-grade dysplasia (LGD) remain debatable, the substantial risk of progression of LGD to CRC in PSC-IBD should prompt a discussion with patients regarding more intensive surveillance or colectomy [75]. A variety of techniques have been evaluated to improve dysplasia detection given the low yield of random biopsies for the detection of dysplasia [76]. There is consensus that high-definition colonoscopy significantly improves dysplasia detection over standard white-light colonoscopy and should be utilized if available [74]. Additionally, chromoendoscopy using intracolonic application of indigo carmine or methylene blue significantly improves dysplasia detection over standard white-light colonoscopy and, to a lesser degree, over high-definition colonoscopy [74] (Fig. 3.2). Because of improved dysplasia detection, chromoendoscopy is frequently utilized for surveillance of high-risk populations, including patients with PSC-IBD, and has been recommended in some society guidelines [71]. Additional image enhancement modalities such as narrow band imaging (NBI) and autofluorescence technology are yet to show significant benefit in dysplasia detection in IBD [74].

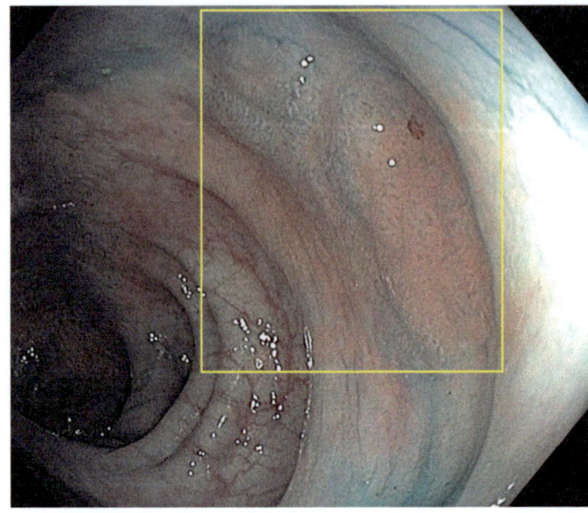

Fig. 3.2 Dysplastic colonic tissue identified with the aid of chromoendoscopy with methylene blue

Colectomy and Pouch Function in PSC-IBD Patients

Up to one-third of PSC-IBD patients will ultimately undergo colectomy [77–79]; however, colectomy rates may be decreasing [80]. Although it has not been studied directly, comparison of colectomy rates among study cohorts from similar time periods suggests that PSC-IBD patients may have a two- to threefold increase in colectomy rates over patients with isolated UC [81–84]. While extensive colitis and associated refractory disease is the most significant risk factor for colectomy among non-PSC-UC patients [85], PSC-IBD patients are much more likely to undergo colectomy for colorectal dysplasia/neoplasia [42, 82, 83]. Hepatic dysfunction is an important risk factor for adverse outcomes from colectomy [84]. In patients with portal hypertension who undergo ileostomies, peristomal varices can occur, and variceal bleeding may be very difficult to control, sometimes necessitating TIPS or liver transplantation (Fig. 3.3) [86–88]. As a consequence, proctocolectomy with formation of an ileal pouch anal anastomosis (IPAA), often called a "J pouch," is the favored procedure for patients requiring colectomy (Fig. 3.4). For patients with poor hepatic reserve, however, concomitant liver transplantation with total colectomy followed subsequently by IPAA may be a preferable approach [89].

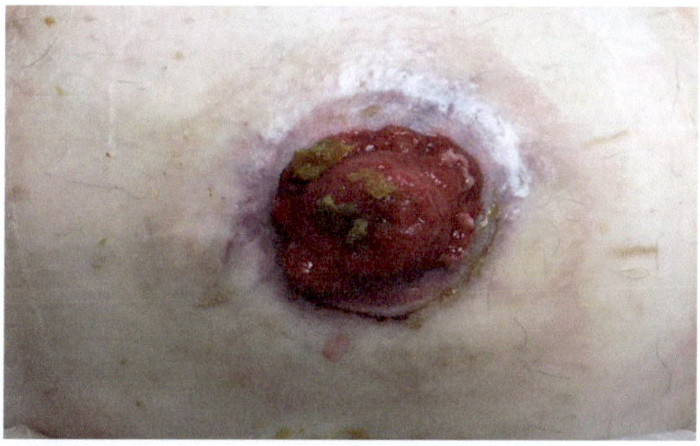

Fig. 3.3 Peristomal varices in a patient with PSC-IBD who underwent colectomy with end ileostomy and subsequently developed cirrhosis (Image courtesy of Hugo R. Rosen, MD)

Patients undergoing proctocolectomy with IPAA can experience a variety of pouch complications. The most common complication is pouchitis, which occurs in approximately 20–45 % of patients, and presents as increased stool frequency and urgency [90]. Pouchitis is thought to be a consequence of microbial dysbiosis and typically responds to a short course of antibiotic therapy, most often with ciprofloxacin and/or metronidazole [91]. A subset of patients will develop chronic antibiotic-refractory pouchitis (CARP) that requires more aggressive immunosuppressive therapy. PSC-IBD patients who undergo IPAA are more likely to develop pouchitis and have higher rates of CARP [92, 93]. This risk does not appear to be affected by liver disease severity [92] or worsen after liver transplantation [94]. De novo CARP appears to occur less frequently if IPAA is performed after liver transplantation (58.3 %) than if IPAA precedes transplantation (100 %; $p=0.047$) [95].

Neoplasia of the pouch or anal transition zone (ATZ) following IPAA has been described [96, 97] and occurs more often in patients undergoing colectomy for dysplasia/CRC [96]. Some studies suggest that PSC-IBD patients are at increased risk for pouch or ATZ neoplasia [98, 99]. The overall rate of pouch/ATZ neoplasia remains low, however, and there is no consensus on the need, or optimal protocol, for surveillance for pouch/ATZ neoplasia following IPAA [98, 100]. PSC

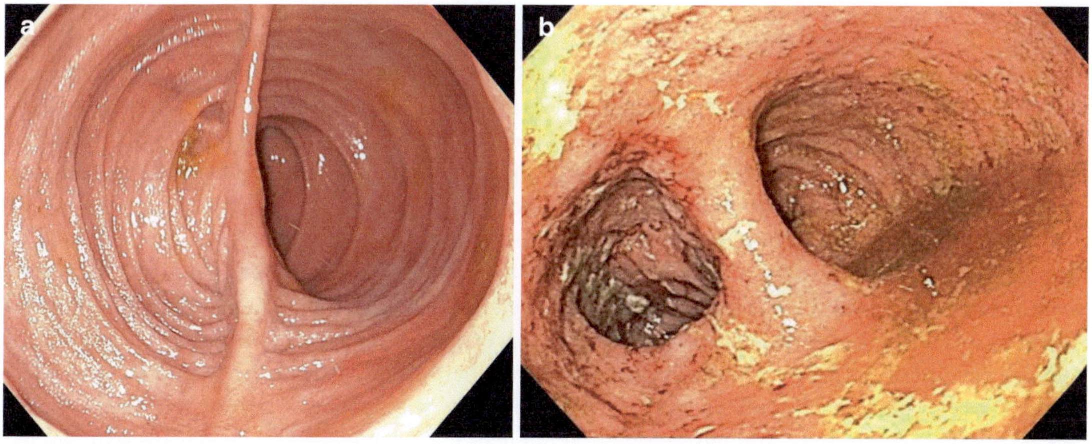

Fig. 3.4 (**a**) Normal pouch with healthy-appearing mucosa and an owl's eye configuration demonstrating a patent pouch inlet leading to the pre-pouch ileum; (**b**) diffuse pouchitis in a patient with PSC-IBD

and/or liver transplant does not appear to be a significant risk factor for other pouch-related complications including infections (*Clostridium difficile* and CMV) [101, 102], irritable pouch syndrome [103], or pouch failure [104].

Effect of IBD on Transplant Outcomes Among PSC-IBD Patients

Concomitant IBD does not appear to significantly affect overall patient survival following liver transplant for PSC; however, it may adversely impact graft function [105, 106]. The presence of IBD and an intact colon appears to be a significant risk factor for recurrence of PSC posttransplant. Pre- or peri-transplant colectomy is associated with much lower rates of recurrent PSC (2–3 %) than those seen among transplanted PSC patients who retain their colon or undergo colectomy following transplant (40–44 %) [107, 108]. PSC-IBD has also been associated with increased rates of acute cellular rejection [109] and chronic ductopenic rejection [106], while active IBD at the time of transplant has been associated with decreased graft survival and hepatic artery thrombosis [110].

Effect of Liver Transplantation on IBD Activity Among PSC-IBD Patients

PSC-IBD activity in patients requiring liver transplantation tends to be mild [83]. IBD activity following transplant follows a more variable course [111]. Some studies describe generally quiescent disease posttransplant [112, 113], while others document predominantly poor disease control and even the development of de novo IBD in approximately one-fifth of PSC patients despite transplant immunosuppression [13, 105, 114–116]. Although it is a well-described clinical phenomenon, the pathogenesis of de novo IBD posttransplant remains unclear. Theories include the unmasking of autoimmunity through suppression of regulatory T cells by transplant immunosuppressive agents, the loss of tolerance to microbial antigens, and the initiation of a chronic inflammatory response by damage-associated molecular pattern molecules and pathogen-associated molecular pattern molecules [117, 118]. Risk factors for poor IBD outcomes posttransplant also remain unclear. Clinically active IBD at the time of transplant may be a risk factor for worse disease after transplant [13], and inactive IBD at transplant has been associated with good disease control afterward [112]; however, as with many other reported predictors of posttransplant disease course, these associations have not been found in all studies. Another relatively common, but not universal, finding is that tacrolimus-based transplant immunosuppressive regimens are associated with higher rates of IBD flares [13, 119, 120] than regimens using azathioprine and cyclosporine [13, 116, 120, 121].

Management of PSC-IBD Following Liver Transplantation

The management of active IBD in the posttransplant setting is complicated by the competing need for antirejection immunosuppressive agents that are not always effective as IBD treatments and may actually promote disease activity. The successive use of calcineurin inhibitors and anti-TNF agents has been associated with a significant risk of infectious complications among patients with severe UC and raises concerns about the use of anti-TNF agents in the posttransplant PSC-IBD population [122]. Although data is very limited, in three small case series, the use of anti-TNF therapies in combination with calcineurin inhibitors and/or mycophenolate mofetil (MMF) in the posttransplant setting appeared to be safe and similarly effective at managing IBD as in the non-transplant population [123–125]. There is a single case report regarding the use of vedolizumab in the posttransplant setting with no adverse reactions observed after 11 months of treatment, during which the frequency of administration was increased to every 4 weeks [126]. There have been only three case reports in adults and a single case series in children assessing the use of mTOR inhibitors for the management of refractory IBD. While there appears to be some efficacy in a very selective population, their use in treating IBD in the posttransplant setting has not been evaluated [127–129].

The relative risk of colorectal cancer following liver transplant for non-PSC indications is approximately twofold that of the general population [130]. PSC-IBD patients with an intact colon posttransplant have a tenfold increased risk of CRC as compared to non-PSC transplant indications and 20-fold increased risk over the general population [110]. Similar to IBD in general, the colorectal cancer risk among PSC-IBD patients following transplant is related to the extent and duration of colitis [131]. Notably, transplant-related factors such as type of immunosuppression, rates of rejection, and CMV infection have not been shown to affect posttransplant CRC risk [132, 133]. Patients undergoing regular colonoscopic surveillance posttransplant are more likely to be diagnosed with early stage cancer, and therefore PSC-IBD patients should continue to undergo surveillance colonoscopy every 1–2 years following transplant [133].

Summary

IBD is present in approximately two-thirds of patients with PSC. The pathogenesis of this close association remains unclear. Although there is a clear genetic link between the two diseases, PSC-associated IBD likely represents a distinct clinical entity. PSC-IBD is often characterized by pancolitis with right colon predominant inflammation and relative rectal sparing. Importantly, these patients harbor a dramatically increased risk of colorectal cancer and thus require rigorous colonoscopic surveillance to minimize unfavorable outcomes related to colonic dysplasia. Liver disease progression and liver transplantation present additional challenges related to colitis management, which can have important effects on graft outcomes. Understanding the unique diagnostic, prognostic, and management considerations of this patient population provides the opportunity for optimization of patient care and improved outcomes.

References

1. Loftus EV, Sandborn WJ, Lindor KD, et al. Interactions between chronic liver disease and inflammatory bowel disease. Inflamm Bowel Dis. 1997;3:288–302.
2. Chapman R, Fevery J, Kalloo A, Nagorney DM, Boberg KM, Shneider B, et al. Diagnosis and management of primary sclerosing cholangitis. Hepatology. 2010;51(2):660–78. Epub 2010/01/27.
3. Takikawa H, Manabe T. Primary sclerosing cholangitis in Japan–analysis of 192 cases. J Gastroenterol. 1997;32(1):134–7. Epub 1997/02/01.
4. Tanaka A, Takamori Y, Toda G, Ohnishi S, Takikawa H. Outcome and prognostic factors of 391 Japanese patients with primary sclerosing cholangitis. Liver Int. 2008;28(7):983–9. Epub 2008/04/10.
5. Tanaka A, Tazuma S, Okazaki K, Tsubouchi H, Inui K, Takikawa H. Nationwide survey for primary sclerosing cholangitis and IgG4-related sclerosing cholangitis in Japan. J Hepatobiliary Pancreat Sci. 2014;21(1):43–50. Epub 2013/12/20.
6. Ang TL, Fock KM, Ng TM, Teo EK, Chua TS, Tan JY. Clinical profile of primary sclerosing cholangitis in Singapore. J Gastroenterol Hepatol. 2002; 17(8):908–13. Epub 2002/08/08.
7. Broome U, Lofberg R, Veress B, Eriksson LS. Primary sclerosing cholangitis and ulcerative colitis: evidence for increased neoplastic potential. Hepatology. 1995;22(5):1404–8. Epub 1995/11/01.
8. Broome U, Olsson R, Loof L, Bodemar G, Hultcrantz R, Danielsson A, et al. Natural history and prognostic factors in 305 Swedish patients with primary sclerosing cholangitis. Gut. 1996;38(4):610–5. Epub 1996/04/01.
9. Cangemi JR, Wiesner RH, Beaver SJ, Ludwig J, MacCarty RL, Dozois RR, et al. Effect of proctocolectomy for chronic ulcerative colitis on the natural history of primary sclerosing cholangitis. Gastroenterology. 1989;96(3):790–4. Epub 1989/03/01.
10. Farrant JM, Hayllar KM, Wilkinson ML, Karani J, Portmann BC, Westaby D, et al. Natural history and prognostic variables in primary sclerosing cholangitis. Gastroenterology. 1991;100(6):1710–7. Epub 1991/06/01.
11. Kornfeld D, Ekbom A, Ihre T. Is there an excess risk for colorectal cancer in patients with ulcerative colitis and concomitant primary sclerosing cholangitis? A population based study. Gut. 1997;41(4):522–5. Epub 1997/12/10.
12. Loftus Jr EV, Harewood GC, Loftus CG, Tremaine WJ, Harmsen WS, Zinsmeister AR, et al. PSC-IBD: a unique form of inflammatory bowel disease associated with primary sclerosing cholangitis. Gut. 2005;54(1):91–6. Epub 2004/12/14.
13. Verdonk RC, Dijkstra G, Haagsma EB, Shostrom VK, Van den Berg AP, Kleibeuker JH, et al. Inflammatory bowel disease after liver transplantation: risk factors for recurrence and de novo disease.

Am J Transplant. 2006;6(6):1422–9. Epub 2006/05/12.
14. Wiesner RH, Grambsch PM, Dickson ER, Ludwig J, MacCarty RL, Hunter EB, et al. Primary sclerosing cholangitis: natural history, prognostic factors and survival analysis. Hepatology. 1989;10(4):430–6. Epub 1989/10/01.
15. Fausa O, Schrumpf E, Elgjo K. Relationship of inflammatory bowel disease and primary sclerosing cholangitis. Semin Liver Dis. 1991;11(1):31–9. Epub 1991/02/01.
16. Bernstein CN, Blanchard JF, Rawsthorne P, Yu N. The prevalence of extraintestinal diseases in inflammatory bowel disease: a population-based study. Am J Gastroenterol. 2001;96(4):1116–22. Epub 2001/04/24.
17. Rasmussen HH, Fallingborg JF, Mortensen PB, Vyberg M, Tage-Jensen U, Rasmussen SN. Hepatobiliary dysfunction and primary sclerosing cholangitis in patients with Crohn's disease. Scand J Gastroenterol. 1997;32(6):604–10. Epub 1997/06/01.
18. Nguyen GC, Torres EA, Regueiro M, Bromfield G, Bitton A, Stempak J, et al. Inflammatory bowel disease characteristics among African Americans, Hispanics, and non-Hispanic Whites: characterization of a large North American cohort. Am J Gastroenterol. 2006;101(5):1012–23. Epub 2006/05/16.
19. Orholm M, Munkholm P, Langholz E, Nielsen OH, Sorensen TI, Binder V. Familial occurrence of inflammatory bowel disease. N Engl J Med. 1991;324(2):84–8. Epub 1991/01/10.
20. Bergquist A, Montgomery SM, Bahmanyar S, Olsson R, Danielsson A, Lindgren S, et al. Increased risk of primary sclerosing cholangitis and ulcerative colitis in first-degree relatives of patients with primary sclerosing cholangitis. Clin Gastroenterol Hepatol. 2008;6(8):939–43. Epub 2008/08/05.
21. Gaya DR, Russell RK, Nimmo ER, Satsangi J. New genes in inflammatory bowel disease: lessons for complex diseases? Lancet. 2006;367(9518):1271–84. Epub 2006/04/25.
22. Karlsen TH, Franke A, Melum E, Kaser A, Hov JR, Balschun T, et al. Genome-wide association analysis in primary sclerosing cholangitis. Gastroenterology. 2010;138(3):1102–11. Epub 2009/12/01.
23. Karlsen TH, Schrumpf E, Boberg KM. Genetic epidemiology of primary sclerosing cholangitis. World J Gastroenterol. 2007;13(41):5421–31. Epub 2007/10/02.
24. Karlsen TH, Boberg KM, Vatn M, Bergquist A, Hampe J, Schrumpf E, et al. Different HLA class II associations in ulcerative colitis patients with and without primary sclerosing cholangitis. Genes Immun. 2007;8(3):275–8. Epub 2007/02/16.
25. Karlsen TH, Hampe J, Wiencke K, Schrumpf E, Thorsby E, Lie BA, et al. Genetic polymorphisms associated with inflammatory bowel disease do not confer risk for primary sclerosing cholangitis. Am J Gastroenterol. 2007;102(1):115–21. Epub 2006/11/15.
26. Ellinghaus D, Folseraas T, Holm K, Ellinghaus E, Melum E, Balschun T, et al. Genome-wide association analysis in primary sclerosing cholangitis and ulcerative colitis identifies risk loci at GPR35 and TCF4. Hepatology. 2013;58(3):1074–83. Epub 2012/07/24.
27. Janse M, Lamberts LE, Franke L, Raychaudhuri S, Ellinghaus E, Muri Boberg K, et al. Three ulcerative colitis susceptibility loci are associated with primary sclerosing cholangitis and indicate a role for IL2, REL, and CARD9. Hepatology. 2011;53(6):1977–85. Epub 2011/03/23.
28. Liu JZ, Hov JR, Folseraas T, Ellinghaus E, Rushbrook SM, Doncheva NT, et al. Dense genotyping of immune-related disease regions identifies nine new risk loci for primary sclerosing cholangitis. Nat Genet. 2013;45(6):670–5. Epub 2013/04/23.
29. Terjung B, Worman HJ. Anti-neutrophil antibodies in primary sclerosing cholangitis. Best Pract Res Clin Gastroenterol. 2001;15(4):629–42. Epub 2001/08/09.
30. Terjung B, Sohne J, Lechtenberg B, Gottwein J, Muennich M, Herzog V, et al. p-ANCAs in autoimmune liver disorders recognise human beta-tubulin isotype 5 and cross-react with microbial protein FtsZ. Gut. 2010;59(6):808–16. Epub 2009/12/03.
31. Terjung B, Spengler U. Atypical p-ANCA in PSC and AIH: a hint toward a "leaky gut"? Clin Rev Allergy Immunol. 2009;36(1):40–51. Epub 2008/07/16.
32. Olsson R, Bjornsson E, Backman L, Friman S, Hockerstedt K, Kaijser B, et al. Bile duct bacterial isolates in primary sclerosing cholangitis: a study of explanted livers. J Hepatol. 1998;28(3):426–32. Epub 1998/04/29.
33. Bjornsson ES, Kilander AF, Olsson RG. Bile duct bacterial isolates in primary sclerosing cholangitis and certain other forms of cholestasis–a study of bile cultures from ERCP. Hepatogastroenterology. 2000;47(36):1504–8. Epub 2001/01/10.
34. Borchers AT, Shimoda S, Bowlus C, Keen CL, Gershwin ME. Lymphocyte recruitment and homing to the liver in primary biliary cirrhosis and primary sclerosing cholangitis. Semin Immunopathol. 2009;31(3):309–22. Epub 2009/06/18.
35. Eksteen B, Grant AJ, Miles A, Curbishley SM, Lalor PF, Hubscher SG, et al. Hepatic endothelial CCL25 mediates the recruitment of CCR9+ gut-homing lymphocytes to the liver in primary sclerosing cholangitis. J Exp Med. 2004;200(11):1511–7. Epub 2004/11/24.
36. Briskin M, Winsor-Hines D, Shyjan A, Cochran N, Bloom S, Wilson J, et al. Human mucosal addressin cell adhesion molecule-1 is preferentially expressed in intestinal tract and associated lymphoid tissue. Am J Pathol. 1997;151(1):97–110. Epub 1997/07/01.
37. Papadakis KA, Prehn J, Moreno ST, Cheng L, Kouroumalis EA, Deem R, et al. CCR9-positive lymphocytes and thymus-expressed chemokine distinguish small bowel from colonic Crohn's disease. Gastroenterology. 2001;121(2):246–54. Epub 2001/08/07.

38. Grant AJ, Lalor PF, Hubscher SG, Briskin M, Adams DH. MAdCAM-1 expressed in chronic inflammatory liver disease supports mucosal lymphocyte adhesion to hepatic endothelium (MAdCAM-1 in chronic inflammatory liver disease). Hepatology. 2001;33(5):1065–72. Epub 2001/05/09.
39. de Vries AB, Janse M, Blokzijl H, Weersma RK. Distinctive inflammatory bowel disease phenotype in primary sclerosing cholangitis. World J Gastroenterol. 2015;21(6):1956–71. Epub 2015/02/17.
40. Joo M, Abreu-e-Lima P, Farraye F, Smith T, Swaroop P, Gardner L, et al. Pathologic features of ulcerative colitis in patients with primary sclerosing cholangitis: a case–control study. Am J Surg Pathol. 2009;33(6):854–62. Epub 2009/03/20.
41. Faubion Jr WA, Loftus EV, Sandborn WJ, Freese DK, Perrault J. Pediatric "PSC-IBD": a descriptive report of associated inflammatory bowel disease among pediatric patients with psc. J Pediatr Gastroenterol Nutr. 2001;33(3):296–300. Epub 2001/10/11.
42. Boonstra K, van Erpecum KJ, van Nieuwkerk KM, Drenth JP, Poen AC, Witteman BJ, et al. Primary sclerosing cholangitis is associated with a distinct phenotype of inflammatory bowel disease. Inflamm Bowel Dis. 2012;18(12):2270–6.
43. Sinakos E, Samuel S, Enders F, Loftus Jr EV, Sandborn WJ, Lindor KD. Inflammatory bowel disease in primary sclerosing cholangitis: a robust yet changing relationship. Inflamm Bowel Dis. 2013;19(5):1004–9. Epub 2013/03/19.
44. Lindstrom L, Lapidus A, Ost A, Bergquist A. Increased risk of colorectal cancer and dysplasia in patients with Crohn's colitis and primary sclerosing cholangitis. Dis Colon Rectum. 2011;54(11): 1392–7. Epub 2011/10/08.
45. Halliday JS, Djordjevic J, Lust M, Culver EL, Braden B, Travis SP, et al. A unique clinical phenotype of primary sclerosing cholangitis associated with Crohn's disease. J Crohns Colitis. 2012;6(2):174–81. Epub 2012/02/14.
46. Lundqvist K, Broome U. Differences in colonic disease activity in patients with ulcerative colitis with and without primary sclerosing cholangitis: a case control study. Dis Colon Rectum. 1997;40(4):451–6. Epub 1997/04/01.
47. Broome U, Bergquist A. Primary sclerosing cholangitis, inflammatory bowel disease, and colon cancer. Semin Liver Dis. 2006;26(1):31–41. Epub 2006/02/24.
48. O'Toole A, Alakkari A, Keegan D, Doherty G, Mulcahy H, O'Donoghue D. Primary sclerosing cholangitis and disease distribution in inflammatory bowel disease. Clin Gastroenterol Hepatol. 2012;10(4):439–41. Epub 2011/11/19.
49. Eaden JA, Abrams KR, Mayberry JF. The risk of colorectal cancer in ulcerative colitis: a meta-analysis. Gut. 2001;48(4):526–35. Epub 2001/03/15.
50. Canavan C, Abrams KR, Mayberry J. Meta-analysis: colorectal and small bowel cancer risk in patients with Crohn's disease. Aliment Pharmacol Ther. 2006;23(8):1097–104. Epub 2006/04/14.
51. Castano-Milla C, Chaparro M, Gisbert JP. Systematic review with meta-analysis: the declining risk of colorectal cancer in ulcerative colitis. Aliment Pharmacol Ther. 2014;39(7):645–59. Epub 2014/03/13.
52. Xie J, Itzkowitz SH. Cancer in inflammatory bowel disease. World J Gastroenterol. 2008;14(3):378–89. Epub 2008/01/18.
53. Ekbom A, Helmick C, Zack M, Adami HO. Ulcerative colitis and colorectal cancer. A population-based study. N Engl J Med. 1990;323(18):1228–33. Epub 1990/11/01.
54. Claessen MM, Vleggaar FP, Tytgat KM, Siersema PD, van Buuren HR. High lifetime risk of cancer in primary sclerosing cholangitis. J Hepatol. 2009;50(1):158–64. Epub 2008/11/18.
55. Soetikno RM, Lin OS, Heidenreich PA, Young HS, Blackstone MO. Increased risk of colorectal neoplasia in patients with primary sclerosing cholangitis and ulcerative colitis: a meta-analysis. Gastrointest Endosc. 2002;56(1):48–54. Epub 2002/06/27.
56. Braden B, Halliday J, Aryasingha S, Sharifi Y, Checchin D, Warren BF, et al. Risk for colorectal neoplasia in patients with colonic Crohn's disease and concomitant primary sclerosing cholangitis. Clin Gastroenterol Hepatol. 2012;10(3):303–8. Epub 2011/11/01.
57. Tsaitas C, Semertzidou A, Sinakos E. Update on inflammatory bowel disease in patients with primary sclerosing cholangitis. World J Hepatol. 2014;6(4): 178–87. Epub 2014/05/07.
58. Claessen MM, Lutgens MW, van Buuren HR, Oldenburg B, Stokkers PC, van der Woude CJ, et al. More right-sided IBD-associated colorectal cancer in patients with primary sclerosing cholangitis. Inflamm Bowel Dis. 2009;15(9):1331–6. Epub 2009/02/21.
59. Hansen JD, Kumar S, Lo WK, Poulsen DM, Halai UA, Tater KC. Ursodiol and colorectal cancer or dysplasia risk in primary sclerosing cholangitis and inflammatory bowel disease: a meta-analysis. Dig Dis Sci. 2013;58(11):3079–87. Epub 2013/07/31.
60. Singh S, Khanna S, Pardi DS, Loftus Jr EV, Talwalkar JA. Effect of ursodeoxycholic acid use on the risk of colorectal neoplasia in patients with primary sclerosing cholangitis and inflammatory bowel disease: a systematic review and meta-analysis. Inflamm Bowel Dis. 2013;19(8):1631–8. Epub 2013/05/15.
61. Farraye FA, Odze RD, Eaden J, Itzkowitz SH, McCabe RP, Dassopoulos T, et al. AGA medical position statement on the diagnosis and management of colorectal neoplasia in inflammatory bowel disease. Gastroenterology. 2010;138(2):738–45. Epub 2010/02/10.
62. Farraye FA, Odze RD, Eaden J, Itzkowitz SH. AGA technical review on the diagnosis and management of colorectal neoplasia in inflammatory bowel disease. Gastroenterology. 2010;138(2):746–74. 74 e1–4; quiz e12–3. Epub 2010/02/10.

63. Matula S, Croog V, Itzkowitz S, Harpaz N, Bodian C, Hossain S, et al. Chemoprevention of colorectal neoplasia in ulcerative colitis: the effect of 6-mercaptopurine. Clin Gastroenterol Hepatol. 2005;3(10):1015–21. Epub 2005/10/20.
64. Velayos FS, Loftus Jr EV, Jess T, Harmsen WS, Bida J, Zinsmeister AR, et al. Predictive and protective factors associated with colorectal cancer in ulcerative colitis: a case–control study. Gastroenterology. 2006;130(7):1941–9. Epub 2006/06/10.
65. Subramanian V, Logan RF. Chemoprevention of colorectal cancer in inflammatory bowel disease. Best Pract Res Clin Gastroenterol. 2011;25(4–5):593–606. Epub 2011/11/30.
66. Gong J, Zhu L, Guo Z, Li Y, Zhu W, Li N, et al. Use of thiopurines and risk of colorectal neoplasia in patients with inflammatory bowel diseases: a meta-analysis. PLoS One. 2013;8(11):e81487. Epub 2013/12/07.
67. Chapman CG, Rubin DT. The potential for medical therapy to reduce the risk of colorectal cancer and optimize surveillance in inflammatory bowel disease. Gastrointest Endosc Clin N Am. 2014;24(3):353–65. Epub 2014/07/01.
68. Baars JE, Looman CW, Steyerberg EW, Beukers R, Tan AC, Weusten BL, et al. The risk of inflammatory bowel disease-related colorectal carcinoma is limited: results from a nationwide nested case–control study. Am J Gastroenterol. 2011;106(2):319–28. Epub 2010/11/04.
69. Nyboe Andersen N, Pasternak B, Basit S, Andersson M, Svanstrom H, Caspersen S, et al. Association between tumor necrosis factor-alpha antagonists and risk of cancer in patients with inflammatory bowel disease. JAMA. 2014;311(23):2406–13. Epub 2014/06/19.
70. Cairns SR, Scholefield JH, Steele RJ, Dunlop MG, Thomas HJ, Evans GD, et al. Guidelines for colorectal cancer screening and surveillance in moderate and high risk groups (update from 2002). Gut. 2010;59(5):666–89. Epub 2010/04/30.
71. Lindor KD, Kowdley KV, Harrison ME. ACG clinical guideline: primary sclerosing cholangitis. Am J Gastroenterol. 2015;110(5):646–59. quiz 60. Epub 2015/04/15.
72. Kornbluth A, Sachar DB. Ulcerative colitis practice guidelines in adults: American College of Gastroenterology Practice Parameters Committee. Am J Gastroenterol. 2010;105(3):501–23. quiz 24. Epub 2010/01/14.
73. Leighton JA, Shen B, Baron TH, Adler DG, Davila R, Egan JV, et al. ASGE guideline: endoscopy in the diagnosis and treatment of inflammatory bowel disease. Gastrointest Endosc. 2006;63(4):558–65. Epub 2006/03/28.
74. Laine L, Kaltenbach T, Barkun A, McQuaid KR, Subramanian V, Soetikno R. SCENIC international consensus statement on surveillance and management of dysplasia in inflammatory bowel disease. Gastroenterology. 2015;148(3):639–51. e28. Epub 2015/02/24.
75. Venkatesh PG, Jegadeesan R, Gutierrez NG, Sanaka MR, Navaneethan U. Natural history of low grade dysplasia in patients with primary sclerosing cholangitis and ulcerative colitis. J Crohns Colitis. 2013;7(12):968–73. Epub 2013/02/26.
76. van den Broek FJ, Stokkers PC, Reitsma JB, Boltjes RP, Ponsioen CY, Fockens P, et al. Random biopsies taken during colonoscopic surveillance of patients with longstanding ulcerative colitis: low yield and absence of clinical consequences. Am J Gastroenterol. 2014;109(5):715–22. Epub 2011/03/24.
77. Loftus Jr EV, Sandborn WJ, Tremaine WJ, Mahoney DW, Zinsmeister AR, Offord KP, et al. Risk of colorectal neoplasia in patients with primary sclerosing cholangitis. Gastroenterology. 1996;110(2):432–40. Epub 1996/02/01.
78. Farmer RG, Easley KA, Rankin GB. Clinical patterns, natural history, and progression of ulcerative colitis. A long-term follow-up of 1116 patients. Dig Dis Sci. 1993;38(6):1137–46. Epub 1993/06/01.
79. Leijonmarck CE, Persson PG, Hellers G. Factors affecting colectomy rate in ulcerative colitis: an epidemiologic study. Gut. 1990;31(3):329–33. Epub 1990/03/01.
80. Targownik LE, Singh H, Nugent Z, Bernstein CN. The epidemiology of colectomy in ulcerative colitis: results from a population-based cohort. Am J Gastroenterol. 2012;107(8):1228–35. Epub 2012/05/23.
81. Block M, Jorgensen KK, Oresland T, Lindholm E, Grzyb K, Cvancarova M, et al. Colectomy for patients with ulcerative colitis and primary sclerosing cholangitis – what next? J Crohns Colitis. 2014;8(5):421–30. Epub 2013/11/19.
82. Marelli L, Xirouchakis E, Kalambokis G, Cholongitas E, Hamilton MI, Burroughs AK. Does the severity of primary sclerosing cholangitis influence the clinical course of associated ulcerative colitis? Gut. 2011;60(9):1224–8. Epub 2011/03/16.
83. Navaneethan U, Venkatesh PG, Mukewar S, Lashner BA, Remzi FH, McCullough AJ, et al. Progressive primary sclerosing cholangitis requiring liver transplantation is associated with reduced need for colectomy in patients with ulcerative colitis. Clin Gastroenterol Hepatol. 2012;10(5):540–6. Epub 2012/01/17.
84. Treeprasertsuk S, Bjornsson E, Sinakos E, Weeding E, Lindor KD. Outcome of patients with primary sclerosing cholangitis and ulcerative colitis undergoing colectomy. World J Gastrointest Pharmacol Ther. 2013;4(3):61–8. Epub 2013/08/07.
85. Solberg IC, Lygren I, Jahnsen J, Aadland E, Hoie O, Cvancarova M, et al. Clinical course during the first 10 years of ulcerative colitis: results from a population-based inception cohort (IBSEN Study). Scand J Gastroenterol. 2009;44(4):431–40. Epub 2008/12/23.
86. Kartheuser AH, Dozois RR, LaRusso NF, Wiesner RH, Ilstrup DM, Schleck CD. Comparison of surgical treatment of ulcerative colitis associated with primary sclerosing cholangitis: ileal pouch-anal

anastomosis versus Brooke ileostomy. Mayo Clin Proc. 1996;71(8):748–56. Epub 1996/08/01.

87. Wiesner RH, LaRusso NF, Dozois RR, Beaver SJ. Peristomal varices after proctocolectomy in patients with primary sclerosing cholangitis. Gastroenterology. 1986;90(2):316–22. Epub 1986/02/01.
88. Peck JJ, Boyden AM. Exigent ileostomy hemorrhage. A complication of proctocolectomy in patients with chronic ulcerative colitis and primary sclerosing cholangitis. Am J Surg. 1985;150(1):153–8. Epub 1985/07/01.
89. Poritz LS, Koltun WA. Surgical management of ulcerative colitis in the presence of primary sclerosing cholangitis. Dis Colon Rectum. 2003;46(2):173–8. Epub 2003/02/11.
90. Gorgun E, Remzi FH. Complications of ileoanal pouches. Clin Colon Rectal Surg. 2004;17(1):43–55. Epub 2004/02/01.
91. Shen B. Pouchitis: what every gastroenterologist needs to know. Clin Gastroenterol Hepatol. 2013;11(12):1538–49. Epub 2013/04/23.
92. Penna C, Dozois R, Tremaine W, Sandborn W, LaRusso N, Schleck C, et al. Pouchitis after ileal pouch-anal anastomosis for ulcerative colitis occurs with increased frequency in patients with associated primary sclerosing cholangitis. Gut. 1996;38(2):234–9. Epub 1996/02/01.
93. Rahman M, Desmond P, Mortensen N, Chapman RW. The clinical impact of primary sclerosing cholangitis in patients with an ileal pouch-anal anastomosis for ulcerative colitis. Int J Colorectal Dis. 2011;26(5):553–9. Epub 2011/02/01.
94. Zins BJ, Sandborn WJ, Penna CR, Landers CJ, Targan SR, Tremaine WJ, et al. Pouchitis disease course after orthotopic liver transplantation in patients with primary sclerosing cholangitis and an ileal pouch-anal anastomosis. Am J Gastroenterol. 1995;90(12):2177–81. Epub 1995/12/01.
95. Freeman K, Shao Z, Remzi FH, Lopez R, Fazio VW, Shen B. Impact of orthotopic liver transplant for primary sclerosing cholangitis on chronic antibiotic refractory pouchitis. Clin Gastroenterol Hepatol. 2008;6(1):62–8. Epub 2007/12/11.
96. Derikx LA, Kievit W, Drenth JP, de Jong DJ, Ponsioen CY, Oldenburg B, et al. Prior colorectal neoplasia is associated with increased risk of ileoanal pouch neoplasia in patients with inflammatory bowel disease. Gastroenterology. 2014;146(1):119–28. e1. Epub 2013/10/01.
97. Kariv R, Remzi FH, Lian L, Bennett AE, Kiran RP, Kariv Y, et al. Preoperative colorectal neoplasia increases risk for pouch neoplasia in patients with restorative proctocolectomy. Gastroenterology. 2010;139(3):806–12. 12 e1–2. Epub 2010/06/12.
98. Imam MH, Eaton JE, Puckett JS, Loftus Jr EV, Mathis KL, Gossard AA, et al. Neoplasia in the ileoanal pouch following colectomy in patients with ulcerative colitis and primary sclerosing cholangitis. J Crohns Colitis. 2014;8(10):1294–9. Epub 2014/04/29.
99. Stahlberg D, Veress B, Tribukait B, Broome U. Atrophy and neoplastic transformation of the ileal pouch mucosa in patients with ulcerative colitis and primary sclerosing cholangitis: a case control study. Dis Colon Rectum. 2003;46(6):770–8. Epub 2003/06/10.
100. McLaughlin SD, Clark SK, Tekkis PP, Ciclitira PJ, Nicholls RJ. Review article: restorative proctocolectomy, indications, management of complications and follow-up–a guide for gastroenterologists. Aliment Pharmacol Ther. 2008;27(10):895–909. Epub 2008/02/13.
101. McCurdy JD, Loftus Jr EV, Tremaine WJ, Smyrk TC, Bruining DH, Pardi DS, et al. Cytomegalovirus infection of the ileoanal pouch: clinical characteristics and outcomes. Inflamm Bowel Dis. 2013;19(11):2394–9. Epub 2013/08/27.
102. Seril DN, Shen B. Clostridium difficile infection in patients with ileal pouches. Am J Gastroenterol. 2014;109(7):941–7. Epub 2014/07/06.
103. Makkar R, Graff LA, Bharadwaj S, Lopez R, Shen B. Psychological factors in irritable pouch syndrome and other pouch disorders. Inflamm Bowel Dis. 2015;21(12):2815–24. Epub 2015/09/24.
104. Gorgun E, Remzi FH, Manilich E, Preen M, Shen B, Fazio VW. Surgical outcome in patients with primary sclerosing cholangitis undergoing ileal pouch-anal anastomosis: a case–control study. Surgery. 2005;138(4):631–7; discussion 7–9. Epub 2005/11/05.
105. Joshi D, Bjarnason I, Belgaumkar A, O'Grady J, Suddle A, Heneghan MA, et al. The impact of inflammatory bowel disease post-liver transplantation for primary sclerosing cholangitis. Liver Int. 2013;33(1):53–61. Epub 2011/11/23.
106. Graziadei IW, Wiesner RH, Marotta PJ, Porayko MK, Hay JE, Charlton MR, et al. Long-term results of patients undergoing liver transplantation for primary sclerosing cholangitis. Hepatology. 1999;30(5):1121–7. Epub 1999/10/26.
107. Alabraba E, Nightingale P, Gunson B, Hubscher S, Olliff S, Mirza D, et al. A re-evaluation of the risk factors for the recurrence of primary sclerosing cholangitis in liver allografts. Liver Transpl. 2009;15(3):330–40. Epub 2009/02/27.
108. Cholongitas E, Shusang V, Papatheodoridis GV, Marelli L, Manousou P, Rolando N, et al. Risk factors for recurrence of primary sclerosing cholangitis after liver transplantation. Liver Transpl. 2008;14(2):138–43. Epub 2008/02/01.
109. Miki C, Harrison JD, Gunson BK, Buckels JA, McMaster P, Mayer AD. Inflammatory bowel disease in primary sclerosing cholangitis: an analysis of patients undergoing liver transplantation. Br J Surg. 1995;82(8):1114–7. Epub 1995/08/01.
110. Singh S, Edakkanambeth Varayil J, Loftus Jr EV, Talwalkar JA. Incidence of colorectal cancer after liver transplantation for primary sclerosing cholangitis: a systematic review and meta-analysis. Liver Transpl. 2013;19(12):1361–9. Epub 2013/09/11.
111. Singh S, Loftus EV, Talwalkar JA. Inflammatory bowel disease after liver transplantation for primary

sclerosing cholangitis. Am J Gastroenterol. 2013;108(9):1417–25.
112. Befeler AS, Lissoos TW, Schiano TD, Conjeevaram H, Dasgupta KA, Millis JM, et al. Clinical course and management of inflammatory bowel disease after liver transplantation. Transplantation. 1998;65(3):393–6. Epub 1998/03/04.
113. Navaneethan U, Choudhary M, Venkatesh PG, Lashner BA, Remzi FH, Shen B, et al. The effects of liver transplantation on the clinical course of colitis in ulcerative colitis patients with primary sclerosing cholangitis. Aliment Pharmacol Ther. 2012;35(9): 1054–63. Epub 2012/03/21.
114. Papatheodoridis GV, Hamilton M, Mistry PK, Davidson B, Rolles K, Burroughs AK. Ulcerative colitis has an aggressive course after orthotopic liver transplantation for primary sclerosing cholangitis. Gut. 1998;43(5):639–44. Epub 1998/11/21.
115. Riley TR, Schoen RE, Lee RG, Rakela J. A case series of transplant recipients who despite immunosuppression developed inflammatory bowel disease. Am J Gastroenterol. 1997;92(2):279–82. Epub 1997/02/01.
116. Jorgensen KK, Lindstrom L, Cvancarova M, Karlsen TH, Castedal M, Friman S, et al. Immunosuppression after liver transplantation for primary sclerosing cholangitis influences activity of inflammatory bowel disease. Clin Gastroenterol Hepatol. 2013; 11(5):517–23. Epub 2013/01/22.
117. Hampton DD, Poleski MH, Onken JE. Inflammatory bowel disease following solid organ transplantation. Clin Immunol. 2008;128(3):287–93. Epub 2008/08/19.
118. Nepal S, Navaneethan U, Bennett AE, Shen B. De novo inflammatory bowel disease and its mimics after organ transplantation. Inflamm Bowel Dis. 2013;19(7):1518–27. Epub 2013/05/10.
119. Dvorchik I, Subotin M, Demetris AJ, Fung JJ, Starzl TE, Wieand S, et al. Effect of liver transplantation on inflammatory bowel disease in patients with primary sclerosing cholangitis. Hepatology. 2002;35(2):380–4. Epub 2002/02/05.
120. Haagsma EB, Van Den Berg AP, Kleibeuker JH, Slooff MJ, Dijkstra G. Inflammatory bowel disease after liver transplantation: the effect of different immunosuppressive regimens. Aliment Pharmacol Ther. 2003;18(1):33–44. Epub 2003/07/10.
121. Cholongitas E, Papatheodoridis GV, Zappoli P, Giannakopoulos A, Patch D, Marelli L, et al. Combined HLA-DR and -DQ disparity is associated with a stable course of ulcerative colitis after liver transplantation for primary sclerosing cholangitis. Liver Transpl. 2007;13(4):552–7. Epub 2007/03/31.
122. Leblanc S, Allez M, Seksik P, Flourie B, Peeters H, Dupas JL, et al. Successive treatment with cyclosporine and infliximab in steroid-refractory ulcerative colitis. Am J Gastroenterol. 2011;106(4):771–7. Epub 2011/03/10.
123. Mohabbat AB, Sandborn WJ, Loftus Jr EV, Wiesner RH, Bruining DH. Anti-tumour necrosis factor treatment of inflammatory bowel disease in liver transplant recipients. Aliment Pharmacol Ther. 2012;36(6):569–74. Epub 2012/07/12.
124. Sandhu A, Alameel T, Dale CH, Levstik M, Chande N. The safety and efficacy of antitumour necrosis factor-alpha therapy for inflammatory bowel disease in patients post liver transplantation: a case series. Aliment Pharmacol Ther. 2012;36(2):159–65. Epub 2012/05/24.
125. Schnitzler F, Friedrich M, Stallhofer J, Schonermarck U, Fischereder M, Habicht A, et al. Solid organ transplantation in patients with Inflammatory Bowel Diseases (IBD): analysis of transplantation outcome and IBD activity in a large single center cohort. PLoS One. 2015;10(8):e0135807. Epub 2015/08/20.
126. Meszaros M, Pageaux GP, Altwegg R. Management of ulcerative colitis using vedolizumab after liver transplantation for primary sclerosing cholangitis. J Crohns Colitis. 2015. Epub 2015/10/10.
127. Dumortier J, Lapalus MG, Guillaud O, Poncet G, Gagnieu MC, Partensky C, et al. Everolimus for refractory Crohn's disease: a case report. Inflamm Bowel Dis. 2008;14(6):874–7. Epub 2008/02/16.
128. Massey DC, Bredin F, Parkes M. Use of sirolimus (rapamycin) to treat refractory Crohn's disease. Gut. 2008;57(9):1294–6. Epub 2008/08/23.
129. Mutalib M, Borrelli O, Blackstock S, Kiparissi F, Elawad M, Shah N, et al. The use of sirolimus (rapamycin) in the management of refractory inflammatory bowel disease in children. J Crohns Colitis. 2014;8(12):1730–4. Epub 2014/09/23.
130. Sint Nicolaas J, de Jonge V, Steyerberg EW, Kuipers EJ, van Leerdam ME, Veldhuyzen-van Zanten SJ. Risk of colorectal carcinoma in post-liver transplant patients: a systematic review and meta-analysis. Am J Transplant. 2010;10(4):868–76. Epub 2010/04/28.
131. Vera A, Gunson BK, Ussatoff V, Nightingale P, Candinas D, Radley S, et al. Colorectal cancer in patients with inflammatory bowel disease after liver transplantation for primary sclerosing cholangitis. Transplantation. 2003;75(12):1983–8. Epub 2003/06/28.
132. Jorgensen KK, Lindstrom L, Cvancarova M, Castedal M, Friman S, Schrumpf E, et al. Colorectal neoplasia in patients with primary sclerosing cholangitis undergoing liver transplantation: a Nordic multicenter study. Scand J Gastroenterol. 2012; 47(8–9):1021–9. Epub 2012/05/15.
133. Loftus Jr EV, Aguilar HI, Sandborn WJ, Tremaine WJ, Krom RA, Zinsmeister AR, et al. Risk of colorectal neoplasia in patients with primary sclerosing cholangitis and ulcerative colitis following orthotopic liver transplantation. Hepatology. 1998;27(3):685–90. Epub 1998/03/21.

4 Overlap Syndromes of Primary Sclerosing Cholangitis

Albert J. Czaja

Primary sclerosing cholangitis (PSC) has characteristic histological findings (concentric periductal fibrosis, portal edema and fibrosis, bile duct loss, and focal bile ductular proliferation) [1–4] and cholangiographic features (focal biliary strictures and dilations) [5–10] that compel its consideration regardless of other clinical findings. The high disease specificity of these features has facilitated the identification of syndromes in which the findings of PSC are intermixed with those reminiscent of other diseases [11–17]. These hybrid syndromes are bound to the diagnosis of PSC by their histological and/or cholangiographic features, but they warrant separate designations as overlap syndromes because of their strong resemblance to autoimmune hepatitis (AIH) [18–31] or primary biliary cholangitis (PBC) [32–37]. Patients with histological features of bile duct injury or loss suggestive of PSC may also have a cholestatic syndrome characterized by normal cholangiography, the absence of antimitochrondrial antibodies (AMA), and inflammatory and serological findings suggestive of AIH [15, 17]. These patients have been variously designated as having AMA-negative PBC, small duct PSC, or autoimmune cholangitis [29, 38–42]. They are probably more accurately regarded as variants of the classical syndromes of PSC and PBC rather than an overlap syndrome [43–46].

The overlap syndromes of PSC are mainly clinical descriptions rather than valid pathological entities [15, 16, 47]. Their diagnostic criteria have not been codified, and their management has not been established by rigorous clinical trial. They have emerged mainly from large cohorts of patients with predominately PSC [18, 22, 23, 26] or AIH [12, 20, 24, 28, 30, 48] and from single-center experiences that have applied diverse diagnostic criteria and empiric management strategies [21, 25]. The overlap syndromes of PSC can confound the diagnosis, behave differently than classical PSC, respond variably to pharmacological interventions, and warrant individualized management strategies adjusted to the predominant disease component [14–17]. They should be considered in all patients with classical features of AIH who have ulcerative colitis, prominent cholestatic features, or recalcitrance to conventional corticosteroid therapy [12, 49]. They should also be considered in patients with histological and/or cholangiographic features of PSC who have prominent liver inflammation and serological markers of immune reactivity [12, 18] and in patients with predominant cholestatic features, AMA, and destructive cholangitis (florid duct lesions) on histological examination [32–37].

The goals of this review are to describe the clinical features and frequency of the overlap syndromes of PSC, review the syndrome of autoimmune cholangitis, speculate on the

A.J. Czaja, MD
Division of Gastroenterology and Hepatology,
Mayo Clinic College of Medicine,
200 First Street S.W., Rochester, MN, USA
e-mail: czaja.albert@mayo.edu

L.M. Forman (ed.), *Primary Sclerosing Cholangitis*, DOI 10.1007/978-3-319-40908-5_4

pathogenesis of the overlap syndromes of PSC, and provide management guidelines based on the composite experience of limited clinical studies and the recommendations of the major liver societies.

Diagnostic Criteria

Overlap syndromes can have features of PSC and AIH or PBC at the time of disease discovery [28, 36], or the overlapping features may develop later [20, 24, 33–35, 37, 50]. The emergence of the overlapping features may reflect an unawareness of the concurrent disease manifestations at the time of presentation (incomplete diagnosis), or they may indicate a transition of the original classical disease to an overlap syndrome during follow-up (evolving diagnosis) [15]. Patients with classical features of AIH [20, 24, 41, 50] or PBC [34, 35, 37] may have unsuspected cholangiographic changes of PSC at presentation, or they may develop PSC later in the course of their disease. Similar apparent or actual transitions of PSC to features of AIH or PBC have been described [23, 33, 37]. The presence of features commonly associated with disparate diseases in the same patient is sufficient for the designation of an overlap syndrome whether these features have been discovered together or sequentially.

Classical PSC can have autoantibodies (smooth muscle antibodies [SMA], antinuclear antibodies [ANA], and atypical perinuclear antineutrophil cytoplasmic antibodies [pANCA]) [18, 51–56], hypergammaglobulinemia [18, 57], and interface hepatitis that may include lymphoplasmacytic infiltration [4, 18, 51, 57, 58]. These features also typify patients with classical AIH [59–63]. The designation of an overlap syndrome between PSC and AIH implies that the features of AIH are so strong in PSC that they extend beyond the boundary acceptable for classical disease. Similarly, the designation of an overlap syndrome between PSC and PBC implies that the clinical, laboratory, and histological findings of PSC and PBC are so disease specific that their occurrence together cannot be accommodated within a conventional diagnostic category.

Diagnostic Scoring System

The revised original diagnostic scoring system of the International Autoimmune Hepatitis Group (IAIHG) [60] has been used to quantify the strength of autoimmune features in patients with PSC, but it has not been validated for this purpose [12, 13, 18, 48] (Table 4.1). It was developed to ensure the inclusion of homogeneous patient populations in clinical trials, and it cannot serve as a discriminative diagnostic index or supersede clinical judgment [60, 64, 65]. The sensitivity of the scoring system for the overlap syndromes has varied from 50 to 62 % using clinical judgment as the gold standard [66, 67], and its application in diagnosing these syndromes has been discouraged by the IAIHG [47].

Patients with the overlap syndromes typically score less than patients with classical AIH. Scores are based on laboratory and histological findings at presentation which may change during the course of the disease, and scores in retrospective studies of the overlap syndromes have varied widely [48]. Cutoff values for the diagnosis of an autoimmune component have not been established, and the scores have not correlated with outcomes. The ratio of the serum alkaline phosphatase (ALP) level to the serum aspartate aminotransferase (AST) level may be the single most valuable component of the scoring system for assessing an overlap syndrome. The ALP/AST ratio can suggest an unusual cholestatic feature in patients with AIH, especially if it exceeds 1.5 [20, 24]. Furthermore, an increased ratio has also been associated with reduced survival [48]. A similar diagnostic scoring system for PBC has been promulgated for assessing the strength of the PBC component in the overlap syndromes, but it has not been validated or widely used [68].

Diagnostic Requisites

Clinical judgment is the principal basis for diagnosing the overlap syndromes of PSC (Table 4.1). The diagnosis of an overlap syndrome between PSC and AIH requires histological and/or cholangiographic features typical of PSC and prominent

Table 4.1 Diagnostic criteria of overlap syndromes associated with PSC

Diagnostic templates	PSC and AIH	PSC and PBC
Clinical criteria	Histological or cholangiographic PSC [15]: Portal tract edema and fibrosis Bile duct loss or periductal fibrosis Focal biliary strictures and dilations Characteristic features of AIH [15, 17]: Markedly increased serum AST level Hypergammaglobulinemia Increased serum IgG level Autoantibodies (ANA, SMA, or LKM1) Interface hepatitis, plasma cells Normal cholangiography in 27 % [29]	Histological or cholangiographic PSC [36]: Small duct PSC possible Characteristic features of PBC [15]: AMA Destructive cholangitis Nonstandard features of PBC [33, 35, 37]: No AMA AMA develop later AMA detected by immunoblotting Antibodies to gp210 and sp100 Diagnostic standard, clinical judgment [15]
Diagnostic scoring systems	Not validated for AIH or overlaps [48, 60] Poor sensitivity (50–62 %) [66, 67] Use discouraged by IAIHG [47] ALP/AST ratio ≥1.5 useful index [48]	Not validated for PBC [68]
Key cholestatic indices	Serum ALP ≥ 4-fold ULN in AIH [71] Serum GGT ≥ 4-fold ULN in AIH [72] Serum ALP/AST ratio ≥1.5-fold ULN [48]	None applicable [15]
Key histological findings	Histological clues of AIH in PSC [74]: Dense lymphoplasmacytic infiltration Moderate interface hepatitis Hepatocyte rosettes Histological clues of PSC in AIH [74]: Portal edema, fibrosis, ductopenia Periductal fibrosis	Histological clues of PBC in PSC [35]: Destructive cholangitis Portal granulomatous changes Histological clues of PSC in PBC [36]: Periductal fibrosis

Numbers in brackets are references
AIH autoimmune hepatitis, *ALP* alkaline phosphatase, *AMA* antimitochondrial antibodies, *ANA* antinuclear antibodies, *AST* aspartate aminotransferase, *GGT* gamma glutamyl transferase, *IAIHG* International Autoimmune Hepatitis Group, *IgG* immunoglobulin G, *LKM1* antibodies to liver kidney microsome type 1, *PBC* primary biliary cholangitis, *PSC* primary sclerosing cholangitis, *SMA* smooth muscle antibodies, *ULN* upper limit of normal range

features of AIH as reflected in characteristic laboratory tests of inflammatory activity, serological tests of immune reactivity (ANA, SMA, and/or antibodies to liver kidney microsome type 1 [anti-LKM1]), hypergammaglobulinemia (especially, increased serum immunoglobulin G [IgG] level), and dense lymphoplasmacytic infiltration of liver tissue with interface hepatitis. Twenty-seven percent of patients with histological overlap between AIH and PSC have small duct PSC, and normal cholangiography does not exclude this overlap syndrome [29].

The diagnosis of the overlap syndrome between PSC and PBC requires histological and/or cholangiographic features typical of PSC, AMA, and characteristic biliary changes of PBC (destructive or granulomatous cholangitis) [15, 17, 33, 34, 37] (Table 4.1). The serum immunoglobulin M (IgM) concentration is increased in 45 % of patients with PSC [57], but AMA are rarely detected (0–8 %) [55, 57, 69]. Antimitochondrial antibodies in patients with histological and/or cholangiographic features of PSC justify histological review and consideration of an overlap syndrome with PBC.

Patients with the overlap syndrome of PSC and PBC may have absent AMA at presentation but compelling histological features of PBC [33, 35] (Table 4.1). These patients may be seronegative for AMA by the indirect immunofluorescence assay (IIF) and seropositive for AMA by the immunoblotting assay [33]. They may also develop AMA later in the course of their disease and express reactivities to gp210 and sp100 [37]. Characteristic cholangiographic changes of PSC may be absent but not invalidate the diagnosis [36, 70]. Histological findings of concentric periductal fibrous (fibrous obliterative cholangitis) may indicate small duct PSC and an overlap syndrome with PBC that is characterized by AMA and antibodies to gp210 and sp100 [36]. The diagnosis of the overlap syndromes by clinical judgment is characterized by the absence of rigid clinical phenotypes.

Key Cholestatic Indices

The serum ALP level can be the sole indication of an overlap syndrome in adults with otherwise classical AIH. The serum ALP level is abnormally increased in 81 % of patients with severe AIH, but it is more than twofold the upper limit of the normal range (ULN) in only 33 % and more than fourfold ULN in only 10 % [71]. A serum ALP level more than twofold ULN in a patient with classical AIH should generate suspicion about the possibility of an overlap syndrome, and the diagnosis should be pursued if the serum ALP level exceeds fourfold ULN.

The serum gamma glutamyl transferase (GGT) level can also be useful in suggesting an unusual cholestatic component in a patient with otherwise classical AIH. Serum GGT levels are commonly increased in adults with AIH, and the mean serum level has ranged from 1.1- to 3.4-fold ULN [72, 73]. Men have significantly higher serum levels of GGT than women [72], and an upper limit of abnormality still compatible with the diagnosis of classical AIH has not been defined. Nevertheless, a serum GGT level exceeding fourfold ULN should suggest the possibility of an overlapping cholestatic process and justify pursuit of this diagnosis.

Histological Examination

Liver tissue examination has been the strongest independent predictor of the overlap syndromes [66, 67, 74] (Table 4.1). Whereas liver tissue examination is seldom necessary in the diagnosis of classical PSC [75, 76], it can direct the diagnosis of an overlap syndrome between PSC and AIH or PBC [20, 28, 33, 35, 66, 67, 74]. Dense lymphoplasmacytic infiltration of the portal tract, moderate-severe interface hepatitis, rosetting of hepatocytes, and lobular hepatitis are atypical of classical PSC, but they are hallmarks of AIH [63, 74, 77]. Similarly, destructive cholangitis (florid duct lesions) compels the consideration of PBC in patients with otherwise classical features of PSC, even in the absence of AMA [35, 76, 78, 79]. Fibrous obliterative cholangitis is the hallmark of PSC, and its presence supports this diagnosis, even in the absence of characteristic cholangiographic abnormalities [36, 70].

Salient Clinical Features of the Overlap Syndrome of PSC and AIH

One hundred thirteen patients with the overlap syndrome of PSC and AIH or PBC have been reported in ten clinical studies, and the publications vary widely in the amount of detail provided [12, 20, 22–26, 28, 30, 48] (Table 4.2). Patients with the overlap syndrome of PSC and AIH are mainly young men with active liver inflammation. Serum AST and alanine aminotransferase (ALT) levels are markedly abnormal, and hypergammaglobulinemia and elevated serum IgG levels attest to the severity of the inflammatory and immunological activity [20, 22, 23, 26, 28, 30, 48] (Table 4.2). Autoantibodies (ANA, SMA, and/or pANCA) are commonly present, and an atypical cholestatic component is commonly suggested by an abnormally increased serum ALP and/or GGT level. Chronic ulcerative colitis is present in 24–89 % [20, 23, 24, 26, 28, 30], and histological examination typically discloses features of AIH (interface hepatitis, lymphoplasmacytic infiltration, or rosetting of hepatocytes) [20, 22, 23] and bile duct changes associated with PSC [20, 22]. This characteristic clinical phenotype is similar between patients discovered in large cohorts of individuals originally diagnosed as having AIH (AIH-predominant overlap syndrome) or in large cohorts of individuals originally diagnosed as having PSC (PSC-predominant overlap syndrome) (Table 4.2).

Table 4.2 Clinical features of overlap syndrome of PSC and autoimmune hepatitis

Clinical features	AIH predominant	PSC predominant
Age (years)	Median, 20–34 (range,14–74) [20, 28, 48]	Median, 21–22 (range, 7–54) [23, 26]
Male gender	55–81 % [12, 20, 28, 48] 45 % (children) [24]	43–67 % [22, 23, 26]
AST	1.6–35-fold ULN [12, 48] >5-fold ULN [20] Lower than in children with normal cholangiography [24]	≥10-fold ULN (median, 18-fold ULN) [23] Same as in PSC [22] Higher than PSC [26]
ALP	>4-fold ULN, 80 % [20] 1.2–9.6-fold ULN [12, 48]	1.2–6-fold ULN (median, 1.8-fold ULN) [23] Similar to PSC [26]
γ-Globulin	>1.5 ULN, 100 % [20] >ULN, 24 % [28]	>ULN, 100 % [23]
IgG	>ULN, 100 % [20] Similar to AIH [48]	>ULN, 61–100 % [23] Higher than in PSC [22, 26]
GGT	>ULN, 100 % [28] Similar to AIH [48]	Similar to PSC [26]
ANA and/or SMA	50–100 % [12, 20, 28, 30, 48]	73–100 % [22, 23, 26]
pANCA	74–81 % [24, 28]	60 % [23]
CUC	24–44 % [20, 24, 28, 30, 48]	28–89 % [23, 26]
Interface hepatitis	100 % [12, 20]	46–100 % [22, 23] Lymphoplasmacytic infiltrate, 75 % [22] Rosetting, 25 % [22]
Bile duct changes	60 % [20]	75 % [22]

Composite of findings reported in ten clinical studies involving 113 patients
Numbers in brackets are references
AIH autoimmune hepatitis, *ALP* alkaline phosphatase, *ALT* alanine aminotransferase, *ANA* antinuclear antibodies, *AST* aspartate aminotransferase, *CUC* chronic ulcerative colitis, *GGT* gamma glutamyl transferase, *IgG* immunoglobulin G, *pANCA* perinuclear anti-neutrophil cytoplasmic antibodies, *PSC* primary sclerosing cholangitis, *SMA* smooth muscle antibodies, *ULN* upper limit of the normal range

The typical clinical phenotype in children with the overlap syndrome of AIH and PSC is different than that in adults [80, 81]. A distinction has been made between the classical PSC common in adults, which may have multiple etiologies and few or no autoantibodies, and "autoimmune sclerosing cholangitis" (ASC) in children. Children with ASC have typical features of AIH and cholangiographic changes of PSC in association with autoantibodies that suggest an immune-mediated process [24, 82]. There is little gender difference in children with the overlap syndrome of AIH and ASC (45 % male versus 55 % female); the serum AST level is lower than in children with classical AIH; and cholestatic features frequently are absent or mild [24]. The serum ALP level is normal in 59 % of these children, and the GGT level is normal in 30 %. An increased serum ALP/AST ratio (3.96 in ASC versus 1.1 in AIH) is the most compelling clinical finding that suggests the presence of ASC [24]. Small duct PSC has been described in a 7-year-old girl with anti-LKM1, and this overlap should be considered in children with normal cholangiography and periductal fibrosis on histological examination [70].

Jaundice is present in as many as 69 % of adults at presentation, but at least 18 % are asymptomatic [48]. The presence of ulcerative colitis in a patient with AIH justifies the performance of endoscopic resonance cholangiography (ERC) or magnetic resonance cholangiography (MRC) regardless of other clinical features. Chronic ulcerative colitis is present in 16 % of adults with AIH, and 42 % of those undergoing cholangiography have PSC [49]. MRC has been preferred in the evaluation of patients with PSC because of its comparability to ERC, lower cost, and relative safety (mainly by avoiding the complication of pancreatitis) [8–10]. The major caveat in ERC and MRC is the misinterpretation of bile duct distortions by fibrosis as indicative of PSC. Hepatic fibrosis has been a strong independent factor associated with bile duct distortions in AIH [83], and it may account for the high (10 %) frequency of presumed PSC in patients with otherwise classical AIH [84]. Routine cholangiography in adults with AIH and no evidence of inflammatory bowel disease has not been recommended [83].

Salient Clinical Features of the Overlap Syndrome of PSC and PBC

Eight patients with the overlap syndrome of PSC and PBC have been reported in six clinical studies [32–37]. The publications vary widely in the amount of detail provided, but the composite findings allow a clinical phenotype to emerge (Table 4.3). The median age has been 52 years (range, 40–72 years), and all but one have been women. Markedly abnormal elevations of the serum ALP and GGT levels are commonly present [32, 33, 35], and serum levels of IgG and IgM have been abnormally increased when measured [32]. ANA have been detected in 62 % (median titer, 1:40; range, 0–1:1280); SMA have been uniformly absent in those patients who were tested; and AMA have been detected by IIF or immunoblotting in 88 % at presentation or during the course of the disease [32–34].

Patients with the overlap syndrome of PSC and PBC commonly have had a past history of gallstones or biliary surgery (50 % occurrence) [33, 34, 37], and biliary pain has been a presenting symptom in 38 % [33, 34]. Chronic ulcerative

Table 4.3 Clinical features of overlap syndrome of PSC and PBC

Clinical features	Findings (N=8)
Age (years)	Median, 52 (range, 40–72) [32–37]
Gender	Women, 7 (88 %) [32–36]
Past history gallstones, biliary surgery	4 (50 %) [33, 34, 37]
Biliary pain as presenting symptom	3 (38 %) [33, 34]
Aspartate aminotransferase (AST)	0–4-fold ULN [32, 33, 37]
Alkaline phosphatase (ALP)	2–20-fold ULN [32, 33, 35]
Gamma glutamyl transferase (GGT)	Fivefold ULN [33]
Antinuclear antibodies (ANA)	5 (62 %) (including patient negative at entry and 1:80 later) [34] Median titer, 1:40 (range, 0–1:1280 [32–37]
Smooth muscle antibodies (SMA)	0 % [33–35, 37]
Antimitochondrial antibodies (AMA)	7 (88 %) (titer range, 0–1:1280) [32–37] Negative at presentation, 3 (38 %) [33, 35] Positive later or by immunoblotting, 2 (25 %) [33, 37] Antibodies to gp210 and sp100 [36, 37]
Chronic ulcerative colitis (CUC)	None [33]
pANCA	Negative [35]
Endoscopic or magnetic resonance cholangiography	Diagnostic, 88 % [32–35, 37] Normal, 12 % [36]
Histological features (7 of 8 patients biopsied)	Destructive (granulomatous) cholangitis, 4 (57 %) [33, 35, 37] Fibrous obliterative cholangitis, 1 (14 %) [36] Nondestructive cholangitis, 1 (14 %) [34] Ductopenia, portal fibrosis, ductular proliferation, 1 (14 %) [32]

Composite of findings reported in six clinical studies involving eight patients
Numbers in brackets are references
pANCA perinuclear anti-neutrophil cytoplasmic antibodies

colitis has been absent in all patients, and atypical pANCA have not been detected in the one patient in whom it was sought [35]. Histological findings have been commonly those of PBC with destructive (granulomatous) cholangitis in four of the seven patients who underwent liver tissue examination (57 %) [33, 35, 37]. Nondestructive cholangitis has been present in one patient (14 %) [34]; one patient (14 %) has had portal fibrosis, ductopenia, nondestructive cholangitis, and mild ductular proliferation [32]; and one patient (14 %) has had fibrous obliterative cholangitis [36]. Cholangiography has been diagnostic of PSC in 88 %. The one patient with normal MRC has had compelling histological features of PSC (fibrous obliterative cholangitis) and small duct PSC [36].

PSC and PBC have been recognized together in one patient [36]; PSC has preceded the diagnosis of PBC in two patients [33, 37], and PBC has preceded the diagnosis of PSC in five patients [32, 34, 35, 37]. The diagnosis should be considered in patients with PSC who have or develop AMA and histological features of PBC, and it should be considered in patients with classical PBC who have or develop biliary pain, fever, or worsening cholestatic features [32, 34, 35, 37].

Frequency

The frequency of the overlap syndrome of PSC and AIH ranges from 0 to 54 %. This variability probably reflects the size and age of the cohort under study, the predominant disease within that cohort, and the diagnostic criteria that are applied. Studies based mainly on the presence of cholestatic features (laboratory or radiographic findings) in patients with AIH have a frequency of PSC that ranges from 0 to 10 % [12, 30, 84, 85]. Studies based mainly on the presence of autoimmune features in patients with PSC determined by the diagnostic scoring systems of the IAIHG have a frequency of AIH that ranges from 4 to 54 % [12, 22, 23, 26, 28, 48].

The high frequency of the overlap syndrome in some studies of PSC attests mainly to the occurrence of inflammatory features shared by AIH in 35–54 % of patients with severe PSC. The nondiscriminative nature of the diagnostic scoring system of the IAIHG between AIH and PSC also contributes to this variability [12, 18, 86]. The 27 individual clinical manifestations that are graded in the scoring system of the IAIHG include nondiscriminative findings such as gender, the absence of drug and alcohol exposure, negative studies for viral infection, the absence of AMA, and concurrent immune diseases including chronic ulcerative colitis [60]. Many patients with classical PSC may have a score close to that required for probable AIH based simply on these findings. Studies assessing cholangiographic changes of PSC in children with AIH estimate the frequency of overlapping features as 49 % [24], and studies in adults suggest that the frequency of the overlap syndrome is best estimated at 4–17 % [22, 23, 28, 37, 48].

The overlap syndrome of PSC and PBC has been reported in only eight patients [32–37], and one of these patients had overlapping features of AIH, PBC, and PSC [34]. The frequency of this rare overlap syndrome between PSC and PBC has been estimated as 0.7 % (two patients) of 261 patients with autoimmune liver disease [34].

Autoimmune Cholangitis

Patients with AIH may have a cholestatic syndrome in the absence of classical clinical features of PSC or PBC [15, 17]. They lack AMA, have normal cholangiograms, and manifest bile duct injury or loss on histological examination. These patients have been classified as having autoimmune cholangitis [39, 43, 87–90], but they probably constitute a heterogeneous population that includes patients with AMA-negative PBC [38, 44, 91] and small duct PSC [41, 42]. The status of these patients as an overlap syndrome is unsettled since the features of AIH that accompany the cholestatic laboratory and histological changes are not disease specific, and autoimmune cholangitis may simply be a variant of PBC or PSC.

Patients with autoimmune cholangitis should be assessed for small duct PSC. Patients with features of AIH and small duct PSC have been described as an overlap syndrome of PSC, and the diagnosis is most secure in the presence of disease-specific histological features of PSC (concentric periductal fibrosis) and otherwise typical features of AIH [29, 36, 70]. The characteristic histological finding of concentric periductal fibrosis is absent in most patients with PSC [79, 92], and candidates for the designation of an overlap syndrome may have histological changes that are graded as indefinite or indicative rather than diagnostic of PSC [29]. Confidence in the diagnosis can be strengthened by the close resemblance of these patients to those with large duct PSC (male predominance, young age at onset, frequent concurrence of ulcerative colitis) and by a poor response to immunosuppressive therapy [29]. The frequency of autoimmune cholangitis (presumed AMA-negative PBC or small duct PSC) in patients with AIH is 11 % [12, 39], and the frequency of small duct PSC in patients with the overlap syndrome of AIH and PSC is 27 % [29].

Patients with autoimmune cholangitis should also be assessed for PBC by testing for AMA with assays other than IIF and by careful reassessment of the liver tissue for features of destructive cholangitis, nondestructive cholangitis, bile duct loss, and granulomatous change. Immunoblotting assays will detect AMA in 15–28 % of patients with PBC who are seronegative by IIF [44, 45], and new laboratory methods based on recombinant antigens for AMA (pMIT3) and PBC-specific antinuclear antigens (gp210 and sp100) promise to further improve the diagnostic yield [93, 94].

The liver tissue from patients with AIH stain positive for IgG4 in 3–35 % of instances [95–97], and PSC has developed 5 years after the diagnosis of IgG4-associated AIH in one patient [15, 97]. Patients with IgG4-associated AIH have had increased serum levels of IgG4 [97], and the number of T lymphocytes, B lymphocytes, and plasma cells has been greater in liver specimens from these patients than from patients without IgG4-associated AIH [96]. These findings suggest that an overlap syndrome could exist between AIH and IgG4-associated PSC or that the liver disease associated with IgG4 cholangitis could be mistaken for AIH and an overlap syndrome. The histological findings in the liver tissue of patients with IgG4-associated cholangitis include dense lymphoplasmacytic infiltrates of the portal tract, sparing of bile ducts, and occasional extension of the inflammatory infiltrate into the perivenular (zone 3) region [98]. These features are sufficiently nonspecific to be compatible with other inflammatory and cholestatic liver diseases, including AIH.

The frequency of IgG4 staining in the liver tissue of patients with AIH and PSC is uncertain, and cholangiopancreatography in patients with IgG4-associated AIH is necessary to establish its association with IgG4 cholangitis. Patients with IgG4-associated AIH respond well to corticosteroid therapy [96] as do patients with IgG4-associated cholangitis and pancreatitis [99–101]. The wide range of responses to immunosuppressive therapy reported in patients with the overlap syndrome of PSC and AIH suggests that a corticosteroid-responsive, IgG4-associated subgroup could exist [12, 20, 26, 29, 48, 49, 102].

Pathogenic Considerations

The pathogenic mechanisms responsible for the occurrence of the overlap syndromes of PSC are uncertain. Since the clinical features of AIH are not disease specific, their presence in patients with PSC could simply represent a vigorous inflammatory form of PSC [12, 15, 18]. This possibility is supported by the rarity that PSC and PBC, which each have highly disease-specific features (cholangiographic changes, AMA, and destructive cholangitis or fibrous obliterative cholangitis on histological examination), have overlapping phenotypes [32, 33, 37]. Indeed, the clinical manifestations of AIH are the most common components of the overlap syndromes [15], and their occurrence in a patient with overlapping features of PSC and PBC [34] underscores the commonality of these findings in diverse inflammatory liver diseases, including virus-related [11, 103], drug-induced [104], and metabolic disorders [105, 106].

Another hypothesis is that AIH, PBC, and PSC have genetic predispositions that favor the occurrence of overlapping clinical manifestations [107]. Autoimmune hepatitis has been associated mainly with HLA DRB1*03, DRB1*04, and the A1-B8-DRB1*03 phenotype [108–110]. Patients with PBC have a similar frequency of HLA DRB1*04 (41 % versus 44 %) as patients with AIH, but a lower occurrence of HLA DRB1*03 (20 % versus 50 %) [107]. In contrast, patients with PSC have a similar frequency of HLA DRB1*03 as patients with AIH (60 % versus 50 %) but significantly lower frequency of HLA DRB1*04 than patients with AIH (10 % versus 44 %) or PBC (10 % versus 41 %) [107]. Classical AIH has also been associated with the allele, *DRB3*0101*, which encodes for DR52a, and this may be another genetic similarity between AIH and PSC [111–113].

Genetic polymorphisms outside the major histocompatibility complex, such as the *cytotoxic T lymphocyte antigen-4* polymorphism, may also be shared between these diseases and contribute to overlapping similarities in their clinical manifestations [114–117]. Shared genetic predispositions imply that patients with AIH, PBC, and PSC can present the same or similar antigens to naïve $CD4^+$ lymphocytes and generate an immune reactivity that is expressed clinically as a mixed phenotype [118–120]. The association of PSC with inflammatory bowel disease may expose the genetically predisposed individual to diverse foreign antigens that mimic self-antigens and trigger a promiscuous immune response that targets different cell populations within the liver [23, 112, 121, 122]. The apparent low frequency of inflammatory bowel disease in patients with the overlap syndromes of PSC challenges this speculation [20, 26].

Other possible explanations for the overlap syndromes are that they are actually transition stages in the emergence of the classical disease [15]. Patients with early stages of PSC and PBC can have histological features compatible with AIH, including interface hepatitis, lymphoplasmacytic infiltration, and nondestructive cholangitis [30, 74], and the transitions that have been described between these diseases may include such patients [20, 23, 28, 50]. Patients may actually have two diseases, and the sequential occurrence of PBC after PSC [33, 37] or PSC after PBC [34, 35, 37] supports this possibility.

A final consideration is that the overlap syndromes are distinct pathological entities with separate genetic predispositions, triggering antigens, and pathogenic pathways that await validation [15]. This possibility is supported by the lower prevalence of CUC in the overlap syndrome of PSC and AIH than in PSC or AIH and the apparent lack of risk for cholangiocarcinoma or colorectal cancer in this population [26, 28]. Furthermore, PSC and AIH have distinctly different mononuclear cell infiltrations within the liver that might make their coexistence as separate entities difficult. Children with AIH have deficiencies in the immune regulatory activity of peripheral T lymphocytes that are normal in children with PSC [121], and patients with classical AIH have abundant natural killer cells in the portal tracts, whereas patients with PSC have abundant cytotoxic T lymphocytes in the portal tracts [122].

Treatment Regimens

There have been no randomized clinical trials evaluating treatment regimens for the overlap syndromes of PSC, and the principal management strategies have been based on the regimens currently used for classical PSC, AIH, and PBC [63, 76, 78, 79, 123]. Conventional pharmacological agents (corticosteroids, azathioprine, and ursodeoxycholic acid) have been administered alone and in combination, and these regimens have had variable success in small single-center experiences [12, 20, 23–25, 28, 29, 37, 48]. These experiences have in turn generated therapeutic recommendations by the major liver societies based on weak clinical evidence [47, 79, 124]. The uncertainties about natural history and the variable success of pharmacological regimens have justified recommendations that the predominant disease component of the overlap syndrome direct the management strategy [47].

Patients with predominant manifestations of AIH and secondary or subsequent features of PSC have been treated mainly with prednisolone, 0.5 mg/kg daily, in conjunction with azathioprine, 1–2 mg/kg daily [26, 48] (Table 4.4). Regimens that have not used weight-based

Table 4.4 Treatment regimens and outcomes in the overlap syndrome of PSC and AIH

PSC/AIH overlap	Induction regimen	Maintenance regimen	Outcomes
AIH predominant			
Floreani et al. *N*=7	Prednisolone, 0.5 mg/kg daily [26] Azathioprine, 2 mg/kg daily [26] UDCA, 15–20 mg/kg daily [26]	Tailored to response [26]: Prednisolone, 10–15 mg daily Azathioprine, 50–75 mg daily UDCA, 15–20 mg/kg daily	ALT better, 100 % [26] GGT unimproved [26] ALP unimproved [26] Survival, 100 % [26]
Al-Chalabi et al. *N*=16	Prednisolone, 0.5 mg/kg daily [48] Azathioprine, 1 mg/kg daily [48] UDCA, limited use [48]	Tailored to response [48]: Azathioprine, 2 mg/kg daily Prednisolone decreased	Tests improved, 85 % [48] Tissue better, 77 % [48] Malignancy, 12 % [48] Death or LT, 44 % [48]
McNair et al. *N*=5	Prednisolone, 15–80 mg daily [20] Azathioprine, 75–100 mg daily [20] UDCA, limited use [20]	Tailored to response [20]: Azathioprine continued Prednisolone, 7.5 mg daily	Tests better, 100 % [20] UDCA ineffective [20]
Luth et al. *N*=16	Prednisolone, unreported dose [28] Azathioprine, unreported dose [28] UDCA, limited use [28]	Schedule unreported [28]	Tests better, 100 % [28] Cirrhosis, 56 % [28] LT, 19 % [28] No malignancy [28]
Gregorio et al. *N*=27 (children)	Prednisolone, 2 mg/kg daily [125] UDCA in most children [24]	Tailored to response [125]: Prednisolone, 2.5–5 mg daily Azathioprine, 1–2 mg/kg daily	Tests normal, 56 % [24] Transplant-free, 65 % [24] ERC worse, 30 % [24] No malignancy [24]
PSC predominant			
van Buuren et al. *N*=9	Prednisone, unreported dose [23] Azathioprine, unreported dose [23] UDCA in 67 % [23]	Schedule unreported [23]	Tests better, 100 % [23] LT, 11 % [23] UDCA weak effect [23]
Olsson et al. *N*=26	Prednisolone, unreported dose [29] Azathioprine in 58 % [29] UDCA in 50 % [29]	Schedule unreported [29]	Small duct PSC good [29] Large duct PSC poor [29] Tests better, 67 % [29]

Numbers in brackets are references
AIH autoimmune hepatitis, *ALP* serum alkaline phosphatase level, *ALT* serum alanine aminotransferase level, *ERC* endoscopic retrograde cholangiography, *GGT* serum gamma glutamyl transferase level, *LT* liver transplantation, *PBC* primary biliary cholangitis, *PSC* primary sclerosing cholangitis, *UDCA* ursodeoxycholic acid

dosing schedules have administered prednisolone, 15–80 mg daily, and azathioprine, 75–100 mg daily [20]. Children with AIH and ASC have been treated with prednisolone, 2 mg/kg daily (maximum dose, 60 mg daily), and the dose has been tapered by 5–10 mg every 2 weeks depending on symptoms and serum AST level [24, 125]. Azathioprine, 1–2 mg/kg daily, has been added if the serum AST level has increased during the steroid taper or steroid intolerance has developed. Ursodeoxycholic acid, 15–20 mg/kg daily, has been administered to all patients in addition to prednisolone and azathioprine in only one study [26]. Its use in other studies has been limited, and the dosing schedules have not been reported [20, 28, 48]. In most children, ursodeoxycholic acid has been used in addition to prednisolone with or without azathioprine [24].

Prednisone or prednisolone has been the principal drug administered to patients with predominant features of PSC and secondary or subsequent features of AIH [23, 29] (Table 4.4). Ursodeoxycholic acid has been added to the regimen in 50–67 % of patients, and azathioprine has been included in 58–100 % of patients, recognizing that these experiences have been small [23, 29]. The major difference between the regimens used for AIH-predominant disease and those for PSC-predominant disease has been the greater tendency to include ursodeoxycholic acid in the regimens with PSC predominance (Table 4.4). Isolated cases of the overlap syndrome of PSC and AIH have been treated with cyclosporine [126] and tacrolimus [29].

The European Association for the Study of the Liver (EASL) has recommended treatment of the overlap syndrome of PSC and AIH with ursodeoxycholic acid and immunosuppressive medications [124], and the American Association for the Study of Liver Diseases (AASLD) has recommended treatment with corticosteroids or other immunosuppressive agents [79]. Importantly, the presence of PSC in the overlap syndrome warrants compliance with all the guidelines for managing classical PSC, especially the same preventive measures for metabolic bone disease and the same screening procedures for the detection of biliary, liver, and non-liver malignancies [76, 79, 124].

Ursodeoxycholic acid has been the principal agent used in the management of the overlap syndrome of PSC and PBC [33–37] (Table 4.5). It has been administered as a fixed dose (750 mg daily) [33, 34] and as a weight-based dose (10 mg/kg daily increased to 15 mg/kg daily if there has been histological progression) [37]. Prednisolone, 40 mg daily tapered to 5 mg daily, and azathioprine, 150 mg daily tapered to 100 mg daily, have been used in one patient who had features of AIH, PBC, and PSC [34]. Prednisolone and azathioprine (doses unreported) have also been used in conjunction with ursodeoxycholic acid (unreported dose) in a patient with concurrent rheumatoid arthritis [35]. One patient with concurrent rheumatoid arthritis has been treated with ursodeoxycholic acid and monoclonal antibodies to tumor necrosis factor-alpha (adalimumab) [37]. The major liver societies have not promulgated a preferred management strategy for the overlap syndrome of PSC and PBC. High-dose ursodeoxycholic acid (28–30 mg/kg daily) has been associated with adverse clinical events, including disease progression, requirement for liver transplantation, and death, and it should be avoided in all patients with PSC [127, 128].

Outcomes

The overlap syndromes of PSC have been insufficiently studied to establish their outcomes with or without therapy and their risk of biliary, liver, and non-liver malignancy. Most studies have emphasized the low frequency of cholangiocarcinoma and colorectal carcinoma in these patients [24, 26, 28], whereas other studies have indicated that malignancies, including hepatocellular carcinoma, may occur [29, 48] (Table 4.4). Furthermore, laboratory tests of liver inflammation may commonly improve and even normalize during immunosuppressive therapy, whereas the histological disease may still progress to cirrhosis in 56 % and warrant liver transplantation in 19 % [28]. In children, immunosuppressive therapy can normalize the tests of liver inflammation in 56 % but still be associated with worsening cholangiographic changes and reduced transplant-free survival at 10 years compared to children with classical AIH (65 % versus 100 %) [24]. The laboratory indices of cholestasis do not respond as readily or as completely to those of liver inflammation, and this dissociation may indicate or contribute to disease progression during therapy [24, 26, 29].

The prognosis of the overlap syndrome between PSC and AIH is also influenced by the distribution of the disease within the biliary system (Table 4.4). Patients with large duct PSC and AIH progress to hepatic failure or cholangiocarcinoma more commonly than patients with small duct PSC and AIH (11 % versus 0 %) [29]. They also require liver transplantation more commonly (26 % versus 0 %) during comparable periods of observation (120 ± 56 versus 71 ± 56 months) [29]. In contrast, patients with large duct PSC and AIH have greater improvement in their serum aminotransferase levels during immunosuppressive therapy than patients with small duct PSC and AIH while maintaining similar serum alkaline phosphatase levels and a more aggressive potential [29]. The prognosis of the overlap syndrome between PSC and AIH appears to be better than classical PSC [26] and worse than classical AIH [48].

Table 4.5 Treatment regimens and outcomes in the overlap syndrome of PSC and PBC

Agent (s)[a]	Dose (s)[a]	Outcomes[a]
UDCA (fixed dose)	UDCA, 750 mg daily [33, 34] UDCA, unreported dose [36]	Normal tests within 4 months (small duct PSC) [36] Survival for 5 years (small duct PSC) [36] Recurrent cholangitis (large duct PSC) [33, 34] Progression to cirrhosis (large duct PSC) [33] Persistent test abnormalities (large duct PSC) [33] Considered for LT (large duct PSC) [33] Improved tests (large duct PSC) [34]
UDCA (weight-based dose) with adalimumab for concurrent arthritis	UDCA, 10 mg/kg daily, increased to 15 mg/kg daily if progression [37] Adalimumab, unreported dose [37]	Normal serum AST and IgG (large duct PSC) [37] Improved GGT and ALP (large duct PSC) [37] Improved arthritis (large duct PSC) [37]
UDCA and corticosteroids with azathioprine for concurrent arthritis	UDCA, unreported dose [35] Prednisolone, unreported dose [35] Azathioprine, unreported dose [35]	Cholangitis (large duct PSC) [35] Persistent cholestatic test abnormalities [35] Stable tests for 17 years [35]
UDCA and corticosteroids with azathioprine for features of AIH	UDCA, unreported dose [34] Prednisolone, 40 mg daily [34] Azathioprine, 100 mg daily [34]	Tests improved after 4 weeks (large duct PSC) [34] Recurrent hepatic encephalopathy [34] Stable improved tests after 3 years [34] Chronic maintenance therapy (prednisolone, 5 mg daily, and azathioprine, 100 mg daily) [34]

Numbers in brackets are references
AIH autoimmune hepatitis, *ALP* serum alkaline phosphatase level, *AST* serum aspartate aminotransferase level, *GGT* serum gamma glutamyl transferase level, *IgG* serum immunoglobulin G level, *LT* liver transplantation, *PBC* primary biliary cholangitis, *PSC* primary sclerosing cholangitis, *UDCA* ursodeoxycholic acid
[a]Isolated cases

The experiences with the overlap syndrome between PSC and PBC have been too limited to project its outcome (Table 4.5). Recurrent episodes of cholangitis have required intravenous antibiotic therapy and prompted consideration of liver transplantation [33, 35]. Concurrent features of rheumatoid arthritis have contributed to morbidity and justified adjunctive therapies, including monoclonal antibodies to tumor necrosis factor-alpha (adalimumab) [37] and prednisolone in combination with azathioprine [35]. Laboratory tests of liver inflammation and cholestasis have improved [37], normalized [36], or remained abnormal during treatment [33, 35], and progression to cirrhosis has occurred [33]. Transplant-free survival has been possible in all reported cases, and one patient has had stable cholestatic enzyme abnormalities for 17 years [35].

Overview

Patients with histological and/or cholangiographic changes typical of PSC may also have inflammatory and immunological features associated with AIH or PBC [15]. These patients have been designated as having the overlap syndromes of PSC and AIH and PSC and PBC. Patients with AIH may have a cholestatic syndrome in the absence of AMA and cholangiographic changes of PSC, and they have been designated as having autoimmune cholangitis [12, 15, 39]. These patients probably include individuals with small duct PSC and AMA-negative PBC, and they are more likely to be variants of classical PSC and PBC than overlap syndromes.

The diagnosis of the overlap syndromes of PSC is based mainly on clinical judgment [15, 47].

Marked laboratory (serum AST and ALT abnormalities, hypergammaglobulinemia, and increased serum IgG levels) and serological (ANA, SMA, or anti-LKM1) manifestations of inflammatory and immune-mediated activity in patients with PSC suggest the overlap syndrome between PSC and AIH [15]. Marked cholestatic laboratory (serum ALP and GGT abnormalities, ALP/AST ratio >1) and histological (cholangitis, ductopenia, periductal fibrosis) features in patients with AIH suggest the overlap syndrome of AIH and PSC [15]. The presence of AMA and histological features of destructive cholangitis in patients with PSC constitute the overlap syndrome of PSC and PBC [15].

The histological assessment is a key determinant of the overlap syndromes of PSC, whereas the use of scoring systems that have been developed by the IAIHG for the diagnosis of AIH has been discouraged [47]. The frequency of the overlap syndrome of PSC and AIH is widely variable, but it is best estimated to be 4–17 % in adults with immune-mediated liver disease [22, 23, 28, 37, 48]. The frequency of PSC and PBC is 0.7 % among a similar cohort [34].

Management strategies have not been established by rigorous comparative clinical trials. Corticosteroids in combination with azathioprine have been the principal regimen in adults with predominant features of AIH and secondary features of PSC, whereas ursodeoxycholic acid in conjunction with prednisolone and azathioprine has been used more commonly in patients with predominant features of PSC and secondary features of AIH [15]. The EASL has endorsed combination treatment with ursodeoxycholic acid and immunosuppressive drugs (presumably corticosteroids and azathioprine) [124], and the AASLD has recommended treatment with corticosteroids or other unspecified immunosuppressive agents [79]. Management strategies of the overlap syndrome of PSC and PBC have been based mainly on ursodeoxycholic acid administered in low dose.

This review did not receive financial support from a funding agency or institution, and Albert J. Czaja, MD has no conflict of interests to declare.

References

1. Ludwig J, Barham SS, LaRusso NF, Elveback LR, Wiesner RH, McCall JT. Morphologic features of chronic hepatitis associated with primary sclerosing cholangitis and chronic ulcerative colitis. Hepatology. 1981;1:632–40.
2. Ludwig J, Czaja AJ, Dickson ER, LaRusso NF, Wiesner RH. Manifestations of nonsuppurative cholangitis in chronic hepatobiliary diseases: morphologic spectrum, clinical correlations and terminology. Liver. 1984;4:105–16.
3. Barbatis C, Grases P, Shepherd HA, Chapman RW, Trowell J, Jewell DP, et al. Histological features of sclerosing cholangitis in patients with chronic ulcerative colitis. J Clin Pathol. 1985;38:778–83.
4. Portmann B, Zen Y. Inflammatory disease of the bile ducts-cholangiopathies: liver biopsy challenge and clinicopathological correlation. Histopathology. 2012;60:236–48.
5. Azizi L, Raynal M, Cazejust J, Ruiz A, Menu Y, Arrive L. MR imaging of sclerosing cholangitis. Clin Res Hepatol Gastroenterol. 2012;36:130–8.
6. Arrive L, Ruiz A, El Mouhadi S, Azizi L, Monnier-Cholley L, Menu Y. MRI of cholangitis: traps and tips. Diagn Interv Imaging. 2013;94:757–70.
7. Ruiz A, Lemoinne S, Carrat F, Corpechot C, Chazouilleres O, Arrive L. Radiologic course of primary sclerosing cholangitis: assessment by three-dimensional magnetic resonance cholangiography and predictive features of progression. Hepatology. 2014;59:242–50.
8. Angulo P, Pearce DH, Johnson CD, Henry JJ, LaRusso NF, Petersen BT, et al. Magnetic resonance cholangiography in patients with biliary disease: its role in primary sclerosing cholangitis. J Hepatol. 2000;33:520–7.
9. Berstad AE, Aabakken L, Smith HJ, Aasen S, Boberg KM, Schrumpf E. Diagnostic accuracy of magnetic resonance and endoscopic retrograde cholangiography in primary sclerosing cholangitis. Clin Gastroenterol Hepatol. 2006;4:514–20.
10. Talwalkar JA, Angulo P, Johnson CD, Petersen BT, Lindor KD. Cost-minimization analysis of MRC versus ERCP for the diagnosis of primary sclerosing cholangitis. Hepatology. 2004;40:39–45.
11. Czaja AJ. The variant forms of autoimmune hepatitis. Ann Intern Med. 1996;125:588–98.
12. Czaja AJ. Frequency and nature of the variant syndromes of autoimmune liver disease. Hepatology. 1998;28:360–5.
13. Czaja AJ. Variant forms of autoimmune hepatitis. Curr Gastroenterol Rep. 1999;1:63–70.
14. Ben-Ari Z, Czaja AJ. Autoimmune hepatitis and its variant syndromes. Gut. 2001;49:589–94.
15. Czaja AJ. The overlap syndromes of autoimmune hepatitis. Dig Dis Sci. 2013;58:326–43.
16. Czaja AJ. Diagnosis and management of the overlap syndromes of autoimmune hepatitis. Can J Gastroenterol. 2013;27:417–23.

17. Czaja AJ. Cholestatic phenotypes of autoimmune hepatitis. Clin Gastroenterol Hepatol. 2014;12:1430–8.
18. Boberg KM, Fausa O, Haaland T, Holter E, Mellbye OJ, Spurkland A, et al. Features of autoimmune hepatitis in primary sclerosing cholangitis: an evaluation of 114 primary sclerosing cholangitis patients according to a scoring system for the diagnosis of autoimmune hepatitis. Hepatology. 1996;23:1369–76.
19. Gohlke F, Lohse AW, Dienes HP, Lohr H, Marker-Hermann E, Gerken G, et al. Evidence for an overlap syndrome of autoimmune hepatitis and primary sclerosing cholangitis. J Hepatol. 1996;24:699–705.
20. McNair AN, Moloney M, Portmann BC, Williams R, McFarlane IG. Autoimmune hepatitis overlapping with primary sclerosing cholangitis in five cases. Am J Gastroenterol. 1998;93:777–84.
21. Koskinas J, Raptis I, Manika Z, Hadziyannis S. Overlapping syndrome of autoimmune hepatitis and primary sclerosing cholangitis associated with pyoderma gangrenosum and ulcerative colitis. Eur J Gastroenterol Hepatol. 1999;11:1421–4.
22. Kaya M, Angulo P, Lindor KD. Overlap of autoimmune hepatitis and primary sclerosing cholangitis: an evaluation of a modified scoring system. J Hepatol. 2000;33:537–42.
23. van Buuren HR, van Hoogstraten HJE, Terkivatan T, Schalm SW, Vleggaar FP. High prevalence of autoimmune hepatitis among patients with primary sclerosing cholangitis. J Hepatol. 2000;33:543–8.
24. Gregorio GV, Portmann B, Karani J, Harrison P, Donaldson PT, Vergani D, et al. Autoimmune hepatitis/sclerosing cholangitis overlap syndrome in childhood: a 16-year prospective study. Hepatology. 2001;33:544–53.
25. Takiguchi J, Ohira H, Rai T, Shishido S, Tojo J, Sato Y, et al. Autoimmune hepatitis overlapping with primary sclerosing cholangitis. Intern Med. 2002;41: 696–700.
26. Floreani A, Rizzotto ER, Ferrara F, Carderi I, Caroli D, Blasone L, et al. Clinical course and outcome of autoimmune hepatitis/primary sclerosing cholangitis overlap syndrome. Am J Gastroenterol. 2005;100:1516–22.
27. Saich R, Chapman R. Primary sclerosing cholangitis, autoimmune hepatitis and overlap syndromes in inflammatory bowel disease. World J Gastroenterol. 2008;14:331–7.
28. Luth S, Kanzler S, Frenzel C, Kasper HU, Dienes HP, Schramm C, et al. Characteristics and long-term prognosis of the autoimmune hepatitis/primary sclerosing cholangitis overlap syndrome. J Clin Gastroenterol. 2009;43:75–80.
29. Olsson R, Glaumann H, Almer S, Broome U, Lebrun B, Bergquist A, et al. High prevalence of small duct primary sclerosing cholangitis among patients with overlapping autoimmune hepatitis and primary sclerosing cholangitis. Eur J Intern Med. 2009;20:190–6.
30. Hunter M, Loughrey MB, Gray M, Ellis P, McDougall N, Callender M. Evaluating distinctive features for early diagnosis of primary sclerosing cholangitis overlap syndrome in adults with autoimmune hepatitis. Ulster Med J. 2011;80:15–8.
31. Rojas CP, Bodicharla R, Campuzano-Zuluaga G, Hernandez L, Rodriguez MM. Autoimmune hepatitis and primary sclerosing cholangitis in children and adolescents. Fetal Pediatr Pathol. 2014;33:202–9.
32. Rubel LR, Seeff LB, Patel V. Primary biliary cirrhosis-primary sclerosing cholangitis overlap syndrome. Arch Pathol Lab Med. 1984;108:360–1.
33. Burak KW, Urbanski SJ, Swain MG. A case of coexisting primary biliary cirrhosis and primary sclerosing cholangitis: a new overlap of autoimmune liver diseases. Dig Dis Sci. 2001;46:2043–7.
34. Kingham JG, Abbasi A. Co-existence of primary biliary cirrhosis and primary sclerosing cholangitis: a rare overlap syndrome put in perspective. Eur J Gastroenterol Hepatol. 2005;17:1077–80.
35. Jeevagan A. Overlap of primary biliary cirrhosis and primary sclerosing cholangitis: a rare coincidence or a new syndrome. Int J Gen Med. 2010;3:143–6.
36. Oliveira EM, Oliveira PM, Becker V, Dellavance A, Andrade LE, Lanzoni V, et al. Overlapping of primary biliary cirrhosis and small duct primary sclerosing cholangitis: first case report. J Clin Med Res. 2012;4:429–33.
37. Floreani A, Motta R, Cazzagon N, Franceschet I, Roncalli M, Del Ross T, et al. The overlap syndrome between primary biliary cirrhosis and primary sclerosing cholangitis. Dig Liver Dis. 2015;47:432–5.
38. Lacerda MA, Ludwig J, Dickson ER, Jorgensen RA, Lindor KD. Antimitochondrial antibody-negative primary biliary cirrhosis. Am J Gastroenterol. 1995;90:247–9.
39. Czaja AJ, Carpenter HA, Santrach PJ, Moore SB. Autoimmune cholangitis within the spectrum of autoimmune liver disease. Hepatology. 2000;31: 1231–8.
40. Kim WR, Ludwig J, Lindor KD. Variant forms of cholestatic diseases involving small bile ducts in adults. Am J Gastroenterol. 2000;95:1130–8.
41. Angulo P, Maor-Kendler Y, Lindor KD. Small-duct primary sclerosing cholangitis: a long-term follow-up study. Hepatology. 2002;35:1494–500.
42. Bjornsson E, Olsson R, Bergquist A, Lindgren S, Braden B, Chapman RW, et al. The natural history of small-duct primary sclerosing cholangitis. Gastroenterology. 2008;134:975–80.
43. Goodman ZD, McNally PR, Davis DR, Ishak KG. Autoimmune cholangitis: a variant of primary biliary cirrhosis. Clinicopathologic and serologic correlations in 200 cases. Dig Dis Sci. 1995;40:1232–42.
44. Invernizzi P, Crosignani A, Battezzati PM, Covini G, De Valle G, Larghi A, et al. Comparison of the clinical features and clinical course of antimitochondrial antibody-positive and -negative primary biliary cirrhosis. Hepatology. 1997;25:1090–5.
45. Nakanuma Y, Harada K, Kaji K, Terasaki S, Tsuneyama K, Moteki S, et al. Clinicopathological

study of primary biliary cirrhosis negative for antimitochondrial antibodies. Liver. 1997;17:281–7.
46. Muratori P, Muratori L, Gershwin ME, Czaja AJ, Pappas G, MacCariello S, et al. 'True' antimitochondrial antibody-negative primary biliary cirrhosis, low sensitivity of the routine assays, or both? Clin Exp Immunol. 2004;135:154–8.
47. Boberg KM, Chapman RW, Hirschfield GM, Lohse AW, Manns MP, Schrumpf E. Overlap syndromes: the International Autoimmune Hepatitis Group (IAIHG) position statement on a controversial issue. J Hepatol. 2011;54:374–85.
48. Al-Chalabi T, Portmann BC, Bernal W, McFarlane IG, Heneghan MA. Autoimmune hepatitis overlap syndromes: an evaluation of treatment response, long-term outcome and survival. Aliment Pharmacol Ther. 2008;28:209–20.
49. Perdigoto R, Carpenter HA, Czaja AJ. Frequency and significance of chronic ulcerative colitis in severe corticosteroid-treated autoimmune hepatitis. J Hepatol. 1992;14:325–31.
50. Abdo AA, Bain VG, Kichian K, Lee SS. Evolution of autoimmune hepatitis to primary sclerosing cholangitis: a sequential syndrome. Hepatology. 2002;36: 1393–9.
51. Wiesner RH, LaRusso NF. Clinicopathologic features of the syndrome of primary sclerosing cholangitis. Gastroenterology. 1980;79:200–6.
52. Zauli D, Schrumpf E, Crespi C, Cassani F, Fausa O, Aadland E. An autoantibody profile in primary sclerosing cholangitis. J Hepatol. 1987;5:14–8.
53. Lo SK, Fleming KA, Chapman RW. Prevalence of anti-neutrophil antibody in primary sclerosing cholangitis and ulcerative colitis using an alkaline phosphatase technique. Gut. 1992;33:1370–5.
54. Seibold F, Weber P, Klein R, Berg PA, Wiedmann KH. Clinical significance of antibodies against neutrophils in patients with inflammatory bowel disease and primary sclerosing cholangitis. Gut. 1992;33:657–62.
55. Angulo P, Peter JB, Gershwin ME, DeSotel CK, Shoenfeld Y, Ahmed AE, et al. Serum autoantibodies in patients with primary sclerosing cholangitis. J Hepatol. 2000;32:182–7.
56. Terjung B, Worman HJ. Anti-neutrophil antibodies in primary sclerosing cholangitis. Best Pract Res Clin Gastroenterol. 2001;15:629–42.
57. Chapman RW, Arborgh BA, Rhodes JM, Summerfield JA, Dick R, Scheuer PJ, et al. Primary sclerosing cholangitis: a review of its clinical features, cholangiography, and hepatic histology. Gut. 1980;21:870–7.
58. Aadland E, Schrumpf E, Fausa O, Elgjo K, Heilo A, Aakhus T, et al. Primary sclerosing cholangitis: a long-term follow-up study. Scand J Gastroenterol. 1987;22:655–64.
59. Targan SR, Landers C, Vidrich A, Czaja AJ. High-titer antineutrophil cytoplasmic antibodies in type-1 autoimmune hepatitis. Gastroenterology. 1995;108: 1159–66.
60. Alvarez F, Berg PA, Bianchi FB, Bianchi L, Burroughs AK, Cancado EL, et al. International Autoimmune Hepatitis Group Report: review of criteria for diagnosis of autoimmune hepatitis. J Hepatol. 1999;31:929–38.
61. Czaja AJ. Autoimmune hepatitis. Part B: diagnosis. Expert Rev Gastroenterol Hepatol. 2007;1:129–43.
62. Czaja AJ. Diagnosis and management of autoimmune hepatitis. Clin Liver Dis. 2015;19:57–79.
63. Manns MP, Czaja AJ, Gorham JD, Krawitt EL, Mieli-Vergani G, Vergani D, et al. Diagnosis and management of autoimmune hepatitis. Hepatology. 2010;51:2193–213.
64. Johnson PJ, McFarlane IG. Meeting report: International Autoimmune Hepatitis Group. Hepatology. 1993;18: 998–1005.
65. Czaja AJ. Performance parameters of the diagnostic scoring systems for autoimmune hepatitis. Hepatology. 2008;48:1540–8.
66. Papamichalis PA, Zachou K, Koukoulis GK, Veloni A, Karacosta EG, Kypri L, et al. The revised international autoimmune hepatitis score in chronic liver diseases including autoimmune hepatitis/overlap syndromes and autoimmune hepatitis with concurrent other liver disorders. J Autoimmune Dis. 2007;4:3.
67. Gatselis NK, Zachou K, Papamichalis P, Koukoulis GK, Gabeta S, Dalekos GN, et al. Comparison of simplified score with the revised original score for the diagnosis of autoimmune hepatitis: a new or a complementary diagnostic score? Dig Liver Dis. 2010;42:807–12.
68. Yamamoto K, Terada R, Okamoto R, Hiasa Y, Abe M, Onji M, et al. A scoring system for primary biliary cirrhosis and its application for variant forms of autoimmune liver disease. J Gastroenterol. 2003;38:52–9.
69. Gur H, Shen G, Sutjita M, Terrberry J, Alosachie I, Barka N, et al. Autoantibody profile of primary sclerosing cholangitis. Pathobiology. 1995;63:76–82.
70. Pratico AD, Salafia S, Barone P, La Rosa M, Leonardi S. Type II autoimmune hepatitis and small duct sclerosing cholangitis in a seven years Old child: an overlap syndrome? Hepat Mon. 2013;13, e14452.
71. Kenny RP, Czaja AJ, Ludwig J, Dickson ER. Frequency and significance of antimitochondrial antibodies in severe chronic active hepatitis. Dig Dis Sci. 1986;31:705–11.
72. Muratori P, Granito A, Quarneti C, Ferri S, Menichella R, Cassani F, et al. Autoimmune hepatitis in Italy: the Bologna experience. J Hepatol. 2009;50:1210–8.
73. Zachou K, Gatselis N, Papadamou G, Rigopoulou EI, Dalekos GN. Mycophenolate for the treatment of autoimmune hepatitis: prospective assessment of its efficacy and safety for induction and maintenance of remission in a large cohort of treatment-naive patients. J Hepatol. 2011;55:636–46.
74. Carpenter HA, Czaja AJ. The role of histologic evaluation in the diagnosis and management of autoim-

mune hepatitis and its variants. Clin Liver Dis. 2002;6:685–705.
75. Burak KW, Angulo P, Lindor KD. Is there a role for liver biopsy in primary sclerosing cholangitis? Am J Gastroenterol. 2003;98:1155–8.
76. Lindor KD, Kowdley KV, Harrison ME. ACG clinical guideline: primary sclerosing cholangitis. Am J Gastroenterol. 2015;110:646–59.
77. Czaja AJ, Carpenter HA. Sensitivity, specificity, and predictability of biopsy interpretations in chronic hepatitis. Gastroenterology. 1993;105:1824–32.
78. Lindor KD, Gershwin ME, Poupon R, Kaplan M, Bergasa NV, Heathcote EJ. AASLD Practice Guidelines. Primary biliary cirrhosis. Hepatology. 2009;50:291–308.
79. Chapman R, Fevery J, Kalloo A, Nagorney DM, Boberg KM, Shneider B, et al. Diagnosis and management of primary sclerosing cholangitis. Hepatology. 2010;51:660–78.
80. Mieli-Vergani G, Vergani D. Autoimmune hepatitis in children: what is different from adult AIH? Semin Liver Dis. 2009;29:297–306.
81. Mieli-Vergani G, Vergani D. Autoimmune liver diseases in children: what is different from adulthood? Best Pract Res Clin Gastroenterol. 2011;25:783–95.
82. Mieli-Vergani G, Vergani D. Unique features of primary sclerosing cholangitis in children. Curr Opin Gastroenterol. 2010;26:265–8.
83. Lewin M, Vilgrain V, Ozenne V, Lemoine M, Wendum D, Paradis V, et al. Prevalence of sclerosing cholangitis in adults with autoimmune hepatitis: a prospective magnetic resonance imaging and histological study. Hepatology. 2009;50:528–37.
84. Abdalian R, Dhar P, Jhaveri K, Haider M, Guindi M, Heathcote EJ. Prevalence of sclerosing cholangitis in adults with autoimmune hepatitis: evaluating the role of routine magnetic resonance imaging. Hepatology. 2008;47:949–57.
85. Gheorghe L, Iacob S, Gheorghe C, Iacob R, Simionov I, Vadan R, et al. Frequency and predictive factors for overlap syndrome between autoimmune hepatitis and primary cholestatic liver disease. Eur J Gastroenterol Hepatol. 2004;16:585–92.
86. Czaja AJ, Carpenter HA. Validation of scoring system for diagnosis of autoimmune hepatitis. Dig Dis Sci. 1996;41:305–14.
87. Ben-Ari Z, Dhillon AP, Sherlock S. Autoimmune cholangiopathy: part of the spectrum of autoimmune chronic active hepatitis. Hepatology. 1993;18:10–5.
88. Michieletti P, Wanless IR, Katz A, Scheuer PJ, Yeaman SJ, Bassendine MF, et al. Antimitochondrial antibody negative primary biliary cirrhosis: a distinct syndrome of autoimmune cholangitis. Gut. 1994;35:260–5.
89. Taylor SL, Dean PJ, Riely CA. Primary autoimmune cholangitis. An alternative to antimitochondrial antibody-negative primary biliary cirrhosis. Am J Surg Pathol. 1994;18:91–9.
90. Sherlock S. Ludwig Symposium on biliary disorders. Autoimmune cholangitis: a unique entity? Mayo Clin Proc. 1998;73:184–90.
91. Romero-Gomez M, Wichmann I, Crespo J, Pares A, Rodrigo L, Alvarez A, et al. Serum immunological profile in patients with chronic autoimmune cholestasis. Am J Gastroenterol. 2004;99:2150–7.
92. Wee A, Ludwig J. Pericholangitis in chronic ulcerative colitis: primary sclerosing cholangitis of the small bile ducts? Ann Intern Med. 1985;102:581–7.
93. Bizzaro N, Covini G, Rosina F, Muratori P, Tonutti E, Villalta D, et al. Overcoming a "probable" diagnosis in antimitochondrial antibody negative primary biliary cirrhosis: study of 100 sera and review of the literature. Clin Rev Allergy Immunol. 2010. doi:10.1007/s12016-010-8234-y.
94. Liu H, Norman GL, Shums Z, Worman HJ, Krawitt EL, Bizzaro N, et al. PBC screen: an IgG/IgA dual isotype ELISA detecting multiple mitochondrial and nuclear autoantibodies specific for primary biliary cirrhosis. J Autoimmun. 2010;35:436–42.
95. Umemura T, Zen Y, Hamano H, Ichijo T, Kawa S, Nakanuma Y, et al. IgG4 associated autoimmune hepatitis: a differential diagnosis for classical autoimmune hepatitis. Gut. 2007;56:1471–2.
96. Chung H, Watanabe T, Kudo M, Maenishi O, Wakatsuki Y, Chiba T. Identification and characterization of IgG4-associated autoimmune hepatitis. Liver Int Off J Int Assoc Study Liver. 2010;30: 222–31.
97. Umemura T, Zen Y, Hamano H, Joshita S, Ichijo T, Yoshizawa K, et al. Clinical significance of immunoglobulin G4-associated autoimmune hepatitis. J Gastroenterol. 2011;46 Suppl 1:48–55.
98. Deshpande V, Sainani NI, Chung RT, Pratt DS, Mentha G, Rubbia-Brandt L, et al. IgG4-associated cholangitis: a comparative histological and immunophenotypic study with primary sclerosing cholangitis on liver biopsy material. Mod Pathol. 2009;22: 1287–95.
99. Ghazale A, Chari ST, Zhang L, Smyrk TC, Takahashi N, Levy MJ, et al. Immunoglobulin G4-associated cholangitis: clinical profile and response to therapy. Gastroenterology. 2008;134:706–15.
100. Bjornsson E, Chari S, Silveira M, Gossard A, Takahashi N, Smyrk T, et al. Primary sclerosing cholangitis associated with elevated immunoglobulin G4: clinical characteristics and response to therapy. Am J Ther. 2011;18:198–205.
101. Bjornsson E, Chari ST, Smyrk TC, Lindor K. Immunoglobulin G4 associated cholangitis: description of an emerging clinical entity based on review of the literature. Hepatology. 2007;45:1547–54.
102. Montano-Loza AJ, Lalor E, Mason AL. Recognizing immunoglobulin G4 related overlap syndromes in patients with pancreatic and hepatobiliary diseases. Can J Gastroenterol. 2008;22:840–6.
103. Czaja AJ. Extrahepatic immunologic features of chronic viral hepatitis. Dig Dis. 1997;15:125–44.
104. Czaja AJ. Drug-induced autoimmune-like hepatitis. Dig Dis Sci. 2011;56:958–76.
105. Loria P, Lonardo A, Leonardi F, Fontana C, Carulli L, Verrone AM, et al. Non-organ-specific auto-

antibodies in nonalcoholic fatty liver disease: prevalence and correlates. Dig Dis Sci. 2003;48: 2173–81.
106. Adams LA, Lindor KD, Angulo P. The prevalence of autoantibodies and autoimmune hepatitis in patients with nonalcoholic fatty liver disease. Am J Gastroenterol. 2004;99:1316–20.
107. Czaja AJ, Santrach PJ, Breanndan Moore S. Shared genetic risk factors in autoimmune liver disease. Dig Dis Sci. 2001;46:140–7.
108. Donaldson PT, Doherty DG, Hayllar KM, McFarlane IG, Johnson PJ, Williams R. Susceptibility to autoimmune chronic active hepatitis: human leukocyte antigens DR4 and A1-B8-DR3 are independent risk factors. Hepatology. 1991;13:701–6.
109. Strettell MD, Donaldson PT, Thomson LJ, Santrach PJ, Moore SB, Czaja AJ, et al. Allelic basis for HLA-encoded susceptibility to type 1 autoimmune hepatitis. Gastroenterology. 1997;112:2028–35.
110. Czaja AJ, Strettell MD, Thomson LJ, Santrach PJ, Moore SB, Donaldson PT, et al. Associations between alleles of the major histocompatibility complex and type 1 autoimmune hepatitis. Hepatology. 1997;25:317–23.
111. Doherty DG, Donaldson PT, Underhill JA, Farrant JM, Duthie A, Mieli-Vergani G, et al. Allelic sequence variation in the HLA class II genes and proteins in patients with autoimmune hepatitis. Hepatology. 1994;19:609–15.
112. Boberg KM, Lundin KE, Schrumpf E. Etiology and pathogenesis in primary sclerosing cholangitis. Scand J Gastroenterol Suppl. 1994;204:47–58.
113. Donaldson PT, Norris S. Evaluation of the role of MHC class II alleles, haplotypes and selected amino acid sequences in primary sclerosing cholangitis. Autoimmunity. 2002;35:555–64.
114. Agarwal K, Czaja AJ, Jones DE, Donaldson PT. Cytotoxic T lymphocyte antigen-4 (CTLA-4) gene polymorphisms and susceptibility to type 1 autoimmune hepatitis. Hepatology. 2000;31: 49–53.
115. Agarwal K, Jones DE, Daly AK, James OF, Vaidya B, Pearce S, et al. CTLA-4 gene polymorphism confers susceptibility to primary biliary cirrhosis. J Hepatol. 2000;32:538–41.
116. Juran BD, Atkinson EJ, Schlicht EM, Fridley BL, Petersen GM, Lazaridis KN. Interacting alleles of the coinhibitory immunoreceptor genes cytotoxic T-lymphocyte antigen 4 and programmed cell-death 1 influence risk and features of primary biliary cirrhosis. Hepatology. 2008;47:563–70.
117. Joshita S, Umemura T, Yoshizawa K, Katsuyama Y, Tanaka E, Nakamura M, et al. Association analysis of cytotoxic T-lymphocyte antigen 4 gene polymorphisms with primary biliary cirrhosis in Japanese patients. J Hepatol. 2010;53:537–41.
118. Czaja AJ. Autoimmune hepatitis. Part A: pathogenesis. Expert Rev Gastroenterol Hepatol. 2007;1: 113–28.
119. Czaja AJ. Genetic factors affecting the occurrence, clinical phenotype, and outcome of autoimmune hepatitis. Clin Gastroenterol Hepatol. 2008;6:379–88.
120. Czaja AJ. Transitioning from idiopathic to explainable autoimmune hepatitis. Dig Dis Sci. 2015. doi:10.1007/s10620-015-3708-7.
121. Mieli-Vergani G, Lobo-Yeo A, McFarlane BM, McFarlane IG, Mowat AP, Vergani D. Different immune mechanisms leading to autoimmunity in primary sclerosing cholangitis and autoimmune chronic active hepatitis of childhood. Hepatology. 1989;9:198–203.
122. Senaldi G, Portmann B, Mowat AP, Mieli-Vergani G, Vergani D. Immunohistochemical features of the portal tract mononuclear cell infiltrate in chronic aggressive hepatitis. Arch Dis Child. 1992;67:1447–53.
123. Gleeson D, Heneghan MA. British Society of Gastroenterology (BSG) guidelines for management of autoimmune hepatitis. Gut. 2011;60:1611–29.
124. Beuers U, Boberg KM, Chapman RW, Chazouilleres O, Invernizzi P, Jones DEJ, et al. EASL Clinical Practice Guidelines: management of cholestatic liver diseases. J Hepatol. 2009;51:237–67.
125. Gregorio GV, Portmann B, Reid F, Donaldson PT, Doherty DG, McCartney M, et al. Autoimmune hepatitis in childhood: a 20-year experience. Hepatology. 1997;25:541–7.
126. Lawrence SP, Sherman KE, Lawson JM, Goodman ZD. A 39 year old man with chronic hepatitis. Semin Liver Dis. 1994;14:97–105.
127. Lindor KD, Kowdley KV, Luketic VA, Harrison ME, McCashland T, Befeler AS, et al. High-dose ursodeoxycholic acid for the treatment of primary sclerosing cholangitis. Hepatology. 2009;50:808–14.
128. Sinakos E, Marschall HU, Kowdley KV, Befeler A, Keach J, Lindor K. Bile acid changes after high-dose ursodeoxycholic acid treatment in primary sclerosing cholangitis: relation to disease progression. Hepatology. 2010;52:197–203.

IgG4-Related Sclerosing Cholangitis

5

Tamsin Cargill, Emma L. Culver, and Roger W. Chapman

Introduction

IgG4-related sclerosing cholangitis (IgG4-SC) is the biliary manifestation of IgG4-related disease (IgG4-RD), a systemic fibro-inflammatory condition that manifests as organ dysfunction or mass lesions.

IgG4-SC often occurs alongside the pancreatic manifestation of IgG4-RD, autoimmune pancreatitis type 1 (AIP). It commonly presents with obstructive jaundice; however it may be found incidentally when liver function tests or imaging suggest biliary involvement in a patient with IgG4-RD in other organs. Once diagnosed, the disease has a good response to steroid therapy in the inflammatory phase, but patients often relapse. Progressive fibrosis and cirrhosis can develop if the disease is not well controlled.

T. Cargill, MBBS, BSc(Hons), MRCP • E.L. Culver, MBChB, BSc(Hons), MRCP, PhD
Translational Gastroenterology Unit, John Radcliffe Hospital, Oxford, UK

Nuffield Department of Medicine, University of Oxford, Oxford, UK

R.W. Chapman, MD, FRCP, FAASLD (✉)
Nuffield Department of Medicine, University of Oxford, Oxford, UK

Nuffield Department of Medicine, Translational Gastroenterology Unit, Level 5, John Radcliffe Hospital, Headley Way, Headington, Oxford OX3 9DU, UK
e-mail: roger.chapman@ndm.ox.ac.uk

Clinicians face several challenges in the diagnosis of IgG4-SC. Firstly, clinical, biochemical, and radiological findings can mimic biliary and pancreatic malignancy (cholangiocarcinoma (CCA) and pancreatic adenocarcinoma) or primary sclerosing cholangitis (PSC). Furthermore, although the majority of IgG4-SC patients will have an increased serum IgG4, this is not specific to the disease and there is no available noninvasive diagnostic test. Finally, if a biopsy specimen is obtained, there is often insufficient material to identify all of the characteristic histological features seen in IgG4-RD lesions. As a result, many patients are not treated appropriately or undergo unnecessary surgical resection for presumed malignancy.

This chapter outlines the clinical, biochemical, radiological, and histological characteristics of IgG4-SC, as well as its treatment, natural history, and pathogenesis.

The Discovery of IgG4-Related Sclerosing Cholangitis

Cases of sclerosing cholangitis associated with fibrosis outside the bile duct in the retroperitoneum or thyroid gland were first reported in 1963 [6]. Subsequently, pancreatitis and sclerosing cholangitis were observed together [96]. Although associations were made between sclerosing cholangitis, chronic pancreatitis, and inflammation in a variety of other organs, they were not considered

L.M. Forman (ed.), *Primary Sclerosing Cholangitis*, DOI 10.1007/978-3-319-40908-5_5

to be a single disease entity and their pathophysiology remained elusive. In 1995 it was proposed that chronic pancreatitis was autoimmune in etiology, based on the observation that the disease was steroid responsive and associated with a serum hypergammaglobulinemia [97]. It was later demonstrated that serum IgG4 in particular was raised in the disease [29].

The concept that AIP was part of a systemic disease was not suggested until 2003. Histopathological data showed the infiltration of T-Cells, and IgG4-positive plasma cells seen in the pancreatic lesions of AIP were also present in the bile ducts of the same patients [37]. Evidence that sclerosing cholangitis and AIP shared a distinct histological phenotype supported the idea that sclerosing cholangitis was the biliary manifestation of IgG4-RD [99]. In 2007, it was proposed that this form of cholangitis should be termed IgG4-associated cholangitis (IAC), and this nomenclature is still recommended in the European Association for Study of the Liver (EASL) clinical practice guidelines [7, 21]. Currently, the term IgG4-related sclerosing cholangitis (IgG4-SC) is used, after a consensus agreement at the International Symposium on IgG4-RD in 2014.

Epidemiology

There is a paucity of good epidemiological data to estimate the true incidence and prevalence of IgG4-SC. Data collected on AIP captures some patients with coexistent IgG4-SC. It suggests that patients with IgG4-SC are likely to have concurrent AIP. In Japan, the most recent population survey of AIP in 2011 estimated the annual incidence rate to be 1.4 per 100,000 population and prevalence to be 4.6 per 100,000 population, an increase on previous estimates from the 2007 survey [42, 43]. In the 2011 cohort of 918 patients with both new and existing diagnoses of AIP, 95 (10.3 %) had IgG4-SC at the porta hepatis, and 216 (23.5 %) had intrahepatic IgG4-SC [43]. In Western Countries data suggests a stronger co-occurrence of AIP and IgG4-SC. One report from the United States found that in a group of 53 patients with IgG4-SC, 49 (92 %) of them had coexistent AIP and only 4 (8 %) had IgG4-SC alone [26]. Recent analysis of a cohort of 115 patients with AIP and/or IgG4-SC in the United Kingdom found that of the 106 patients with AIP, 60 (56 %) had concurrent IgG4-SC and 9 patients (8 %) had isolated IgG4-SC [32].

Previous data suggested that IgG4-SC is second only to AIP as the most common site of IgG4-RD. This is being challenged by more recent data from several IgG4-RD cohorts, depending on the referral practices and specialists involved (Table 5.1). As IgG4-RD is diagnosed more frequently, differences in patterns of organ involvement between geographical locations may become more apparent.

Disease Pathogenesis

The pathological mechanisms underlying IgG4-SC are not yet fully understood. The raised serum IgG4, lymphoplasmacytic infiltration seen

Table 5.1 Reported frequency of IgG4-SC and AIP

Study	Country	Cohort	N. of patients	IgG4-SC N (%)	AIP N (%)
Kanno et al. [43]	Japan	AIP	91 8	311 (33.8)	918 (100)
Ghazale et al. [26]	USA	IgG4-SC and AIP	53	53 (100)	49 (92)
Huggett et al. [32]	UK	AIP and IgG4-SC	115	69 (60)	106 (92)
Lin et al. [53]	China	IgG4-RD	118	21 (17.9)	45 (38.1)
Inoue et al. [34]	Japan	IgG4-RD	235	(13)	142 (60)
Fernandez-Codina et al. [22]	Spain	IgG4-RD	55	30 (4)	142 (60)
Campochiaro et al. [10]	Italy	IgG4-RD	41	4 (10)	17 (41)

Key: *N* number, *AIP* autoimmune pancreatitis, *IgG4-SC* IgG4-sclerosing cholangitis in disease lesions, and the response to steroids and immunosuppressive agents indicate that aberration of the immune response is central. What triggers and sustains the inflammatory process is not clear, but several mechanisms have been proposed including autoimmunity against a self-antigen, molecular mimicry, or chronic antigen exposure triggering immune dysregulation. Advances in our understanding of the genetic background and the immunological environment of patients, are beginning to unravel disease pathogenesis.

Genetic Susceptibility

No studies to date have focused on the genetics of IgG4-SC patients specifically. Evidence is growing that AIP patients have a genetic background that makes them susceptible to disease development. Single nucleotide polymorphisms in genes encoding immune factors including cytotoxic T lymphocyte-associated antigen 4 (CTLA-4) and Fc receptor-like 3 (FcR-3) have been reported to be associated with AIP development or recurrence [14, 88, 90]. Class II human leukocyte antigen (HLA) alleles HLA DRB1_0405 and DQB1_0401 were identified to be associated with AIP [44]. A Korean study found that substitution on position 57 on HLA DQB1 was associated with disease relapse in AIP [71]. It is likely that variation in class II alleles involved in antigen presentation can influence predisposition to disease and its course.

Autoantigens

A role for autoimmunity is supported by the presence of a T-Cell, B cell, and antibody-rich infiltrate in disease lesions. Multiple candidate autoantibodies and autoantigens have been investigated in AIP, although none have been found to be specific for the disease. Antibodies against carbonic anhydrase II and lactoferrin, which are expressed widely in exocrine organs, have been reported in 73 % and 54 % of AIP patients, respectively [4, 69]. Anti-carbonic anhydrase II antibodies were found to correlate with serum IgG4 levels [4]. Another purported mechanism of disease pathogenesis is molecular mimicry between sequences found in alpha-carbonic anhydrase of the bacterium *Heliobacter pylori* and carbonic anhydrase II [28]. Other candidate antibodies detected at lower levels in AIP include anti-carbonic anhydrase IV, pancreatic secretory trypsin inhibitor, amylase IV, heat-shock protein 10 and plasminogen binding protein [5, 19, 23, 52, 82].

The Role of B Cells and the IgG4 Molecule

The presence of IgG4-positive plasma cells in disease lesions and raised serum IgG4 levels seen in the majority of patients are indications that B cells and antibody production are important in IgG4-SC pathogenesis. The B lymphocyte-depleting agent rituximab has been used with success to treat IgG4-SC patients refractory to steroids and conventional immunosuppressants [11, 12, 45, 46, 55]. Recent work has identified circulating oligoclonal IgG4-positive plasmablasts in patients with active IgG4-RD, which remit after treatment with rituximab and re-expand during relapse [56, 57, 94, 95]. Relapse of IgG4-RD after B-cell depletion with rituximab infers that the reemergence of IgG4-positive plasmablasts are derived from either a subset of memory B cells that survive rituximab therapy or newly generated naïve B cells that interact with a yet unidentified antigen or pathogenic T-Cell repertoire, unaffected by rituximab.

An important question in understanding IgG4-RD pathogenesis is why IgG4 immunoglobulin and IgG4-positive plasma cells are expanded in a great majority of patients. Although it has been postulated that autoantibodies might induce an inappropriate immune response, candidates thus far are of the IgG1 rather than IgG4 subclass. Oligoclonal IgG4-positive clones have been identified in sequencing of whole blood in IgG4-SC patients, suggesting that only specific B cells are expanded [54]. However a generalized polyclonal IgG4 response to multiple common antigens has been demonstrated in IgG4-RD patients. This supports the alternative theory that increased IgG4 is an epiphenomenon, occurring as a result of the expansion of preexisting IgG4-switched B cells rather than being driven by a specific autoantigen [13].

It is unknown as to whether the IgG4 immunoglobulin is directly involved in driving the inflammation seen in disease lesions. IgG4 has anti-inflammatory properties due to its unique structure that allows exchange of its Fab arm, producing functional monomers that are unable to form large immune complexes [91]. Unlike the other gamma immunoglobulin subclasses, IgG4 is unable to activate complement [92]. Under physiological conditions, specific IgG4 responses occur to generate humoral tolerance after repetitive antigen stimulation, for example, in beekeepers that are repeatedly exposed to bee venom [1]. These tolerogenic properties argue that IgG4 molecules themselves are unlikely to be intrinsically harmful.

However, in other immune conditions including pemphigus vulgaris and myasthenia gravis, IgG4 antibodies are thought to be directly pathogenic [24, 33]. In a small study, IgG4 in sera from AIP patients bound with normal pancreatic and biliary epithelial tissue, indicating an interaction between IgG4 antibodies with a yet unidentified antigen [3].

T-Cell Immunological Response

CD4-positive T-Cells are necessary to support and coordinate IgG4-switched B-cell responses, but their role in IgG4-SC pathogenesis has not been fully elucidated. T-Cells are a component of the lymphoplasmacytic infiltrate in disease lesions and are likely to interact with the B cells when in close proximity.

T-helper type 2 (Th2) cells have been implicated in IgG4-RD pathogenesis. The Th2 cytokines IL-4, IL-5, and IL-13 have been detected at the messenger RNA level in IgG4-RD disease lesions, blood CD4-positive T-Cells in IgG4-RD patients, and in the bile of IgG4-SC patients [41, 60, 83, 100, 101]. A skew of circulating CD4-positive T-Cells towards a Th2 phenotype has also been reported [73]. It has been suggested that Th2 cells in IgG4-RD promote peripheral eosinophilia, raised serum immunoglobulin E (IgE), and IgG4 predominance, as Th2-associated cytokines IL-4 and IL-13 have been shown to promote immunoglobulin class switch toward the IgG4 subtype [72, 87]. However a recent report that blood Th2 cell expansion is restricted to IgG4-RD patients with atopy challenges the hypothesis of a Th2-driven response in IgG4-RD [56, 57]. Mast cells have been suggested as an alternative source of Th2 cytokines, based on their colocalization with IL-4 and IL-13 in IgG4-RD lesions from salivary glands [79, 80].

T follicular helper cells, which support B-cell differentiation into antigen-secreting cells in germinal centers, have also been implicated in IgG4-RD pathogenesis. Next-generation sequencing of the B-cell receptor immunoglobulin heavy chain repertoire of circulating plasmablasts in IgG4-RD patients has shown they have undergone extensive somatic hypermutation, a process for which T follicular helper cells are integral [56, 57]. A recent study has shown that circulating type 2 T follicular helper (Tfh2) cells are expanded in patients with IgG4-RD [2]. Tfh2 cells preferentially secrete Th2 cytokines [59] and could be the driver of the B-cell differentiation to IgG4-positive plasmablasts and plasma cells.

The T regulatory (Treg) cell-associated cytokine IL-10 and tumor growth factor beta (TGF-β) have been found in IgG4-RD lesions [87, 100, 101]. There is also evidence that Tregs are expanded in the circulation and tissue lesions in IgG4-SC and AIP [49, 51, 61]. IL-10 has been shown to preferentially switch immunoglobulin toward IgG4 rather than IgE, and TGF-β has been purported to contribute to the fibrosis seen in late stage disease [36, 78].

Regional Factors Promoting Lymphocyte Recruitment

It has been suggested that factors local to the pancreatobiliary system may be at play in IgG4-SC, as it often occurs alongside AIP. Pathological specimens of IgG4-SC show severe inflammation in the peribiliary glands, which contain pancreatic acini [27]. In tissue specimens from AIP and IgG4-SC, the chemokine CCL1 was expressed highly at the messenger RNA level and was localized to the peribiliary glands and pancreatic duct epithelium. The expression of CCR8, the receptor for CCL1 found on Th2 and Treg lymphocytes, was also upregulated in IgG4-SC disease lesions [102]. Another study found that CXCR5, expressed on Tfh cells, and its ligand CXCL13 were upregulated in AIP tissue [20]. A variety of other chemokines have been found to be overexpressed in AIP and IgG4-SC tissue including CCL1, CXCL13, CCL17, CCL19, and CCL21, but their role in the disease is not yet clear [74].

Clinical Features and Natural History

Clinical Presentation

Patients with IgG4-SC are predominantly males in their seventh decade and most commonly present with obstructive jaundice, weight loss, and abdominal pain. Patients with concomitant pancreatic involvement can present with steatorrhea, indicative of exocrine insufficiency and/or diabetes [26, 32]. In others, biliary involvement might be found incidentally on cross-sectional imaging performed for another reason.

Patients should be asked about previous occupational exposure, especially "blue-collar work" and history of allergy and/or atopy. Both have been observed at increased rates in IgG4-RD, although their significance in disease pathogenesis remains unclear [16, 17, 38, 39].

Laboratory Findings

There is no single laboratory test that can accurately diagnose IgG4-SC. Liver function tests are often deranged. An obstructive pattern of raised alkaline phosphatase, gamma-glutamyltransferase, and bilirubin is most commonly observed. In addition, patients can also have a polyclonal hypergammaglobulinemia and raised serum IgG.

Serum IgG4 is raised in 70–74 % of patients at time of diagnosis [26, 32]. However, an elevated serum IgG4 is not specific to IgG4-RD and can also be raised in PSC and pancreatobiliary malignancy, which mimic IgG4-SC both clinically and radiologically [11, 12, 58, 70, 94, 95]. Several studies have investigated whether using a higher cutoff value for serum IgG4 increases its ability to distinguish IgG4-SC from PSC or CCA. Using a higher IgG4 value over four times the upper limit of normal increases the specificity or positive predictive value (PPV) to almost 100 % for IgG4-SC. Alternatively when serum IgG4 is raised between one and two times the upper limit of normal, using an IgG4 to IgG1 ratio rather than IgG4 in isolation has been shown to increase PPV and sensitivity for IgG4-SC in Dutch and UK cohorts [8, 70]. However these methods do not detect the group of IgG4-SC patients with a normal serum IgG4.

Serum IgE levels are raised in between 35 and 95 % of IgG4-RD patients. Furthermore, 25–30 % of patients have a peripheral blood eosinophilia. There is conflicting evidence as to whether patients with a history of allergy are more likely to have a raised IgE and/or eosinophilia, compared to nonallergic patients [17, 38, 39, 98].

No autoantibody has been found to be specific to IgG4-SC [76]. The tumor marker CA19-9 can be raised in both pancreatobiliary malignancy and IgG4-SC, making it a poor differentiator between the conditions [26]. Although bile IgG4 levels can be elevated in patients with IgG4-SC compared to other biliary disorders including PSC and CCA, it is not specific [93].

Imaging Features

Imaging alone is unable to make a firm diagnosis of IgG4-SC as features can mimic PSC, CCA, and pancreatic carcinoma. Imaging of the biliary tree via magnetic resonance cholangiopancreatography (MRCP) or endoscopic retrograde cholangiopancreatography (ERCP) can reveal IgG4-SC biliary strictures.

Four patterns of strictures have been recognized [66]. Type 1 describes a single distal common bile duct (CBD) stricture which can mimic pancreatic carcinoma or CCA. This appearance commonly occurs in IgG4-SC, particularly in association with AIP where the stricture may be caused by inflammation of both the pancreas and biliary wall [31]. Type 2 lesions can be divided into type 2a intrahepatic strictures with

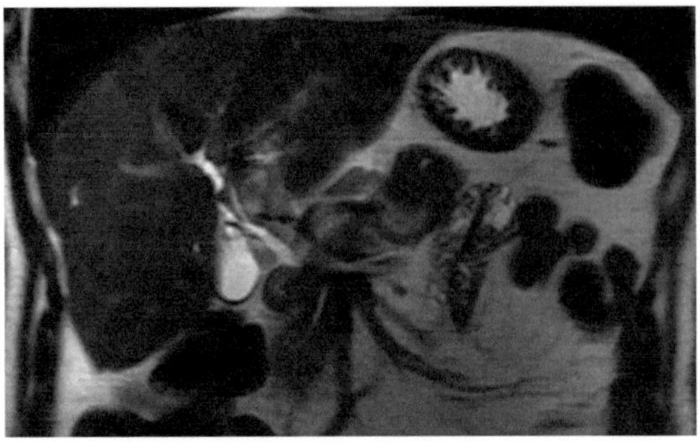

Fig. 5.1 MRCP of a patient with type 2 IgG4-SC with intra- and extrahepatic biliary dilatation

prestenotic dilatation and type 2b intrahepatic strictures without prestenotic dilatation and reduced bile duct branching. Both type 2 patterns can exhibit additional extrahepatic strictures, and appearances can be similar to PSC (Fig. 5.1). Unlike PSC, IgG4-SC strictures often show biliary dilation of over 10 mm proximal to a confluent narrowing in the distal CBD. Characteristic PSC features such as a beaded and pruned-tree appearance of the bile ducts are often absent in IgG4-SC [65]. A recent study of biliary appearance using MRI found continuous rather than skip lesions, and a single wall CBD thickness of over 2.5 mm favored IgG4-SC over PSC [85].

Type 3 IgG4-SC describes a distal CBD stricture and hilar hepatic stricture. Type 4 strictures involve the hilum only (Fig. 5.2). In a Japanese survey of IgG4-SC patients without pancreatic lesions, this was the commonest subtype [84]. Both type 3 and type 4 can mimic hilar CCA.

Other characteristic features of IgG4-SC lesions include symmetrical biliary wall thickening, smooth inner and outer margins, and a homogenous echo appearance of the internal bile duct wall. These can be characterized using conventional abdominal ultrasound, computed tomography (CT), endoscopic ultrasound (EUS), and intraductal ultrasonography (IDUS). Lesions can occur in regions where there is no identifiable biliary stricture on cholangiography [35, 50, 62]. Cross-sectional imaging can identify mass lesions in other organs caused by systemic IgG4-RD. CT pancreas can show a characteristic sausage-shaped appearance or mass lesions within the pancreatic parenchyma representative of AIP [35]. In one series, pancreatic abnormalities were the strongest predictor of correctly distinguishing IgG4-SC from PSC and malignancy [25].

Histopathological Features

Inflammatory lesions in IgG4-SC are usually distributed in the extrahepatic, hilar, and perihilar bile ducts but can also affect the small intrahepatic ducts and gallbladder.

Macroscopically the affected areas of the bile duct are diffusely thickened, with stenotic lumens, and in some cases appear as tumorous lesions [64, 100, 101]. In contrast to PSC, the biliary epithelium is relatively well preserved but inflammation can extend into local veins, glands, and nerves [99].

Microscopically, classical IgG4-SC lesions share the lymphoplasmacytic infiltrate, obliterative phlebitis, and storiform pattern of fibrosis seen in other IgG4-RD conditions [26, 99]. The lymphoplasmacytic infiltrate is T-Cell predominant with scattered B-cell aggregates (Fig. 5.3 left). Germinal centers are sometimes seen and many specimens have an eosinophilia. The presence of IgG4-positive plasma cells, however, is not sufficient for diagnosis, as they can be seen in other conditions. A biopsy specimen with a mean of >10 IgG4 plasma cells per high-power field (HPF) (Fig. 5.3 right) or an IgG4/IgG plasma cell ration of >40 % is suggestive and incorporated into diagnostic guidelines for IgG4-RD and IgG4-SC [15, 68, 75]. It should also be noted that some classical histopathological features might not be present on biopsy if insufficient amounts of tissue are obtained. In one series of transpapillary biopsy specimens collected from IgG4-SC strictures using IDUS, obliterative phlebitis was absent and >10 IgG4-positive cells per HPF was only observed in a minority [62].

Liver biopsy can demonstrate small duct involvement in IgG4-SC in up to 26 % of cases. Specimens typically show portal inflammation and IgG4-positive plasma cell infiltration [63, 89]. Some specimens also have portal-based micro-inflammatory nodules of lymphocytes,

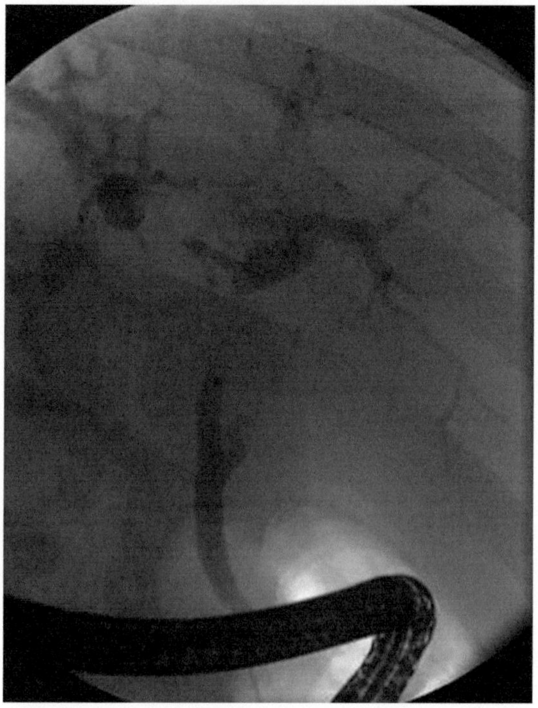

Fig. 5.2 MRCP of a patient with type 4 IgG4-SC with a hilar stricture, which is difficult to differentiate from hilar CCA

plasma cells, eosinophils, and a myxoid stroma, a feature not present in PSC [18].

Diagnosis

There is no single diagnostic test to confirm IgG4-SC. Therefore, diagnosis should be based on a combination of clinical, radiological, laboratory, and histological findings. Several guidelines have been developed. These include the HISORt criteria (histology, imaging, serology, other organ involvement and response to therapy), originally developed for AIP and adapted for IgG4-SC (Table 5.2; [15, 26]). In Japan, clinical diagnostic criteria for IgG4-SC classify the diagnosis as being definite, probable, or possible depending on the features of the case [68]. For definitive diagnosis both guidelines include typical imaging findings of a thickened bile duct wall with segmental or diffuse biliary strictures, raised serum IgG4 titers, coexistence of other organ involvement, and the typical histological features (lymphoplasmacytic infiltrate, >10/HPF IgG4-positive plasma cells, storiform fibrosis, and obliterative phlebitis). If steroid therapy has been effective in improving clinical, radiological, or histological features, this is supportive for diagnosis, although improvement with steroids can also occur in other malignant and inflammatory conditions. It is imperative to exclude malignancy.

Table 5.2 HISORt diagnostic criteria for IgG4-SC

Histology	(i) Lymphoplasmacytic infiltrate
	(ii) >10 IgG4-positive cells per high-power field
	(iii) Obliterative phlebitis
	(iv) Storiform fibrosis
Imaging	Strictures of the biliary tree including
	(i) Intrahepatic ducts
	(ii) Extrahepatic ducts
	(iii) Intrapancreatic ducts
Serology	Serum IgG4 levels above the upper limit of normal
Other organ involvement	Including
	(i) Pancreas
	(ii) Retroperitoneal fibrosis
	(iii) Kidney
	(iv) Salivary or lacrimal gland
Response to steroid treatment	Defined as
	(i) Normalization of liver enzymes (ii) Stricture resolution)

Adapted from Ghazale et al. [26]

Treatment

The aims of treatment in IgG4-SC are to alleviate symptoms and prevent disease complications and irreversible fibrosis. Spontaneous resolution of IgG4-SC lesions without treatment has been described. However, oral steroids have been shown consistently to hasten the resolution of clinical jaundice, itch and abdominal discomfort, radiological strictures, serum IgG4, and microscopic inflammation ([26, 32, 48, 67, 81]; Fig. 5.4). Japanese guidelines recommend biliary drainage in patients with obstructive jaundice prior to the commencement of steroid therapy [40]. A recent international consensus of experts on the

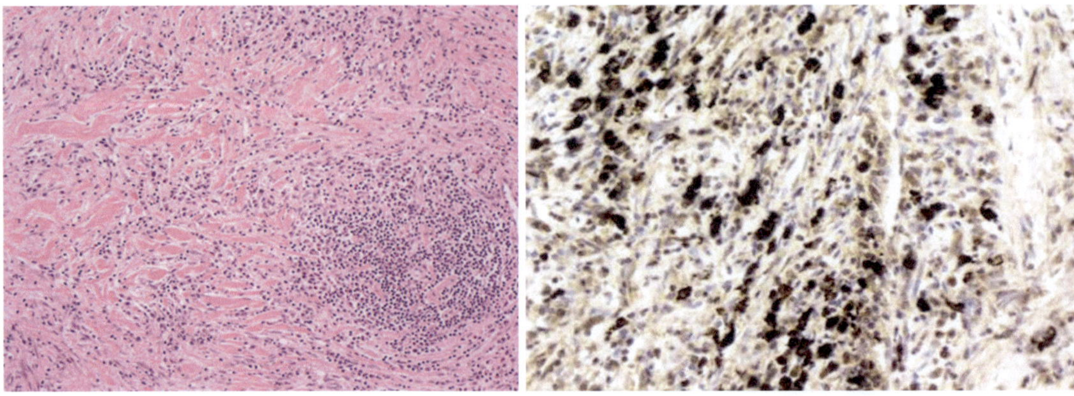

Fig. 5.3 Microscopic appearance of IgG4-SC showing a lymphoplasmacytic infiltrate (*left panel*) and IgG4-positive plasma cells >50/HPF (*right panel*)

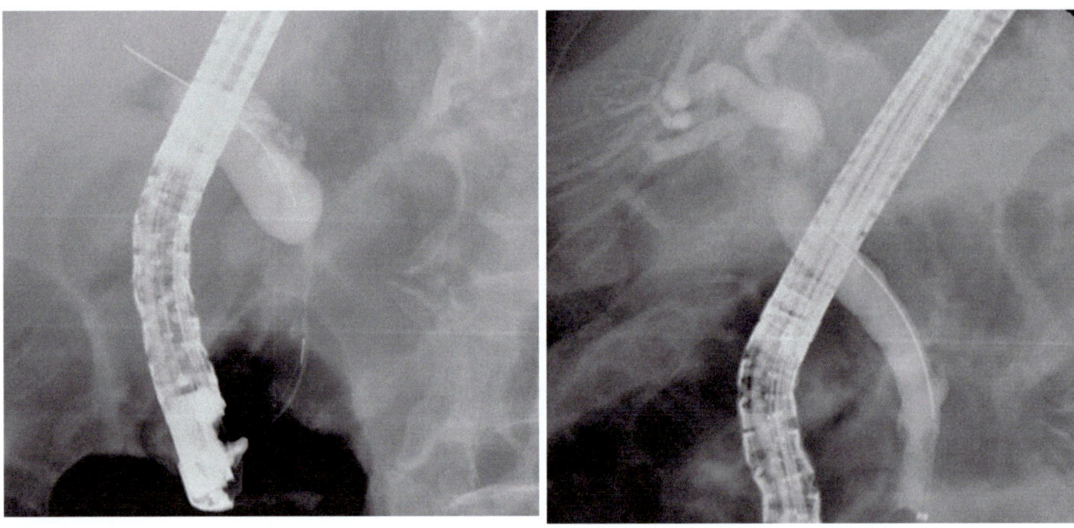

Fig. 5.4 ERCP showing a distal CBD stricture before (*left image*) and after treatment with biliary stenting and corticosteroid therapy (*right image*)

management of IgG4-RD concluded that urgent treatment is appropriate in biliary disease even when asymptomatic, to prevent infectious cholangitis and permanent fibrosis that may complicate untreated disease [47].

No randomized clinical trial has been conducted to determine the dose or duration of steroid treatment, and regimes are based on published clinical experience. Starting doses range from 30 to 40 mg of prednisolone or 0.6 mg/kg once a day for 2–4 weeks; after which the dose is tapered. Tapering regimes vary, but a dose reduction by 5 mg every 1–2 weeks depending on clinical response with a total treatment period of between 3 and 6 months is typical. In Japan guidelines recommend tapering to a maintenance dose between 5 and 10 mg per day to continue for up to 3 years.

Remission, defined as normalization of liver enzymes or stricture resolution, is achieved in 82–100 % of patients after steroid treatment. The diagnosis of IgG4-SC should be reconsidered in steroid nonresponders, but some long-standing strictures may be only partially responsive or unresponsive to treatment if fibrosis has developed, and in these patients, biliary stenting can be used to improve symptoms.

After withdrawal of steroid therapy, relapse rates between 50 and 57 % have been reported; the majority of which occur within 6 months of discontinuation of steroid treatment. In Japan it is commonplace to maintain low-dose steroid for up to 3 years after remission induction. This is based on evidence that relapse rates are significantly lower while on low-dose steroid compared to complete cessation of therapy [38, 39]. The presence of IgG4-SC as opposed to AIP in isolation is a risk factor for relapse [32, 77]. Proximal strictures are more likely to reoccur than distal strictures [26].

For the minority of patients who do not achieve remission on initial treatment induction and for those who relapse after withdrawal of therapy, further treatment is necessary. Steroids can be reintroduced or the dose increased, but long-term high-dose steroid therapy is associated with an adverse side-effect profile. For this reason, steroid-sparing agents including azathioprine, mycophenolate mofetil, 6-mercaptopurine, methotrexate, and tacrolimus have all been used to maintain remission in patients who relapse during steroid tapering or are at high risk of relapse [9, 26, 30, 32, 77]. There is no randomized evidence to support the use of these agents or the type or duration of treatment.

More recently the B-cell-depleting agent rituximab has been shown to be effective in inducing remission in patients with IgG4-RD relapse with promising results [86]. In an open-label trial where two doses of 1 g of intravenous rituximab were administered to IgG4-RD patients, 97 % achieved disease response by 6 months, and 77 % saw an improvement in disease activity, did not need to use oral steroid and did not exhibit any evidence of disease relapse by the end of 6 months. Remission, defined as no use of steroid and no evidence of disease activity, was achieved by 47 % at 6 months and 46 % at 12 months after rituximab therapy [11, 12].

Side effects associated with treatment are largely unexplored in IgG4-SC. In a cohort of 56 patients with IgG4-RD, over 50 % of patients receiving drug treatment reported adverse effects. Most were steroid related including weight gain, hyperglycemia, and cataracts, which are of particular relevance in the older male demographic at risk of IgG4-RD (unpublished data). Side effects in IgG4-RD patients treated with azathioprine and 6-merceptopurine have been reported and include nausea, vomiting, transaminitis, rash, and myelosuppression [30]. In the recent trial of rituximab therapy for IgG4-RD, two patients were hospitalized for bacterial infection [11, 12].

Prognosis

The long-term natural history of IgG4-SC is not yet well defined due to a paucity of cohorts with sufficient follow-up. It is clear that relapse in the bile duct or in another organ is likely to occur despite treatment. In a series of 53 patients with IgG4-SC, three treatment-naïve patients and one nonresponder developed cirrhosis and portal hypertension between 9 and 62 months after IgG4-SC diagnosis [26]. In a UK cohort of 115 patients with AIP and/or IgG4-SC, 5 % developed liver cirrhosis. There is also an increased incidence of all cancers, and all cause mortality compared to the general population [32].

Summary

IgG4-SC remains a diagnostic challenge with the key issue remaining differentiation from pancreatobiliary malignancy and other forms of sclerosing cholangitis. Current therapy follows an international expert consensus but is not supported by randomized controlled trials. More recently, the B-cell-depleting agent rituximab has given clues into disease pathogenesis as well as providing an option in those experiencing adverse effects with, or becoming refractory to, conventional therapy. The longer-term consequences of irreversible fibrosis, cirrhosis, and an increased risk of malignancy are now becoming apparent. Studies have implicated both dysregulation of the immune system and genetic susceptibility in IgG4-SC disease pathogenesis. Further work to establish risk factors and determinants of fibrotic disease and the mechanisms underlying this is essential.

References

1. Aalberse RC, van der Gaag R, van Leeuwen J. Serologic aspects of IgG4 antibodies. I. Prolonged immunization results in an IgG4-restricted response. J Immunol. 1983;130(2):722–6.
2. Akiyama M, Suzuki K, Yamaoka H, Yasuoka H, Takeshita M, Kaneko Y, Kondo H, Kassai Y, Miyazaki T, Morita R, Yoshimura A, Takeuchi T. Number of circulating T follicular helper 2 cells correlates with IgG4 and IL-4 levels and plasmablast numbers in IgG4-related disease. Arthritis Rheumatol. 2015; 67(9):2476–81.
3. Aoki S, Nakazawa T, Ohara H, Sano H, Nakao H, Joh T, Murase T, Eimoto T, Itoh M. Immunohistochemical study of autoimmune pancreatitis using anti-IgG4 antibody and patients' sera. Histopathology. 2005; 47(2):147–58.
4. Aparisi L, Farre A, Gomez-Cambronero L, Martinez J, De Las Heras G, Corts J, Navarro S, Mora J, Lopez-Hoyos M, Sabater L, Ferrandez A, Bautista D, Perez-Mateo M, Mery S, Sastre J. Antibodies to carbonic anhydrase and IgG4 levels in idiopathic chronic pancreatitis: relevance for diagnosis of autoimmune pancreatitis. Gut. 2005;54(5):703–9.
5. Asada M, Nishio A, Uchida K, Kido M, Ueno S, Uza N, Kiriya K, Inoue S, Kitamura H, Ohashi S, Tamaki H, Fukui T, Matsuura M, Kawasaki K, Nishi T, Watanabe N, Nakase H, Chiba T, Okazaki K. Identification of a novel autoantibody against pancreatic secretory trypsin inhibitor in patients with autoimmune pancreatitis. Pancreas. 2006;33(1):20–6.
6. Bartholomew LG, Cain JC, Woolner LB, Utz DC, Ferris DO. Sclerosing cholangitis: its possible association with Riedel's struma and fibrous retroperitonitis. Report of two cases. N Engl J Med. 1963; 269:8–12.
7. Björnsson E, Chari ST, Smyrk TC, Lindor K. Immunoglobulin G4 associated cholangitis: description of an emerging clinical entity based on review of the literature. Hepatology. 2007;45(6):1547–54.
8. Boonstra K, Culver EL, de Buy Wenniger LM, van Heerde MJ, van Erpecum KJ, Poen AC, van Nieuwkerk KM, Spanier BW, Witteman BJ, Tuynman HA, van Geloven N, van Buuren H, Chapman RW, Barnes E, Beuers U, Ponsioen CY. Serum immunoglobulin G4 and immunoglobulin G1 for distinguishing immunoglobulin G4-associated cholangitis from primary sclerosing cholangitis. Hepatology. 2014;59(5):1954–63.
9. Buechter M, Klein CG, Kloeters C, Schlaak JF, Canbay A, Gerken G, Kahraman A. Tacrolimus as a reasonable alternative in a patient with steroid-dependent and thiopurine-refractory autoimmune pancreatitis with IgG4-associated cholangitis. Z Gastroenterol. 2014;52(6):564–8.
10. Campochiaro C, Ramirez GA, Bozzolo EP, Lanzillotta M, Berti A, Baldissera E, Dagna L, Praderio L, Scotti R, Tresoldi M, Roveri L, Mariani A, Balzano G, Castoldi R, Doglioni C, Sabbadini MG, Della-Torre E. IgG4-related disease in Italy: clinical features and outcomes of a large cohort of patients. Scand J Rheumatol. 2015;23:1–11.
11. Carruthers MN, Khosroshahi A, Augustin T, Deshpande V, Stone J. The diagnostic utility of serum IgG4 concentrations in IgG4-related disease. Ann Rheum Dis. 2015;74(1):14–8.
12. Carruthers MN, Topazian MD, Khosroshahi A, Witzig TE, Wallace ZS, Hart PA, Deshpande V, Smyrk TC, Chari S, Stone JH. Rituximab for IgG4-related disease: a prospective, open-label trial. Ann Rheum Dis. 2015;74(6):1171–7.
13. Culver EL, Vermeulen E, Makuch M, van Leeuwen A, Sadler R, Cargill T, Klenerman P, Aalberse RC, van Ham SM, Barnes E, Rispens T. Increased IgG4 responses to multiple food and animal antigens indicate a polyclonal expansion and differentiation of pre-existing B cells in IgG4-related disease. Ann Rheum Dis. 2015;74(5):944–7.
14. Chang MC, Chang YT, Tien YW, Liang PC, Jan IS, Wei SC, Wong JM. T-cell regulatory gene CTLA-4 polymorphism/haplotype association with autoimmune pancreatitis. Clin Chem. 2007;53(9):1700–5.
15. Chari ST, Smyrk TC, Levy MJ, Topazian MD, Takahashi N, Zhang L, Clain JE, Pearson RK, Petersen BT, Vege SS, Farnell MB. Diagnosis of autoimmune pancreatitis: the Mayo Clinic experience. Clin Gastroenterol Hepatol. 2006;4(8):1010–6.
16. de Buy Wenniger LJ, Culver EL, Beuers U. Exposure to occupational antigens might predispose to IgG4-related disease. Hepatology. 2014;60(4):1453–4.
17. Della Torre E, Mattoo H, Mahajan VS, Carruthers M, Pillai S, Stone JH. Prevalence of atopy, eosinophilia, and IgE elevation in IgG4-related disease. Allergy. 2014;69(2):269–72.
18. Deshpande V, Sainani NI, Chung RT, Pratt DS, Mentha G, Rubbia-Brandt L, Lauwers GY. IgG4-associated cholangitis: a comparative histological and immunophenotypic study with primary sclerosing cholangitis on liver biopsy material. Mod Pathol. 2009;22(10):1287–95.
19. Endo T, Takizawa S, Tanaka S, Takahashi M, Fujii H, Kamisawa T, Kobayashi T. Amylase alpha-2A autoantibodies: novel marker of autoimmune pancreatitis and fulminant type 1 diabetes. Diabetes. 2009;58(3):732–7.
20. Esposito I, Born D, Bergmann F, Longerich T, Welsch T, Giese NA, Büchler MW, Kleeff J, Friess H, Schirmacher P. Autoimmune pancreatocholangitis, non-autoimmune pancreatitis and primary sclerosing cholangitis: a comparative morphological and immunological analysis. PLoS One. 2008;3(7):e2539.
21. European Association for the Study of the Liver. EASL Clinical Practice Guidelines: management of cholestatic liver diseases. J Hepatol. 2009;51(2):237–67.
22. Fernández-Codina A, Martínez-Valle F, Pinilla B, López C, DeTorres I, Solans-Laqué R, Fraile-Rodríguez G, Casanovas-Martínez A, López-Dupla M, Robles-Marhuenda Á, Barragán-González MJ,

Cid MC, Prieto-González S, Brito-Zerón P, Cruces-Moreno MT, Fonseca-Aizpuru E, López-Torres M, Gil J, Núñez-Fernández MJ, Pardos-Gea J, Salvador-Cervelló G. IgG4-related disease: results from a multicenter Spanish registry. Medicine (Baltimore). 2015;94(32), e1275.
23. Frulloni L, Lunardi C, Simone R, Dolcino M, Scattolini C, Falconi M, Benini L, Vantini I, Corrocher R, Puccetti A. Identification of a novel antibody associated with autoimmune pancreatitis. N Engl J Med. 2009;361(22):2135–42.
24. Futei Y, Amagai M, Ishii K, Kuroda-Kinoshita K, Ohya K, Nishikawa T. Predominant IgG4 subclass in autoantibodies of pemphigus vulgaris and foliaceus. J Dermatol Sci. 2001;26(1):55–61.
25. Gardner CS, Bashir MR, Marin D, Nelson RC, Choudhury KR, Ho LM. Diagnostic performance of imaging criteria for distinguishing autoimmune cholangiopathy from primary sclerosing cholangitis and bile duct malignancy. Abdom Imaging. 2015;40(8):3052–61.
26. Ghazale A, Chari ST, Zhang L, Smyrk TC, Takahashi N, Levy MJ, Topazian MD, Clain JE, Pearson RK, Petersen BT, Vege SS, Lindor K, Farnell MB. Immunoglobulin G4-associated cholangitis: clinical profile and response to therapy. Gastroenterology. 2008;134(3):706–15.
27. Graham RPD, Smyrk TC, Chari ST, Takahashi N, Zhang L. Isolated IgG4-related sclerosing cholangitis: a report of 9 cases. Hum Pathol. 2014;45(8):1722–9.
28. Guarneri F, Guarneri C, Benvenga S. Helicobacter pylori and autoimmune pancreatitis: role of carbonic anhydrase via molecular mimicry? J Cell Mol Med. 2005;9(3):741–4.
29. Hamano H, Kawa S, Horiuchi A, Unno H, Furuya N, Akamatsu T, Fukushima M, Nikaido T, Nakayama K, Usuda N, Kiyosawa K. High serum IgG4 concentrations in patients with sclerosing pancreatitis. N Engl J Med. 2001;344(10):732–8.
30. Hart PA, Topazian MD, Witzig TE, Clain JE, Gleeson FC, Klebig RR, Levy MJ, Pearson RK, Petersen BT, Smyrk TC, Sugumar A, Takahashi N, Vege SS, Chari ST. Treatment of relapsing autoimmune pancreatitis with immunomodulators and rituximab: the Mayo Clinic experience. Gut. 2013; 62(11):1607–15.
31. Hirano K, Tada M, Isayama H, Yamamoto K, Mizuno S, Yagioka H, Yashima Y, Sasaki T, Kogure H, Togawa O, Arizumi T, Matsubara S, Nakai Y, Sasahira N, Tsujino T, Kawabe T, Omata M. Endoscopic evaluation of factors contributing to intrapancreatic biliary stricture in autoimmune pancreatitis. Gastrointest Endosc. 2010;71(1):85–90.
32. Huggett MT, Culver EL, Kumar M, Hurst JM, Rodriguez-Justo M, Chapman MH, Johnson GJ, Pereira SP, Chapman RW, Webster GJ, Barnes E. Type 1 autoimmune pancreatitis and IgG4-related sclerosing cholangitis is associated with extrapancreatic organ failure, malignancy, and mortality in a prospective UK cohort. Am J Gastroenterol. 2014;109(10):1675–83.
33. Huijbers MG, Zhang W, Klooster R, Niks EH, Friese MB, Straasheijm KR, Thijssen PE, Vrolijk H, Plomp JJ, Vogels P, Losen M, Van der Maarel SM, Burden SJ, Verschuuren JJ. MuSK IgG4 autoantibodies cause myasthenia gravis by inhibiting binding between MuSK and Lrp4. Proc Natl Acad Sci USA. 2013;110(51):20783–8.
34. Inoue D, Yoshida K, Yoneda N, Ozaki K, Matsubara T, Nagai K, Okumura K, Toshima F, Toyama J, Minami T, Matsui O, Gabata T, Zen Y. IgG4-related disease: dataset of 235 consecutive patients. Medicine (Baltimore). 2015;94(15):e680.
35. Itoh S, Nagasaka T, Suzuki K, Satake H, Ota T, Naganawa S. Lymphoplasmacytic sclerosing cholangitis: assessment of clinical, CT, and pathological findings. Clin Radiol. 2009;64(11):1104–14.
36. Jeannin P, Lecoanet S, Delneste Y, Gauchat JF, Bonnefoy JY. IgE versus IgG4 production can be differentially regulated by IL-10. J Immunol. 1998;160(7):3555–61.
37. Kamisawa T, Funata N, Hayashi Y, Eishi Y, Koike M, Tsuruta K, Okamoto A, Egawa N, Nakajima H. A new clinicopathological entity of IgG4-related autoimmune disease. J Gastroenterol. 2003;38(10):982–4.
38. Kamisawa T, Anjiki H, Egawa N, Kubota N. Allergic manifestations in autoimmune pancreatitis. Eur J Gastroenterol Hepatol. 2009;21(10):1136–9.
39. Kamisawa T, Shimosegawa T, Okazaki K, Nishino T, Watanabe H, Kanno A, Okumura F, Nishikawa T, Kobayashi K, Ichiya T, Takatori H, Yamakita K, Kubota K, Hamano H, Okamura K, Hirano K, Ito T, Ko SB, Omata M. Standard steroid treatment for autoimmune pancreatitis. Gut. 2009;58(11):1504–7.
40. Kamisawa T, Okazaki K, Kawa S, Ito T, Inui K, Irie H, Nishino T, Notohara K, Nishimori I, Tanaka S, Nishiyama T, Suda K, Shiratori K, Tanaka M, Shimosegawa T, Working Committee of the Japan Pancreas Society and the Research Committee for Intractable Pancreatic Disease supported by the Ministry of Health, Labour and Welfare of Japan. Amendment of the Japanese Consensus Guidelines for Autoimmune Pancreatitis, 2013 III. Treatment and prognosis of autoimmune pancreatitis. J Gastroenterol. 2014;49(6):961–70.
41. Kanari H, Kagami S, Kashiwakuma D, Oya Y, Furuta S, Ikeda K, Suto A, Suzuki K, Hirose K, Watanabe N, Okamoto Y, Yamamoto S, Iwamoto I, Nakajima H. Role of Th2 cells in IgG4-related lacrimal gland enlargement. Int Arch Allergy Immunol. 2010;152 Suppl 1:47–53.
42. Kanno A, Nishimori I, Masamune A, Kikuta K, Hirota M, Kuriyama S, Tsuji I, Shimosegawa T, Research Committee on Intractable Diseases of Pancreas. Nationwide epidemiological survey of autoimmune pancreatitis in Japan. Pancreas. 2012;41(6):835–9.
43. Kanno A, Masamune A, Okazaki K, Kamisawa T, Kawa S, Nishimori I, Tsuji I, Shimosegawa T,

Research Committee of Intractable Diseases of the Pancreas. Nationwide epidemiological survey of autoimmune pancreatitis in Japan in 2011. Pancreas. 2015;44(4):535–9.
44. Kawa S, Ota M, Yoshizawa K, Horiuchi A, Hamano H, Ochi Y, Nakayama K, Tokutake Y, Katsuyama Y, Saito S, Hasebe O, Kiyosawa K. HLA DRB10405-DQB10401 haplotype is associated with autoimmune pancreatitis in the Japanese population. Gastroenterology. 2002;122(5):1264–9.
45. Khosroshahi A, Bloch DB, Deshpande V, Stone JH. Rituximab therapy leads to rapid decline of serum IgG4 levels and prompt clinical improvement in IgG4-related systemic disease. Arthritis Rheum. 2010;62(6):1755–62.
46. Khosroshahi A, Carruthers MN, Deshpande V, Unizony S, Bloch DB, Stone JH. Rituximab for the treatment of IgG4-related disease: lessons from 10 consecutive patients. Medicine (Baltimore). 2012; 91(1):57–66.
47. Khosroshahi A, Wallace ZS, Crowe JL, Akamizu T, Azumi A, Carruthers MN, Chari ST, Della-Torre E, Frulloni L, Goto H, Hart PA, Kamisawa T, Kawa S, Kawano M, Kim MH, Kodama Y, Kubota K, Lerch MM, Löhr M, Masaki Y, Matsui S, Mimori T, Nakamura S, Nakazawa T, Ohara H, Okazaki K, Ryu JH, Saeki T, Schleinitz N, Shimatsu A, Shimosegawa T, Takahashi H, Takahira M, Tanaka A, Topazian M, Umehara H, Webster GJ, Witzig TE, Yamamoto M, Zhang W, Chiba T, Stone JH, Second International Symposium on IgG4-Related Disease. International consensus guidance statement on the management and treatment of IgG4-related disease. Arthritis Rheumatol. 2015;67(7):1688–99.
48. Kojima E, Kimura K, Noda Y, Kobayashi G, Itoh K, Fujita N. Autoimmune pancreatitis and multiple bile duct strictures treated effectively with steroid. J Gastroenterol. 2003;38(6):603–7.
49. Koyabu M, Uchida K, Miyoshi H, Sakaguchi Y, Fukui T, Ikeda H, Takaoka M, Hirohara J, Nishio A, Uemura Y, Uemoto S, Okazaki K. Analysis of regulatory T cells and IgG4-positive plasma cells among patients of IgG4-related sclerosing cholangitis and autoimmune liver diseases. J Gastroenterol. 2010; 45(7):732–41.
50. Koyama R, Imamura T, Okuda C, Sakamoto N, Honjo H, Takeuchi K. Ultrasonographic imaging of bile duct lesions in autoimmune pancreatitis. Pancreas. 2008;37(3):259–64.
51. Kusuda T, Uchida K, Miyoshi H, Koyabu M, Satoi S, Takaoka M, Shikata N, Uemura Y, Okazaki K. Involvement of inducible costimulator- and interleukin 10-positive regulatory T cells in the development of IgG4-related autoimmune pancreatitis. Pancreas. 2011;40(7):1120–30.
52. Löhr JM, Faissner R, Koczan D, Bewerunge P, Bassi C, Brors B, Eils R, Frulloni L, Funk A, Halangk W, Jesenofsky R, Kaderali L, Kleeff J, Krüger B, Lerch MM, Lösel R, Magnani M, Neumaier M, Nittka S, Sahin-Tóth M, Sänger J, Serafini S, Schnölzer M, Thierse HJ, Wandschneider S, Zamboni G, Klöppel G. Autoantibodies against the exocrine pancreas in autoimmune pancreatitis: gene and protein expression profiling and immunoassays identify pancreatic enzymes as a major target of the inflammatory process. Am J Gastroenterol. 2010;105(9):2060–71.
53. Lin W, Lu S, Chen H, Wu Q, Fei Y, Li M, Zhang X, Tian X, Zheng W, Leng X, Xu D, Wang Q, Shen M, Wang L, Li J, Wu D, Zhao L, Wu C, Yang Y, Peng L, Zhou J, Wang Y, Sha Y, Huang X, Jiao Y, Zeng X, Shi Q, Li P, Zhang S, Hu C, Deng C, Li Y, Zhang S, Liu J, Su J, Hou Y, Jiang Y, You X, Zhang H, Yan L, Zhang W, Zhao Y, Zeng X, Zhang F, Lipsky PE. Clinical characteristics of immunoglobulin G4-related disease: a prospective study of 118 Chinese patients. Rheumatology (Oxford). 2015;54(11):1982–90.
54. de Buy Wenniger LJ M, Doorenspleet ME, Klarenbeek PL, Verheij J, Baas F, Elferink RP, Tak PP, de Vries N, Beuers U. Immunoglobulin G4+ clones identified by next-generation sequencing dominate the B cell receptor repertoire in immunoglobulin G4 associated cholangitis. Hepatology. 2013;57(6):2390–8.
55. Maritati F, Corradi D, Versari A, Casali M, Urban ML, Buzio C, Vaglio A. Rituximab therapy for chronic periaortitis. Ann Rheum Dis. 2012;71(7):1262–4.
56. Mattoo H, Mahajan VS, Della-Torre E, Sekigami Y, Carruthers M, Wallace ZS, Deshpande V, Stone JH, Pillai S. De novo oligoclonal expansions of circulating plasmablasts in active and relapsing IgG4-related disease. J Allergy Clin Immunol. 2014;134(3): 679–87.
57. Mattoo H, Della-Torre E, Mahajan VS, Stone JH, Pillai S. Circulating Th2 memory cells in IgG4-related disease are restricted to a defined subset of subjects with atopy. Allergy. 2014;69(3):399–402.
58. Mendes FD, Jorgensen R, Keach J, Katzmann JA, Smyrk T, Donlinger J, Chari S, Lindor KD. Elevated serum IgG4 concentration in patients with primary sclerosing cholangitis. Am J Gastroenterol. 2006;101(9):2070–5.
59. Morita R, Schmitt N, Bentebibel SE, Ranganathan R, Bourdery L, Zurawski G, Foucat E, Dullaers M, Oh S, Sabzghabaei N, Lavecchio EM, Punaro M, Pascual V, Banchereau J, Ueno H. Human blood CXCR5(+)CD4(+) T cells are counterparts of T follicular cells and contain specific subsets that differentially support antibody secretion. Immunity. 2011;34(1):108–21.
60. Müller T, Beutler C, Picó AH, Otten M, Dürr A, Al-Abadi H, Guckelberger O, Meyer Zum Büschenfelde D, Jöhrens K, Volkmann M, Lankisch T, Voigtländer T, Anders M, Shibolet O, Jefferson DM, Podolsky DK, Fischer A, Veltzke-Schlieker W, Adler A, Baumgart DC, Sturm A, Wiedenmann B, Schott E, Berg T. Increased T-helper 2 cytokines in bile from patients with IgG4-related cholangitis disrupt the tight junction-associated biliary epithelial cell barrier. Gastroenterology. 2013;144(5):1116–28.
61. Miyoshi H, Uchida K, Taniguchi T, Yazumi S, Matsushita M, Takaoka M, Okazaki K. Circulating naïve and CD4+CD25 high regulatory T cells in

patients with autoimmune pancreatitis. Pancreas. 2008;36(2):133–40.
62. Naitoh I, Nakazawa T, Ohara H, Andoh T, Hayashi K, Tanaka H, Okumura F, Takahashi S, Joh T. Endoscopic transpapillary intraductal ultrasonography and biopsy in the diagnosis of IgG4-related sclerosing cholangitis. J Gastroenterol. 2009;44(11):1147–55.
63. Naitoh I, Zen Y, Nakazawa T, Ando T, Hayashi K, Okumura F, Miyabe K, Yoshida M, Nojiri S, Kanematsu T, Ohara H, Joh T. Small bile duct involvement in IgG4-related sclerosing cholangitis: liver biopsy and cholangiography correlation. J Gastroenterol. 2011;46(2):269–76.
64. Nakanuma Y, Zen Y. Pathology and immunopathology of immunoglobulin G4-related sclerosing cholangitis: the latest addition to the sclerosing cholangitis family. Hepatol Res. 2007;37 Suppl 3:S478–86.
65. Nakazawa T, Ohara H, Sano H, Aoki S, Kobayashi S, Okamoto T, Imai H, Nomura T, Joh T, Itoh M. Cholangiography can discriminate sclerosing cholangitis with autoimmune pancreatitis from primary sclerosing cholangitis. Gastrointest Endosc. 2004;60(6):937–44.
66. Nakazawa T, Ohara H, Sano H, Ando T, Joh T. Schematic classification of sclerosing cholangitis with autoimmune pancreatitis by cholangiography. Pancreas. 2006;32(2):229.
67. Nishino T, Toki F, Oyama H, Oi I, Kobayashi M, Takasaki K, Shiratori K. Biliary tract involvement in autoimmune pancreatitis. Pancreas. 2005;30(1): 76–82.
68. Ohara H, Okazaki K, Tsubouchi H, Inui K, Kawa S, Kamisawa T, Tazuma S, Uchida K, Hirano K, Yoshida H, Nishino T, Ko SB, Mizuno N, Hamano H, Kanno A, Notohara K, Hasebe O, Nakazawa T, Nakanuma Y, Takikawa H, Research Committee of IgG4-related Diseases; Research Committee of Intractable Diseases of Liver and Biliary Tract; Ministry of Health, Labor and Welfare, Japan; Japan Biliary Association. Clinical diagnostic criteria of IgG4-related sclerosing cholangitis 2012. J Hepatobiliary Pancreat Sci. 2012;19(5):536–42.
69. Okazaki K, Uchida K, Ohana M, Nakase H, Uose S, Inai M, Matsushima Y, Katamura K, Ohmori K, Chiba T. Autoimmune-related pancreatitis is associated with autoantibodies and a Th1/Th2-type cellular immune response. Gastroenterology. 2000; 118(3):573–81.
70. Oseini AM, Chaiteerakij R, Shire AM, Ghazale A, Kaiya J, Moser CD, Aderca I, Mettler TA, Therneau TM, Zhang L, Takahashi N, Chari ST, Roberts LR. Utility of serum immunoglobulin G4 in distinguishing immunoglobulin G4-associated cholangitis from cholangiocarcinoma. Hepatology. 2011;54(3): 940–8.
71. Park DH, Kim MH, Oh HB, Kwon OJ, Choi YJ, Lee SS, Lee TY, Seo DW, Lee SK. Substitution of aspartic acid at position 57 of the DQbeta1 affects relapse of autoimmune pancreatitis. Gastroenterology. 2008; 134(2):440–6.
72. Punnonen J, Aversa G, Cocks BG, McKenzie AN, Menon S, Zurawski G, de Waal Malefyt R, de Vries JE. Interleukin 13 induces interleukin 4-independent IgG4 and IgE synthesis and CD23 expression by human B cells. Proc Natl Acad Sci U S A. 1993;90(8):3730–4.
73. Saito Y, Kagami S, Kawashima S, Takahashi K, Ikeda K, Hirose K, Oshitari T, Yamamoto S, Okamoto Y, Nakajima H. Roles of CRTH2+ CD4+ T cells in immunoglobulin G4-related lacrimal gland enlargement. Int Arch Allergy Immunol. 2012;158 Suppl 1:42–6.
74. Seleznik GM, Reding T, Romrig F, Saito Y, Mildner A, Segerer S, Sun LK, Regenass S, Lech M, Anders HJ, McHugh D, Kumagi T, Hiasa Y, Lackner C, Haybaeck J, Angst E, Perren A, Balmer ML, Slack E, MacPherson A, Manz MG, Weber A, Browning JL, Arkan MC, Rülicke T, Aguzzi A, Prinz M, Graf R, Heikenwalder M. Lymphotoxin β receptor signaling promotes development of autoimmune pancreatitis. Gastroenterology. 2012;143(5):1361–74.
75. Shimosegawa T, Chari ST, Frulloni L, Kamisawa T, Kawa S, Mino-Kenudson M, Kim MH, Klöppel G, Lerch MM, Löhr M, Notohara K, Okazaki K, Schneider A, Zhang L, International Association of Pancreatology. International consensus diagnostic criteria for autoimmune pancreatitis: guidelines of the International Association of Pancreatology. Pancreas. 2011;40(3):352–8.
76. Sah RP, Chari ST. Serologic issues in IgG4-related systemic disease and autoimmune pancreatitis. Curr Opin Rheumatol. 2011;23(1):108–13.
77. Sandanayake NS, Church NI, Chapman MH, Johnson GJ, Dhar DK, Amin Z, Deheragoda MG, Novelli M, Winstanley A, Rodriguez-Justo M, Hatfield AR, Pereira SP, Webster GJ. Presentation and management of post-treatment relapse in autoimmune pancreatitis/immunoglobulin G4-associated cholangitis. Clin Gastroenterol Hepatol. 2009;7(10):1089–96.
78. Satoguina JS, Weyand E, Larbi J, Hoerauf A. T regulatory-1 cells induce IgG4 production by B cells: role of IL-10. J Immunol. 2005;174(8):4718–26.
79. Takeuchi M, Sato Y, Ohno K, Tanaka S, Takata K, Gion Y, Orita Y, Ito T, Tachibana T, Yoshino T. T helper 2 and regulatory T-cell cytokine production by mast cells: a key factor in the pathogenesis of IgG4-related disease. Mod Pathol. 2014;27(8): 1126–36.
80. Takeuchi M, Ohno K, Takata K, Gion Y, Tachibana T, Orita Y, Yoshino T, Sato Y. Interleukin 13-positive mast cells are increased in immunoglobulin G4-related sialadenitis. Sci Rep. 2015;5:7696.
81. Takikawa H, Takamori Y, Tanaka A, Kurihara H, Nakanuma Y. Analysis of 388 cases of primary sclerosing cholangitis in Japan; Presence of a subgroup without pancreatic involvement in older patients. Hepatol Res. 2004;29(3):153–9.
82. Takizawa S, Endo T, Wanjia X, Tanaka S, Takahashi M, Kobayashi T. HSP 10 is a new autoantigen in both autoimmune pancreatitis and fulminant type 1

diabetes. Biochem Biophys Res Commun. 2009; 386(1):192–6.

83. Tanaka A, Moriyama M, Nakashima H, Miyake K, Hayashida JN, Maehara T, Shinozaki S, Kubo Y, Nakamura S. Th2 and regulatory immune reactions contribute to IgG4 production and the initiation of Mikulicz disease. Arthritis Rheum. 2012;64(1):254–63.
84. Tanaka A, Tazuma S, Okazaki K, Tsubouchi H, Inui K, Takikawa H. Nationwide survey for primary sclerosing cholangitis and IgG4-related sclerosing cholangitis in Japan. J Hepatobiliary Pancreat Sci. 2014;21(1):43–50.
85. Tokala A, Khalili K, Menezes R, Hirschfield G, Jhaveri KS. Comparative MRI analysis of morphologic patterns of bile duct disease in IgG4-related systemic disease versus primary sclerosing cholangitis. AJR Am J Roentgenol. 2014;202(3):536–43.
86. Topazian M, Witzig TE, Smyrk TC, Pulido JS, Levy MJ, Kamath PS, Chari ST. Rituximab therapy for refractory biliary strictures in immunoglobulin G4-associated cholangitis. Clin Gastroenterol Hepatol. 2008;6(3):364–6.
87. Tsuboi H, Matsuo N, Iizuka M, Tsuzuki S, Kondo Y, Tanaka A, Moriyama M, Matsumoto I, Nakamura S, Sumida T. Analysis of IgG4 class switch-related molecules in IgG4-related disease. Arthritis Res Ther. 2012;14(4):R171.
88. Umemura T, Ota M, Hamano H, Katsuyama Y, Kiyosawa K, Kawa S. Genetic association of Fc receptor-like 3 polymorphisms with autoimmune pancreatitis in Japanese patients. Gut. 2006;55(9): 1367–8.
89. Umemura T, Zen Y, Hamano H, Kawa S, Nakanuma Y, Kiyosawa K. Immunoglobin G4-hepatopathy: association of immunoglobin G4-bearing plasma cells in liver with autoimmune pancreatitis. Hepatology. 2007;46(2):463–71.
90. Umemura T, Ota M, Hamano H, Katsuyama Y, Muraki T, Arakura N, Kawa S, Kiyosawa K. Association of autoimmune pancreatitis with cytotoxic T-lymphocyte antigen 4 gene polymorphisms in Japanese patients. Am J Gastroenterol. 2008;103(3):588–94.
91. van der Neut KM, Schuurman J, Losen M, Bleeker WK, Martínez-Martínez P, Vermeulen E, den Bleker TH, Wiegman L, Vink T, Aarden LA, De Baets MH, van de Winkel JG, Aalberse RC, Parren PW. Anti-inflammatory activity of human IgG4 antibodies by dynamic Fab arm exchange. Science. 2007; 317(5844):1554–7.
92. van der Zee JS, van Swieten P, Aalberse RC. Inhibition of complement activation by IgG4 antibodies. Clin Exp Immunol. 1986;64(2):415–22.
93. Vosskuhl K, Negm AA, Framke T, Weismüller T, Manns MP, Wedemeyer H, Plentz RR, Wedemeyer J, Lankisch TO. Measurement of IgG4 in bile: a new approach for the diagnosis of IgG4-associated cholangiopathy. Endoscopy. 2012;44(1):48–52.
94. Wallace ZS, Deshpande V, Mattoo H, Mahajan VS, Kulikova M, Pillai S, Stone JH. IgG4-related disease: clinical and laboratory features in one hundred twenty-five patients. Arthritis Rheumatol. 2015; 67(9):2466–75.
95. Wallace ZS, Mattoo H, Carruthers M, Mahajan VS, Della Torre E, Lee H, Kulikova M, Deshpande V, Pillai S, Stone JH. Plasmablasts as a biomarker for IgG4-related disease, independent of serum IgG4 concentrations. Ann Rheum Dis. 2015;74(1): 190–5.
96. Waldram R, Tsantoulas D, Kopelman H, Williams R. Chronic pancreatitis, sclerosing cholangitis and sicca complex in two siblings. Lancet. 1975; 305(7906):550–2.
97. Yoshida K, Toki F, Takeuchi T, Watanabe S, Shiratori K, Hayashi N. Chronic pancreatitis caused by an autoimmune abnormality. Proposal of the concept of autoimmune pancreatitis. Dig Dis Sci. 1995; 40(7):1561–8.
98. Zhang L, Guo L, Huang Y, Wang T, Shi X, Chang H, Yao W, Huang X. Allergic diseases, immunoglobulin E, and autoimmune pancreatitis: a retrospective study of 22 patients. Chin Med J (Engl). 2014; 127(23):4104–9.
99. Zen Y, Harada K, Sasaki M, Sato Y, Tsuneyama K, Haratake J, Kurumaya H, Katayanagi K, Masuda S, Niwa H, Morimoto H, Miwa A, Uchiyama A, Portmann BC, Nakanuma Y. IgG4-related sclerosing cholangitis with and without hepatic inflammatory pseudotumor, and sclerosing pancreatitis-associated cholangitis: do they belong to a spectrum of sclerosing pancreatitis? Am J Surg Pathol. 2004;28(9): 1193–203.
100. Zen Y, Fujii T, Sato Y, Masuda S, Nakanuma Y. Pathological classification of hepatic inflammatory pseudotumor with respect to IgG4-related disease. Mod Pathol. 2007;20(8):884–94.
101. Zen Y, Fujii T, Harada K, Kawano M, Yamada K, Takahira M, Nakanuma Y. Th2 and regulatory immune reactions are increased in immunoglobin G4-related sclerosing pancreatitis and cholangitis. Hepatology. 2007;45(6):1538–46.
102. Zen Y, Liberal R, Nakanuma Y, Heaton N, Portmann B. Possible involvement of CCL1-CCR8 interaction in lymphocytic recruitment in IgG4-related sclerosing cholangitis. J Hepatol. 2013;59(5):1059–64.

Pediatric Primary Sclerosing Cholangitis

6

Dania Molla-Hosseini and Cara L. Mack

Abbreviations

AIH	Autoimmune hepatitis
ALP	Alkaline phosphatase
ALT	Alanine aminotransferase
ANA	Antinuclear antibody
ASC	Autoimmune sclerosing cholangitis
ASMA	Anti-smooth muscle antibody
AST	Aspartate aminotransferase
CCA	Cholangiocarcinoma
CD	Crohn's disease
ERCP	Endoscopic retrograde cholangiopancreatography
GGTP	Gamma-glutamyl transpeptidase
IBD	Inflammatory bowel disease
LCH	Langerhans cell histiocytosis
LKM	Liver-kidney microsomal antibody
MRCP	Magnetic resonance cholangiopancreatography
OV	Oral vancomycin
PSC	Primary sclerosing cholangitis
SSC	Secondary sclerosing cholangitis
UC	Ulcerative colitis
UDCA	Ursodeoxycholic acid

D. Molla-Hosseini, MD (✉) • C.L. Mack, MD
Section of Pediatric Gastroenterology, Hepatology and Nutrition, Children's Hospital Colorado, University of Colorado School of Medicine, 13123 E. 16th Ave., B290, Aurora, CO 80045, USA
e-mail: dania.mollahosseini@childrenscolorado.org; cara.mack@childrenscolorado.org

Introduction

Primary sclerosing cholangitis (PSC) is a rare disorder of the hepatobiliary system characterized by chronic diffuse inflammation and obliterative fibrosis of the intrahepatic and/or extrahepatic bile ducts that subsequently progresses to liver cirrhosis and end-stage liver disease in the majority of patients [1]. This chapter will detail unique aspects of pediatric PSC, including the use of gamma-glutamyl transpeptidase as a biomarker of bile duct injury, the higher rate of autoimmune sclerosing cholangitis and small duct PSC, and the lower incidence of PSC and cholangiocarcinoma in children compared to adults.

Epidemiology

The incidence of PSC in children, similar to the overall incidence of PSC at large, is estimated based on a limited number of population-based studies. The incidence of PSC in children in Canada was reported as 0.23 cases per 100,000 person-years compared with 1.11 per 100,000 in adults [2]. An epidemiology study in the United States estimated the incidence and prevalence of pediatric PSC at 0.2 and 1.5 cases per 100,000 children [3]. Table 6.1 summarizes the largest retrospective studies on pediatric PSC in the United States, revealing that the median age at diagnosis was 11.7 ± 2.5 years old, with a

L.M. Forman (ed.), *Primary Sclerosing Cholangitis*, DOI 10.1007/978-3-319-40908-5_6

Table 6.1 Summary of pediatric PSC studies

First author	Wilschanski [7]	Gregorio [5]		Feldstein [4]	Miloh [6]	Deneau [3]		All studies
Year published	1995	2001		2003	2009	2013		1995–2013
# Patients (n)	32 PSC	9 PSC	27 ASC	52 PSC/ASC	47 PSC/ASC	29 PSC	12 ASC	208
Median age at diagnosis (year) (range)	13 (0.5–18)	6.6 (2–14.5)	11.8 (2.3–16)	14.7 (1.5–19.6)	12 (2–20)	13.0 (5.3–18)	11.3 (3.1–17.6)	11.7 ± 2.5
Mean follow-up (year) (range)	3.8 (0–15)	6 (5–15)	6 (2–16)	6.6 (0.2–16.0037)	6.5 (0.5–19)	5.6 (0.4–14)	6.4 (0.6–13.3)	5.8 ± 1.0
Gender (% male)	72 %	66 %	45 %	65 %	62 %	76 %	50 %	62 ± 11 %
IBD overall	53 %	33 %	30 %	73 %	59 %	96.6 %	75 %	60 ± 24 %
UC	44 %	33 %	18.5 %	58 %	42 %	–		39 ± 14 %
Crohn's disease	9 %	0 %	11 %	15 %	17 %	–		10.4 ± 6.6 %
Overlap syndrome/ASC	28 %	75 %		35 %	25 %	29 %		38.4 ± 20.8 %
PSC/ASC preceded IBD	25 %	–		15 %	15 %	12 %		16.8 ± 5.7 %
Mean ± SD labs at diagnosis:								
AST (U/L)	156.7 ± 195	[a]90	102	271 ± 310	236 ± 245	[a]76	167	155 ± 82.6
ALT (U/L)	–	–		331 ± 336	233 ± 327	72	160	199 ± 110
GGTP (U/L)	–	141	129	536 ± 376	553 ± 676	221	275	267.5 ± 223.5
Alk. Phos. (U/L)	589.8 ± 399	474	303	913 ± 652	610 ± 340	316	292	569.8 ± 257.2
Liver transplantation	31 %	0 %	14.8 %	21 %	19 %	17 %		17.1 ± 10 %

[a]Mean only (no standard deviations reported)

62 ± 11 % male predominance. Associated diseases include inflammatory bowel disease (IBD) in 60 ± 24 % and concurrent autoimmune hepatitis (AIH) (or autoimmune sclerosing cholangitis) in 38.4 ± 20.8 % of PSC patients [3–7]. The rising awareness for this disease alongside the growing use of magnetic resonance cholangiopancreatography (MRCP) for biliary imaging will likely lead to an increased frequency of diagnosis.

Diagnosis of PSC

The majority of cases of pediatric PSC are symptomatic at presentation. Asymptomatic patients are often diagnosed after routine screening of liver biochemistries in the setting of preexisting IBD [4, 6, 7]. The most common symptoms of pediatric PSC are fatigue, abdominal pain, anorexia, and pruritus. Other signs include fever, jaundice, weight loss, delayed growth, and fat-soluble vitamin deficiencies. Approximately 20 % of pediatric PSC patients have pruritus at presentation, of whom ~4 % have extremely debilitating pruritus [4, 6]. Intractable pruritus and fatigue can lead to sleep disturbance, depression, and impairment of quality of life in adults [8–10]. There is only one published health-related quality of life assessment on children with autoimmune liver diseases which revealed that symptoms of abdominal pain, fatigue, and psychological distress were associated with impaired physical activity and school functioning [11]. Physical exam at presentation may reveal hepatomegaly and splenomegaly.

The diagnosis of PSC relies on the combined clinical findings of a cholestatic liver biochemistry profile, imaging (MRCP or endoscopic retrograde cholangiopancreatography [ERCP]), and/or liver histological findings consistent with PSC [12]. In the past decade, great advances in MRCP imaging for infants and children have occurred, and MRCP has an 84 % accuracy rate in the diagnosis of pediatric PSC [13]. Children with PSC have significantly higher levels of serum gamma-glutamyl transpeptidase (GGTP), alanine aminotransferase (ALT), and aspartate aminotransferase (AST) compared to their adult counterparts [12] (see Table 6.1). Reports from large cohorts of adults with PSC have shown that serum alkaline phosphatase (ALP) is of prognostic importance in PSC [14–16]. The incidence of cirrhosis and cholangiocarcinoma has been found to be higher in adult PSC patients with persistently elevated serum ALP levels compared to those who achieve normalization of serum ALP [14–16]. In pediatric PSC, serum GGTP should be considered as a more accurate measure of bile duct injury compared to ALP for the following reasons: First, in four large retrospective reviews of pediatric PSC, only 53–81 % of patients had an elevated ALP at diagnosis compared to 94–100 % of patients with elevated GGTP [3, 4, 6, 17] Second, the range of normal ALP levels substantially increases during times of rapid bone growth in children, making any single elevated ALP level difficult to interpret in children [18]. For example, the upper limit of normal for ALP in a 13-year-old male is 587 U/L, a value that is five-fold higher than the upper limit of normal in adults (mayomedicallaboratories.com). Lastly, serum GGTP levels have been found to be of prognostic importance in pediatric patients with other cholestatic diseases including total parenteral nutrition-related liver disease [19], idiopathic neonatal hepatitis [20, 21], and pediatric sepsis-related cholestasis [22]. A small study on the use of ursodeoxycholic acid for pediatric PSC revealed that GGTP significantly decreased in response to therapy; however changes in ALP were less impressive [23]. Further research into the use of GGTP as a biomarker of disease severity or treatment response in pediatric PSC is warranted.

Natural History and Outcomes in Pediatric PSC

PSC carries significant morbidity in children. Approximately 30–40 % of pediatric PSC patients will suffer from consequences of chronic biliary disease, including significant pruritus, recurrent bacterial cholangitis, and complications of portal hypertension. The largest pediatric PSC study encompassed 52 children who were seen over a 20-year period and followed for up to 16.7 years [4]. Pediatric PSC often progressed to end-stage liver disease, with approximately one-fifth requiring liver transplantation in childhood. The median transplant-free survival in the population studied was 12.7 years, and the mean time from diagnosis of PSC to liver transplantation was 6.6 years [4]. Miloh et al. analyzed the outcome in 47 children with PSC and found that 65 % had significant fibrosis (>grade II) on liver histology at diagnosis. Patients were followed on average for 6.5 years (range 0.5–19), and 19 % required liver transplant [6]. In children, PSC-autoimmune hepatitis (AIH) overlap syndrome (or autoimmune sclerosing cholangitis) seems to have a more favorable outcome than PSC alone, with an estimated 5-year transplant-free survival of 90 % in children with overlap syndrome compared to 78 % in children with PSC alone [3]. Lastly, cholangiocarcinoma (CCA) is a well-known complication of PSC in adults with incidences ranging from 5 to 36 % [24]. Only three cases of CCA have been reported in the setting of pediatric PSC. The range of ages at presentation of the CCA was 14–18 years old, and the CCA was diagnosed 1.2–6 years after the onset of PSC [25]. Clues to the diagnosis of CCA in pediatric PSC include rapid onset of jaundice and abdominal pain, newly diagnosed dominant stricture, and CA19-9 levels consistently >100 U/mL [26].

Subtypes of Pediatric PSC

Autoimmune Sclerosing Cholangitis (PSC-AIH Overlap Syndrome)

Autoimmune sclerosing cholangitis (ASC) was first described by Gregorio et al. in reference to pediatric patients with AIH and cholangiographic or histological features consistent with sclerosing cholangitis [5]. The combination of concurrent PSC with AIH is also known as "overlap syndrome" in children and adults [27]. ASC is much more common in children, with prevalence rates of ~38 % (range 25–75 %) in pediatric PSC patients compared to only 1–4 % of adult patients [3, 4, 6, 7, 28]. The fact that the incidence of ASC is substantially lower in adults may be due to the possibility that the autoimmune-mediated inflammation of ASC subsides or "burns out" by adulthood. A summary of the incidence of ASC in children is provided in Table 6.1. The study by Gregorio et al. was a prospective analysis of biliary disease in all patients with AIH, which may explain why the majority of patients (75 %) had ASC (data on newly diagnosed PSC cases was also collected during the study time frame). Due to the high prevalence of ASC in children, it is recommended that all children with PSC be screened for concurrent AIH with serum autoantibodies (antinuclear antibody (ANA), anti-smooth muscle antibody (ASMA), liver-kidney microsomal antibody (LKM), total IgG), followed by a liver biopsy for histology if any of the autoantibodies are positive. Similarly, for all children with AIH, screening MRCP or ERCP should be performed to determine if ASC is the accurate diagnosis. In addition, because the diagnosis of PSC and ASC can precede the diagnosis of IBD, it is recommended that all children diagnosed with PSC or ASC undergo surveillance upper endoscopy and colonoscopy.

Pediatric ASC patients tend to have higher levels of AST, ALT, and GGTP at presentation compared to PSC only patients [3, 6], and total IgG levels are often >2,000 mg/dL [4, 6]. The vast majority of pediatric ASC cases have positivity for ANA and/or ASMA; to date only two cases of LKM positivity in ASC have been reported [3, 5]. Interestingly, treatment of the AIH component of ASC with immunosuppressive therapy is associated with normalization of AST, ALT, GGTP, and ALP in >70 % of cases. However, this most likely reflects remission of the AIH component, as repeat cholangiographic studies or liver biopsies performed at a median of 5 years after diagnosis revealed that the majority of cases had static disease or progression of biliary disease and fibrosis [5].

Small Duct PSC

Small duct PSC is defined as biochemical cholestasis and liver histology consistent with PSC in the absence of bile duct abnormalities on standard biliary imaging (ERCP or MRCP) [1]. The occurrence of small duct PSC in children ranges from 34 to 42 % of all pediatric PSC cases, a rate that is fourfold higher than that found in adults [4, 6]. Advanced liver fibrosis is less prominent in small duct PSC pediatric patients compared to large duct PSC (44 % versus 65 %), and in general small duct PSC is associated with a more benign course [6]. Interestingly, pediatric small duct PSC patients have a higher prevalence of Crohn's disease than ulcerative colitis [6].

PSC and Inflammatory Bowel Disease

Inflammatory bowel disease (IBD) is strongly associated with the diagnosis of PSC and was noted in 53–96 % of all pediatric PSC cases (Table 6.1). The more common IBD phenotype associated with pediatric PSC is ulcerative colitis (UC), found in 39 ± 14 % of all cases published, compared to 10.4 ± 6.6 % of pediatric PSC cases with Crohn's disease (CD) [3–7, 17]. A large study on the incidence of liver disease in pediatric IBD patients revealed that PSC occurred in 28 of 607 IBD patients (4.6 % overall). The majority of the pediatric PSC cases were associated with UC – 26 of 262 UC patients had PSC (9.9 %), compared to only 2 of 317 CD patients with concurrent PSC (0.6 %) [3]. Adult studies show that the severity of PSC does not correlate to the severity of the associated IBD, and the treatment of IBD does not affect the course of PSC [29]. Similar to adults with IBD and PSC, the symptoms and diagnosis of liver disease in children may precede, coincide with, or follow the diagnosis of IBD. Data from all published studies on pediatric PSC estimate that PSC will be diagnosed before IBD in 16.8 ± 5.7 % of cases (Table 6.1).

Secondary Sclerosing Cholangitis

Many diseases can have biliary manifestations that mimic the histological and cholangiographic findings of PSC, suggesting that widely different insults may cause similar patterns of biliary injury [30]. The presence of sclerosing cholangitis as a result of another underlying disorder is collectively known as secondary sclerosing cholangitis (SSC). In pediatrics the spectrum of diseases that can be associated with SSC is broad and includes diseases resulting in mechanical obstruction or injury of the biliary tree, infections, immunodeficiencies, neoplastic disorders, and congenital diseases such as cystic fibrosis (see Table 6.2). Two of the more common causes of SSC in children include Langerhans cell histiocytosis (LCH) and hyper-IgM syndrome-CD40 ligand deficiency [31]. LCH is a rare, multisystem disorder characterized by clonal expansion of Langerhans cells predominantly within the skin and bone but can infiltrate the liver in up to 35 % of cases. SSC develops in ~30 % of pediatric patients with LCH, and the SSC can occur despite chemotherapy and persist after remission of the LCH. The estimated prevalence of SSC in children with congenital immunodeficiencies and elevated liver tests is ~15 %. Patients with hyper-IgM syndrome-CD40 ligand deficiency and SSC usually have associated infection of the biliary tree with *Cryptosporidium parvum*, which can exacerbate the biliary injury [32]. Other immunodeficiencies are also associated with concurrent biliary infections as described in Table 6.2.

Therapies for PSC

There are presently no effective therapies that are known to delay the progression of pediatric PSC. Two therapies highlighted in the literature for possible use in pediatric PSC include ursodeoxycholic acid (UDCA) and oral vancomycin (OV). UDCA is thought to exert its beneficial effects on cholestatic diseases through many different mechanisms including: (1) inhibition of intestinal absorption of endogenous "hepatotoxic" bile acids; (2) stimulation of biliary secretion of bile acids, thus limiting cellular injury from excess hydrophobic bile acids; and (3) anti-inflammatory and immunomodulatory effects, resulting in decreased inflammatory-mediated

Table 6.2 Causes of secondary sclerosing cholangitis

Mechanical	Choledocholithiasis
	Idiopathic
	Sickle-cell anemia Parenteral nutrition-associated liver disease
Infection	Bacterial cholangitis
	E. coli O157:H7 enterocolitis
	Cryptosporidium
	Septic shock
Immunodeficiency	X-linked hyper-IgM syndrome-CD40 ligand deficiency and *Cryptosporidium*
	Wiskott-Aldrich syndrome
	Natural killer cell deficiency and *Trichosporon*
	Agammaglobulinemia and *Cryptosporidium*
	Combined variable immunodeficiency and *Cryptosporidium*
	AIDS-associated cholangiopathy and *Cytomegalovirus* and *Cryptosporidium*
Neoplastic	Langerhans cell histiocytosis
	Hodgkin lymphoma
	Ductal cancer, gallbladder cancer
	Reticulum cell sarcoma
Congenital	Cystic fibrosis
	Congenital hepatic fibrosis
	Ductal plate abnormalities
	Caroli disease
Injury	Postsurgical stenosis
	Trauma
	Caustic injury

injury [33]. UDCA use in adults is detailed in a separate chapter and will not be reviewed in this section. UDCA has been extensively utilized as a therapeutic option for the treatment of many pediatric cholestatic liver diseases, including Alagille syndrome, progressive familial intrahepatic cholestasis, and biliary atresia [34–39]. Gilger et al. analyzed UDCA treatment in ten pediatric PSC patients and found that UDCA had significant reductions of liver chemistries, including GGTP [23]. Data from pediatric PSC case series have shown that treatment with UDCA improves liver biochemistries and cholestatic parameters [4, 6]; however the impact of UDCA on long-term clinical outcomes has not been studied. In order to determine the effectiveness of UDCA for the treatment of pediatric PSC, a multicentered, randomized comparative effectiveness or placebo-controlled clinical trial would be necessary.

Vancomycin is a glycopeptide antibiotic commonly used for the treatment of infections caused by gram-positive bacteria [40]. Oral vancomycin is poorly absorbed from the intestines [41], and so it remains active in the gastrointestinal tract and has minimal to no systemic side effects [42–49]. OV may eliminate the enteric pathogens that produce toxins which can be absorbed through the enteroportal circulation and cause periportal inflammation, including activation of the innate immune system [50]. In addition, OV may have direct anti-inflammatory effects through inhibition of TNF-α production [51]. Cox et al. reported the response to OV in 14 pediatric PSC patients with concurrent active IBD. The use of OV was associated with significant improvement in GGTP, ALT, and erythrocyte sedimentation rate levels within 3 months of therapy, and 57 % of patients had normalization of GGTP [52, 53]. Half of the patients were kept on long-term therapy, with a mean duration on OV use of 19 ± 24 months (range 4–56 months). When OV was stopped, the liver biochemistries worsened, suggesting that OV was directly responsible for decreased biliary injury [52, 53]. Potential immunoregulatory effects of prolonged use of OV in pediatric PSC include increased production of transforming growth factor-β, an anti-inflammatory protein, and regulatory T cells, which are responsible for controlling autoimmune responses [54]. This study also showed improvement in liver histology and MRCP findings after 6–12 months of OV therapy. Limitations of these studies include the small sample sizes (~10–14 patients) and the lack of a control group (i.e., other therapy or placebo). Furthermore, all of the pediatric reports on the use of OV are based on PSC patients who have concurrent evidence of active colitis. A recent randomized trial on the use of OV in adults with PSC resulted in a significant reduction of serum ALP and a trend toward significant reduction of total bilirubin [55]. Again, this study analyzed a small number of patients per group. Collectively, these data suggest that long-term treatment with OV may be of therapeutic benefit in PSC patients but requires further investigation through a large multicentered study.

Liver transplantation is a viable option for end-stage liver disease secondary to pediatric PSC and accounts for ~2 % of all pediatric liver transplants in the United States (https://www.unos.org) [25]. Calculated 10-year transplant-free survival rates in pediatric PSC and ASC range from 65 to 90 %. On average, 17 % (range 0–31 %) of PSC and ASC patients will have a liver transplant in childhood (Table 6.1) [3–5]. The largest published series characterizing pediatric PSC patients who underwent liver transplantation originates from the Studies of Pediatric Liver Transplantation registry. Seventy-nine pediatric PSC patients in the United States and Canada underwent liver transplantation between 1995 and 2008 (2.6 % of all liver transplants) [56]. At the time of transplant, 46 % of patients had IBD, and an additional 9.8 % developed IBD post transplant. The pediatric PSC cohort had similar patient and graft survival rates compared to patients transplanted for indications other than PSC. Posttransplant recurrent PSC occurred in 9.8 % of patients at a mean of 18.7 ± 13.8 months after transplant. Other studies report recurrent PSC in up to 30 % of pediatric liver transplant patients [57].

Summary

In summary, pediatric PSC is a rare disease that is associated with significant morbidity and often leads to liver transplantation for survival. Unique aspects of pediatric PSC compared to adults include the high incidence of ASC and small duct PSC and the rarity of development of CCA in childhood. There is no medical therapy that is known to prevent progression of the disease. Research efforts should focus on deciphering the immunopathogenesis of PSC in order to identify potential therapeutic targets to halt progression of the disease.

References

1. Hirschfield GM, et al. Primary sclerosing cholangitis. Lancet. 2013;382(9904):1587–99.
2. Kaplan GG, et al. The burden of large and small duct primary sclerosing cholangitis in adults and children: a population-based analysis. Am J Gastroenterol. 2007;102(5):1042–9.
3. Deneau M, et al. Primary sclerosing cholangitis, autoimmune hepatitis, and overlap in Utah children: epidemiology and natural history. Hepatology. 2013; 58(4):1392–400.
4. Feldstein AE, et al. Primary sclerosing cholangitis in children: a long-term follow-up study. Hepatology. 2003;38(1):210–7.
5. Gregorio GV, et al. Autoimmune hepatitis/sclerosing cholangitis overlap syndrome in childhood: a 16-year prospective study. Hepatology. 2001;33(3): 544–53.
6. Miloh T, et al. A retrospective single-center review of primary sclerosing cholangitis in children. Clin Gastroenterol Hepatol. 2009;7(2):239–45.
7. Wilschanski M, et al. Primary sclerosing cholangitis in 32 children: clinical, laboratory, and radiographic features, with survival analysis. Hepatology. 1995;22(5):1415–22.
8. Benito de Valle M, et al. Factors that reduce health-related quality of life in patients with primary sclerosing cholangitis. Clin Gastroenterol Hepatol. 2012; 10(7):769–775.e2.
9. Younossi ZM, et al. Cholestatic liver diseases and health-related quality of life. Am J Gastroenterol. 2000;95(2):497–502.
10. Bjornsson E, et al. Fatigue in patients with primary sclerosing cholangitis. Scand J Gastroenterol. 2004; 39(10):961–8.
11. Gulati R, et al. Health-related quality of life in children with autoimmune liver disease. J Pediatr Gastroenterol Nutr. 2013;57(4):444–50.
12. Chapman R, et al. Diagnosis and management of primary sclerosing cholangitis. Hepatology. 2010;51(2): 660–78.
13. Chavhan GB, et al. Primary sclerosing cholangitis in children: utility of magnetic resonance cholangiopancreatography. Pediatr Radiol. 2008;38(8):868–73.
14. Al Mamari S, et al. Improvement of serum alkaline phosphatase to <1.5 upper limit of normal predicts better outcome and reduced risk of cholangiocarcinoma in primary sclerosing cholangitis. J Hepatol. 2013;58(2):329–34.
15. Lindstrom L, et al. Association between reduced levels of alkaline phosphatase and survival times of patients with primary sclerosing cholangitis. Clin Gastroenterol Hepatol. 2013;11(7):841–6.
16. Stanich PP, et al. Alkaline phosphatase normalization is associated with better prognosis in primary sclerosing cholangitis. Dig Liver Dis. 2011;43(4):309–13.
17. Debray D, et al. Sclerosing cholangitis in children. J Pediatr. 1994;124(1):49–56.

18. Cabrera-Abreu JC, Green A. Gamma-glutamyltransferase: value of its measurement in paediatrics. Ann Clin Biochem. 2002;39(Pt 1):22–5.
19. Spagnuolo MI, et al. Ursodeoxycholic acid for treatment of cholestasis in children on long-term total parenteral nutrition: a pilot study. Gastroenterology. 1996;111(3):716–9.
20. Wang J, Wang ZL, Zhu QR, Wang XH, Zheng S. The prognostic value of serum gamma glutamyltransferase activity in Chinese infants with previously diagnosed idiopathic neonatal hepatitis. HK J Paediatr (new series). 2008;13:39–45.
21. Wang JS, Tan N, Dhawan A. Significance of low or normal serum gamma glutamyl transferase level in infants with idiopathic neonatal hepatitis. Eur J Pediatr. 2006;165(11):795–801.
22. Oswari H, et al. Prognostic value of biochemical liver parameters in neonatal sepsis-associated cholestasis. J Paediatr Child Health. 2013;49(1):E6–11.
23. Gilger MA, et al. Efficacy of ursodeoxycholic acid in the treatment of primary sclerosing cholangitis in children. J Pediatr Gastroenterol Nutr. 2000;31(2):136–41.
24. Burak K, et al. Incidence and risk factors for cholangiocarcinoma in primary sclerosing cholangitis. Am J Gastroenterol. 2004;99(3):523–6.
25. Mieli-Vergani G, Vergani D. Sclerosing cholangitis in children and adolescents. Clin Liver Dis. 2016;20(1):99–111.
26. Deneau M, et al. Cholangiocarcinoma in a 17-year-old boy with primary sclerosing cholangitis and inflammatory bowel disease. J Pediatr Gastroenterol Nutr. 2011;52(5):617–20.
27. Beuers U, Rust C. Overlap syndromes. Semin Liver Dis. 2005;25(3):311–20.
28. Ibrahim SH, Lindor KD. Current management of primary sclerosing cholangitis in pediatric patients. Paediatr Drugs. 2011;13(2):87–95.
29. LaRusso NF, et al. Primary sclerosing cholangitis: summary of a workshop. Hepatology. 2006;44(3):746–64.
30. Abdalian R, Heathcote EJ. Sclerosing cholangitis: a focus on secondary causes. Hepatology. 2006;44(5):1063–74.
31. Girard M, et al. Specificities of sclerosing cholangitis in childhood. Clin Res Hepatol Gastroenterol. 2012;36(6):530–5.
32. Rodrigues F, et al. Liver disease in children with primary immunodeficiencies. J Pediatr. 2004;145(3):333–9.
33. Ali A, Carey EJ, Lindor KD. An overview of current and future strategies for the treatment of primary sclerosing cholangitis. Expert Opin Orphan Drugs. 2014;2(6):545–56.
34. Kelly DA, Davenport M. Current management of biliary atresia. Arch Dis Child. 2007;92(12):1132–5.
35. Nousia-Arvanitakis S, et al. Long-term prospective study of the effect of ursodeoxycholic acid on cystic fibrosis-related liver disease. J Clin Gastroenterol. 2001;32(4):324–8.
36. O'Leary JG, Pratt DS. Cholestasis and cholestatic syndromes. Curr Opin Gastroenterol. 2007;23(3):232–6.
37. Paumgartner G, Beuers U. Ursodeoxycholic acid in cholestatic liver disease: mechanisms of action and therapeutic use revisited. Hepatology. 2002;36(3):525–31.
38. Willot S, et al. Effect of ursodeoxycholic acid on liver function in children after successful surgery for biliary atresia. Pediatrics. 2008;122(6):e1236–41.
39. Beuers U. Drug insight: mechanisms and sites of action of ursodeoxycholic acid in cholestasis. Nat Clin Pract Gastroenterol Hepatol. 2006;3(6):318–28.
40. Moellering Jr RC. Vancomycin: a 50-year reassessment. Clin Infect Dis. 2006;42 Suppl 1:S3–4.
41. Armstrong CJ, Wilson TS. Systemic absorption of vancomycin. J Clin Pathol. 1995;48(7):689.
42. Appel GB, et al. Vancomycin and the kidney. Am J Kidney Dis. 1986;8(2):75–80.
43. Bryan CS, White WL. Safety of oral vancomycin in functionally anephric patients. Antimicrob Agents Chemother. 1978;14(4):634–5.
44. Cooper G, Given DB. Vancomycin: a comprehensive review of 30 years clinical experience. New York: John Wiley & Sons; 1986. p. 84.
45. Dudley MN, et al. Absorption of vancomycin. Ann Intern Med. 1984;101(1):144.
46. Matzke GR, et al. Systemic absorption of oral vancomycin in patients with renal insufficiency and antibiotic-associated colitis. Am J Kidney Dis. 1987;9(5):422–5.
47. Matzke GR, Zhanel GG, Guay DR. Clinical pharmacokinetics of vancomycin. Clin Pharmacokinet. 1986;11(4):257–82.
48. Rybak MJ, et al. Nephrotoxicity of vancomycin, alone and with an aminoglycoside. J Antimicrob Chemother. 1990;25(4):679–87.
49. Tange RA, et al. An experimental study of vancomycin-induced cochlear damage. Arch Otorhinolaryngol. 1989;246(2):67–70.
50. Hobson CH, et al. Enterohepatic circulation of bacterial chemotactic peptide in rats with experimental colitis. Gastroenterology. 1988;94(4):1006–13.
51. Howden BP, et al. Different bacterial gene expression patterns and attenuated host immune responses are associated with the evolution of low-level vancomycin resistance during persistent methicillin-resistant Staphylococcus aureus bacteraemia. BMC Microbiol. 2008;8:39.
52. Cox KL, Cox KM. Oral vancomycin: treatment of primary sclerosing cholangitis in children with inflammatory bowel disease. J Pediatr Gastroenterol Nutr. 1998;27(5):580–3.
53. Davies YK, et al. Long-term treatment of primary sclerosing cholangitis in children with oral vancomycin: an immunomodulating antibiotic. J Pediatr Gastroenterol Nutr. 2008;47(1):61–7.
54. Abarbanel DN, et al. Immunomodulatory effect of vancomycin on Treg in pediatric inflammatory bowel

disease and primary sclerosing cholangitis. J Clin Immunol. 2013;33(2):397–406.
55. Tabibian JH, et al. Randomised clinical trial: vancomycin or metronidazole in patients with primary sclerosing cholangitis – a pilot study. Aliment Pharmacol Ther. 2013;37(6):604–12.
56. Miloh T, et al. Pediatric liver transplantation for primary sclerosing cholangitis. Liver Transpl. 2011;17(8):925–33.
57. Venkat VL, Ranganathan S, Sindhi R. The challenges of liver transplantation in children with primary sclerosing cholangitis. Expert Rev Gastroenterol Hepatol. 2015;9(3):289–94.

Cholangiocyte Biology

7

Lorena Loarca, María José Lorenzo Pisarello, Leslie Morton, Bing Q. Huang, Steven O'Hara, Patrick Splinter, and Nicholas LaRusso

Abbreviations

ADP	Adenosine diphosphate
AE2	Anion exchanger 2
APM	Apical plasma membrane
AQP	Aquaporin
ARPKD	Autosomal recessive polycystic kidney disease
ASBT	Apical Na^+-dependent bile salt uptake transporter
ATP	Adenosine triphosphate
BA	Bile acids
BDL	Bile duct ligation
BPM	Basolateral plasma membrane
C. parvum	*Cryptosporidium parvum*
Ca^{2+}	Calcium
cAMP	Cyclic adenosine 3′, 5′- monophosphate
CCA	Cholangiocarcinoma
CFTR	Cystic fibrosis transmembrane conductance regulator
CK19	Cytokeratin 19
Cl^-	Chloride
COX-2	Cyclooxygenase-2
ECVs	Extracellular vesicles
EGFR	Epidermal growth factor receptor
ERK1/2	Extracellular signal-regulated protein kinases 1 and 2
HBD2	Human β-defensin 2
HCO_3^-	Bicarbonate
Hh	Hedgehog
HSC	Hepatic stellate cell
IGFBP	Insulin-like growth factor-binding protein
IL-6	Interleukin 6
IL-8	Interleukin 8
ILV	Intraluminal vesicles
iNOs	Inducible nitric oxide synthase
K^+	Potassium
LPS	Lipopolysaccharide
MCP	Monocyte chemoattractant protein
MRP	Multidrug resistance protein
MVB	Multivesicular bodies
MyD88	Myeloid differentiation protein 88
Na^+	Sodium
SGLT1	Na^+-glucose cotransporter
NF-kB	Nuclear factor kappa B
NKCC1	$Na^+/K^+/Cl^-$ cotransporter 1
NO	Nitric oxide
PDFG-BB	Platelet-derived growth factor-BB
PKA	Protein kinase A

This work was supported by grants awarded to NFL: NIH NIDDK DK 24031 (R01), Pathobiology of Hepatic Epithelia; NIH NIDDK DK 57993 (R01), Pathophysiology of Biliary Disease; and NIH NIDDK DK 84567 (P30), Mayo Center for Cell Signaling in Gastroenterology

L. Loarca • M.J.L. Pisarello • L. Morton • B.Q. Huang • S. O'Hara • P. Splinter • N. LaRusso (✉)
Division of Gastroenterology and Hepatology, Mayo Clinic Center for Signaling in Gastroenterology, Mayo Clinic, Rochester, MN 55905, USA
e-mail: Loarca.Lorena@mayo.edu; Pisarello.Maria@mayo.edu; Morton.Leslie@mayo.edu; Huang.Bing@mayo.edu; Ohara.Steven@mayo.edu; Splinter.Patrick@mayo.edu; LaRusso.Nicholas@mayo.edu

L.M. Forman (ed.), *Primary Sclerosing Cholangitis*, DOI 10.1007/978-3-319-40908-5_7

PSC	Primary sclerosing cholangitis
SASP	Senescence-associated secretory phenotype
SR	Secretin receptor
t-ASBT	Truncated ASBT
TGF-β	Transforming growth factor beta
TJ	Tight junction
TLR	Toll-like receptors
TRPV4	Transient receptor potential 4

Introduction

The biliary system consists of a network of tubular structures, or bile ducts, inside (intrahepatic bile ducts) and outside of the liver (extrahepatic bile ducts). This system facilitates the flow of bile from the liver to the gallbladder for storage before being secreted into the small intestine after meals to aid in the digestion of dietary fats [1]. Bile ducts are lined by epithelial cells, known as cholangiocytes, that vary in morphology and function. Cholangiocytes are best known for their role in bile modification and secretion; however, over the past decades, other functions have been attributed to these cells. For instance, cholangiocytes are key contributors to the function of the innate and adaptive immune systems, as they are "the first line of defense" in the biliary tract against harmful, gut-derived molecules [2]. These cells express receptors on their apical surface that recognize endogenous and exogenous pathogens, chemicals, microbial products, and xenobiotics present in bile. Upon recognition of potentially injurious agents, cholangiocytes may become activated, secreting pro-inflammatory factors necessary for the recruitment of a variety of different cells, including immune cells, to the site of injury [3] (Table 7.1) (Fig. 7.1). Moreover, activated cholangiocytes secrete profibrotic molecules, such as transforming growth factor beta (TGF-β) [4] and platelet-derived growth factor-BB (PDGF-BB), that can activate myofibroblasts, the main mediators of the wound-healing response [5]. Another mechanism of defense for damaged cholangiocytes against stressors, particularly oncogenic agents, is the termination of cellular replication via the process of cellular senescence [6] (Fig. 7.1). Further, when cholangiocytes become senescent, they can transition to a senescence-associated secretory phenotype (i.e., SASP) characterized by the robust secretion of an array of soluble and intravesical factors that affect neighboring cells. For example, the cholangiocyte SASP is characterized by high secretion levels of pro-inflammatory cytokines, such as interleukins 6 (IL-6) and 8 (IL-8) [6] (Table 7.1) (Fig. 7.1). Importantly, IL-6 may play a role in malignant transition of cholangiocytes [7].

In this chapter we review selected aspects related to cholangiocyte biology with a particular emphasis on cholangiocyte adaptability to changes in their microenvironment as a mechanistic response to injury. The pathways involved in this cholangiocyte plasticity are also reviewed.

Cholangiocyte Biology

Structural Features

Biliary Tree Anatomy The biliary tree network consists of intrahepatic and extrahepatic ducts [8]. The intrahepatic ducts can be described from four perspectives according to luminal diameter, area, morphology, and physiology [8, 9]. The small ducts (<15 μm) originate from the Canals of Hering and, when combined, give rise to interlobular ducts (10–100 μm) [8]. The merging of two or more septal ducts (100–300 μm) results in the development of large ducts (300–400 μm) [8]. The large ducts combine to form segmental ducts (400–800 μm) and left and right hepatic ducts (>800 μm) from which the extrahepatic ducts emerge. The gallbladder connected to the extrahepatic portion of the biliary tree functions as a storage of bile [8] (Fig. 7.2).

Cholangiocytes along the biliary tree are morphologically heterogeneous [8]. The small ducts are lined by 4–5 cholangiocytes, termed small cholangiocytes, which exhibit a cuboidal or flattened shape and possess a basement membrane on their basolateral domain. On their apical domain, microvilli and primary cilia face the bile duct

Table 7.1 Cholangiocyte plasticity table. A summary of the markers and phenotypic characteristics of cholangiocytes as they evolve from normal to activated, senescent, and transformed phenotypes [3, 5, 8, 89–91]

Normal		Activated		Senescent/SASP		Malignant	
Markers	Phenotypic characteristic	Markers	Phenotypic characteristic	Markers	Phenotypic characteristic	Markers	Phenotypic characteristic
AE2	Transports intracellular Cl^-/HCO_3^-	αvβ6 integrin	Induces proliferation and migration	SA-β-Gal	Large, flat cells	IL-6	Induces cholangiocyte proliferation and controls methylation of tumor suppressor genes in CCA
AQP1	Transports water	Secrete Hh ligands, ET-1, TGF-β, PDGF-BB, and CFTG	Perpetuation of the activated phenotype, activation of myofibroblasts	p16INK4a	Inhibits CDK4 and CDK6 functions, blocking the cell cycle in G1	CEA	Increases migration, invasion, and proliferation
GGT	Catabolizes extracellular glutathione	Pathogen recognition receptors such as TLRs and NODs when injury is caused by microbes	Secrete IL-6, IL-8, NO, TNF-α, IFN-γ, and MCP-1	p21Waf1	Increases cytoplasm granules and vacuoles	ENO2	Induces apoptosis and chemotherapy resistance
ASBT	Trafficking of conjugated BAs	Secrete neurocrine molecules such as secretin, histamine, and estrogens, etc.	Induce cholangiocyte proliferation	p53	Tumor suppression or oncogenesis	ErbB-2/Neu	Activates the AKT pathway. Increases production of COX-2, prostaglandin 2, and telomerase activity.
CFTR	Transports Cl-	VEGF	Promotes cholangiocyte cystogenesis	SASP (IL-6, IL-8, CCL2, PAI1, MMPs, TGF-β, IGFBP)	SASP hypersecretion	MUC1	Stimulates cholangiocyte proliferation

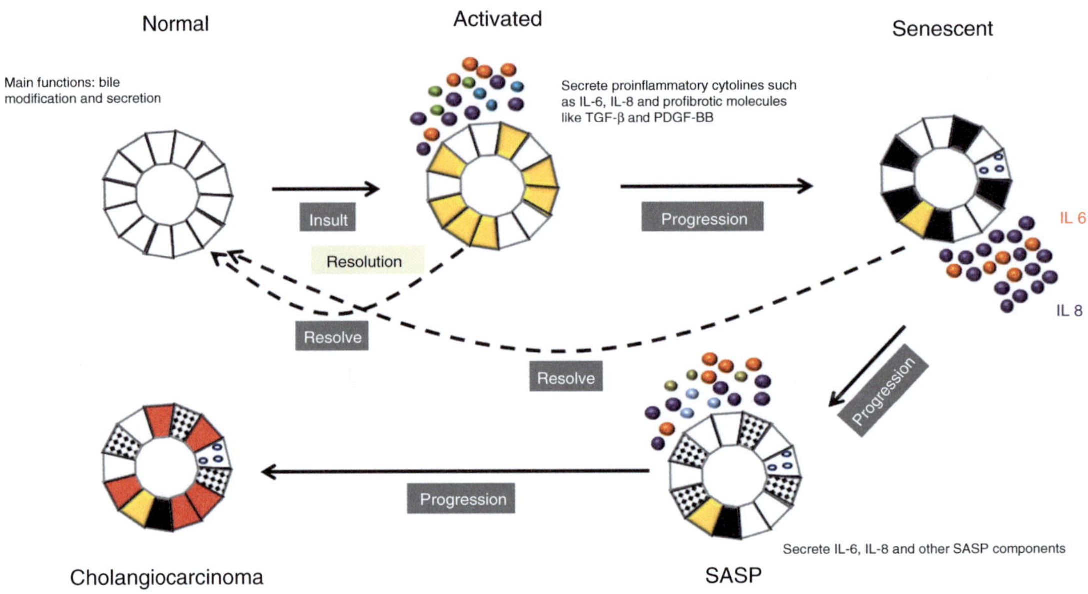

Fig. 7.1 Cholangiocyte plasticity model. Schematic representation of the proposed model of the plasticity of cholangiocytes during biliary injury. The *solid arrow* lines indicate the transition of normal cholangiocytes through the various disease phenotypes. The *dashed arrows* suggest that activated or senescent cholangiocytes could resolve back to the normal phenotype. The major key molecules and pathways that participate in each stage are also shown [3, 89]

Fig. 7.2 Biliary tract anatomy. The biliary tree is depicted from the finest branches at the Canals of Hering to the small, interlobular, septal, and large ducts. Also shown, the right and left intrahepatic ducts that merge to form the extrahepatic ducts, from where the gallbladder emerges [8]

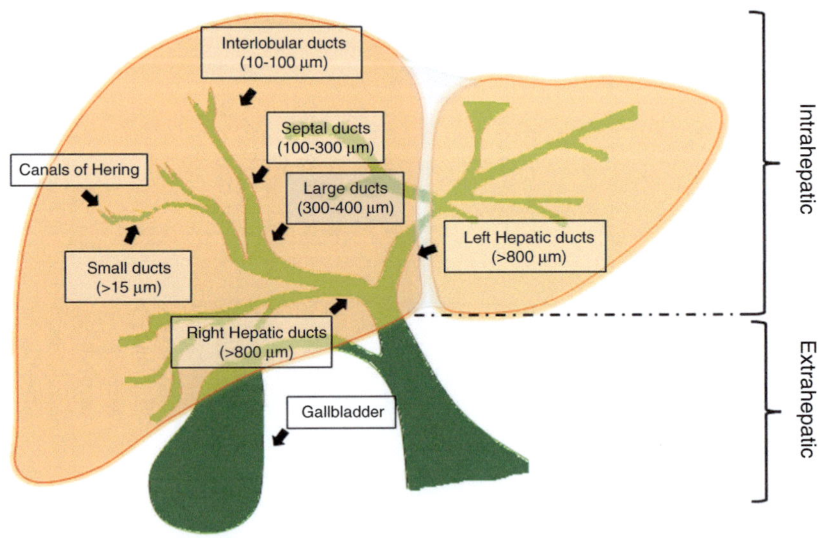

lumen. Large bile ducts are lined by columnar-shaped cells known as large cholangiocytes that also express both microvilli and cilia on their apical domain [8]. When compared to small cholangiocytes, large cholangiocytes have a smaller nuclear to cytoplasmic ratio with a higher content of rough endoplasmic reticulum [1]. This feature implies that large cholangiocytes are more differentiated and have less plasticity relative to small cholangiocytes [8].

Cholangiocytes are connected to each other via tight junctions that maintain cholangiocyte polarity through cell-to-cell adhesion [8]. The apical plasma membrane domain faces the ductal

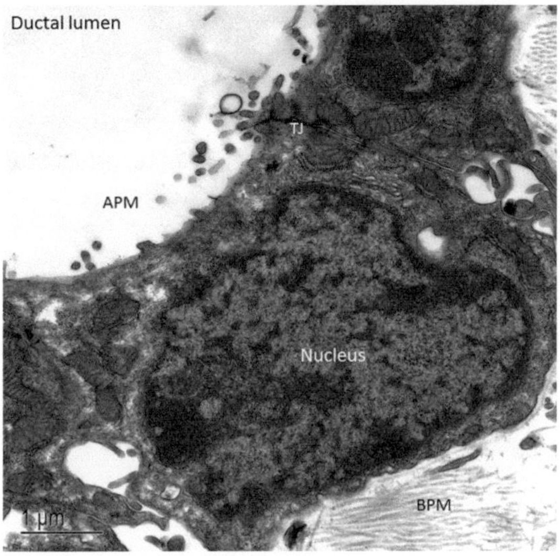

Fig. 7.3 Cholangiocyte ultrastructure. Transmission electron micrograph of a small mouse cholangiocyte, showing the apical plasma membrane (APM) that faces the ductal lumen. The nucleus, a tight junction (TJ) between two cholangiocytes, and the basolateral plasma membrane (BPM) are also shown

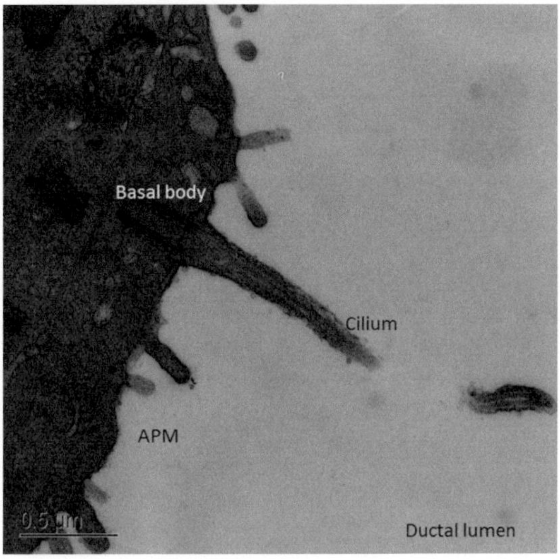

Fig. 7.4 Cholangiocyte cilium. Transmission electron micrograph of a small mouse cholangiocyte showing a primary cilium facing the ductal lumen. The basal body of the primary cilium and the apical plasma membrane (APM) are also shown

lumen, which functions as the secretory pole for ductal bile formation; the basolateral plasma membrane domain faces the extracellular matrix and underlying connective tissue [10], Fig. 7.3.

Cholangiocyte Cilia Each small and large cholangiocyte possesses a primary cilium (~7 μm in length) extending from the apical cholangiocyte membrane into the ductal lumen. Primary cilia are nonmotile, microtubule-based organelles consisting of a membrane-bound axoneme composed of microtubules and a basal body (Fig. 7.4). The axoneme contains a 9+0 microtubule arrangement, i.e., nine peripheral microtubule doublets lacking a central pair of microtubules [11, 12]; in contrast, motile cilia have a similar structure but contain two central microtubules (i.e., 9+2 structure). The existence of primary cilia was originally reported in various mitotically quiescent mammalian cells by Sergei Sorokin in 1968 [13]. In 2006, primary cilia were described in mouse and rat small and large cholangiocytes [11]. However, their physiological importance was not appreciated until recently when it was demonstrated that primary cilia are involved in mechano-, chemo-, and osmo-sensation [14–18].

Functional Features

The main function of intrahepatic cholangiocytes is to modify bile via a series of secretory/absorptive events. These are regulated by several gastrointestinal peptides/hormones including gastrin, endothelin-1, somatostatin, TGR-5, and secretin, which display inhibitory and stimulatory effects on water and bicarbonate (HCO_3^-) secretion. These modifications ultimately influence the bile volume, content, tonicity, and alkalinity [8, 14]. While there is considerable species variation, intrahepatic cholangiocytes directly generate up to 40 % of daily bile secretion [2]. Secretory functions are performed mainly by large intrahepatic cholangiocytes via a mechanism dependent on cAMP activation. Large cholangiocytes abundantly express the appropriate ion transport systems and hormone receptors for these functions. For example, cholangiocytes in the large ducts are the major functional anatomic sites for expression of secretin and somatostatin receptors necessary for bile modification and secretion. In contrast, cholangiocytes lining small bile ducts, including the finest branches of the biliary system, do not express the secretin and somatostatin receptors exerting secretory activities independent of cAMP activation [19, 20]. For instance, during injury of large bile ducts, small cholangiocytes, which lack the cystic fibrosis transmembrane conductance regulator (CFTR), activate an alternative pathway for water and electrolyte secretion dependent of Ca^{+} signaling [21].

Small cholangiocytes, which are mitotically quiescent, proliferate via activation of Ca^{+2} signaling in response to liver injury and toxins [19, 20]. For instance, small cholangiocytes may replicate upon stimulation with histamine or secretin or injury by α-naphthylisothiocyanate or acute carbon tetrachloride. Le Sage et al. demonstrated that acute administration of carbon tetrachloride to rats induces apoptosis of large cholangiocytes and proliferation of small cholangiocytes. Furthermore, small cholangiocytes acquired de novo expression of secretin receptors. Stimulation of small cholangiocytes with secretin-induced activation of cAMP suggests that upon injury small cholangiocyte may acquire secretory features of large cholangiocytes. This suggested that small cholangiocytes compensated for the functions of the injured large cholangiocytes [22]. Also, after partial hepatectomy, rat small cholangiocytes function as a niche for hepatobiliary progenitor cells. Studies performed in human cholestatic livers and in human-regenerating liver after alcohol-induced injury suggest that human cholangiocytes behave in a similar manner [23]. Thiese et al. reported that acetaminophen-induced hepatic massive necrosis stimulates a niche of stem cells containing small cells positive for the cholangiocyte marker cytokeratin 19 (CK19) within the Canals of Hering [24]. Thus, the main biological properties of small cholangiocytes are their ability to proliferate, to acquire features of large cholangiocytes, to differentiate into hepatocytes, and to be a cell reservoir upon injury [1, 25].

Bile Formation Ninety-five percent of bile is water with the remaining 5% consisting of organic solutes such as bile salts, phospholipids, cholesterol, as well as inorganic salts such as Na^+, K^+, and HCO_3^- [26, 27]. Bile is first formed (i.e., primary bile) by hepatocytes and then secreted into the canaliculi via osmotic-dependent excretion of organic solutes across the canalicular membrane drawing water via aquaporin water channels [28]. The principal driver of hepatocyte bile secretion is bile acids (i.e., bile acid-dependent bile flow) [29]. Bile is then modified via absorptive and secretory processes initially by large cholangiocytes via transport of chloride (Cl^-), HCO_3^-, bile acids (BAs), amino acids, and glucose to modify the water content and alkalinity of bile through a series of hormone-regulated, Ca^{2+} (calcium)- or cyclic adenosine 3′, 5′-monophosphate (cAMP)-dependent intracellular processes [8, 26].

Moreover, cAMP and/or Ca^{2+}-sensitive basolateral potassium (K^+) channels, expressed in cholangiocytes, mediate K^+ release which leads to membrane hyperpolarization to maintain the electrical driving force for continued apical Cl^- secretion [30]. Under basal conditions, the permeability of the apical membrane is low but can be increased several fold following cAMP stimulation [31, 32]. Furthermore, Cl^- secretion and subsequent reuptake is required for HCO_3^- secretion by the Cl^-/HCO_3^- anion exchanger 2 (AE2). Cl^- uptake is mediated by the sodium (Na^+)/K^+/Cl^- cotransporter NKCC1, which is localized in the basolateral membrane of rat cholangiocytes. In an electrically neutral manner with stoichiometry of $1Na^+{:}1\ K^+{:}2Cl^-$, a gradient is established, which maintains a high concentration of intracellular Cl^- [33]. This is important as HCO_3^- is secreted in exchange for luminal Cl^-. The movement of ions across the cholangiocyte apical and basolateral membranes promotes osmotic-driven bile secretion [34].

The absorption of ions, BAs, amino acids, and glucose are additional processes that contribute to ductal bile modification [8]. Glucose is removed from bile in a Na^+-dependent manner by the Na^+-glucose cotransporter, SGLT1, localized in the apical plasma membrane of the bile ducts. Conjugated BAs enter cholangiocytes through the apical Na^+ -dependent bile salt uptake transporter (ASBT) [35]. This is a 48 kDa integral membrane protein, localized on the cholangiocyte apical membrane. A truncated form of this transporter (t-ASBT), responsible for the final reabsorption of bile salts from the bile into the blood, is found on the basolateral membrane [36, 37]. To prevent the cytotoxic effects of intracellular BA accumulation, basolateral extrusion of bile salts is mediated by MRP3, a member of the multidrug resistance protein (MRP) subfamily of transporters. MRP3 substrates include the organic anions estradiol-17-glucuronide, bilirubin glucuronide, monovalent bile salts taurocholate and glycocholate, as well as divalent sulfated bile salts [8, 38].

Hepatocytes secrete glutathione into the bile. After glutathione in bile is hydrolyzed, the amino acids, glutamate, cysteine, and glycine are produced and then absorbed by cholangiocytes for the resynthesis of glutathione, which mediates bile salt-independent secretion of canalicular bile. Additionally, taurine and glycine play a key role in the formation of conjugated BAs, preventing the reabsorption of the conjugated BAs as they traffick through the biliary tract [28].

Water Secretion Water not only plays a major role as the main constituent in bile, but is also involved in the flow of bile and of cholangiocyte signaling pathways via ciliary transduction mechanisms [28]. Osmosis-dependent excretion of ions, organic solutes, and water into the canaliculi establishes osmotic gradients necessary to stimulate bile formation and secretion [8, 26]. Water transport, which is mediated by water channels known as aquaporins (AQPs), plays a key role in ductal bile formation [39]. AQPs are a family of ubiquitously expressed membrane proteins first discovered in the 1980s [35, 36] that form channels allowing the transport of water and small solutes such as glycerol to cross the plasma membrane. The permeability of water across the cell plasma membrane lipid bilayer is increased up to 50 times when AQPs are present relative to plasma membranes lacking AQPs [40]. At least 13 types of AQPs (AQP 0–12) have been described in mammalian cells and have been grouped into three categories according to their functions. Orthodox AQPs (i.e., AQPs 0,1,2,4, and 5) selectively mediate water flow through plasma membranes. Aquaglyceroporins (i.e., AQPs 3,7,9, and 10) allow the passage of water in addition to glycerol and urea. Unorthodox AQPs (i.e., AQPs 6,8,11, and 12) were only recently identified, and their functions remain uncertain [41–43]. AQPs 0, 1, 4, 5, 8, 9, and 11 are all expressed in cholangiocytes [44]. In cholangiocytes, water movement likely occurs principally via a shuttle mechanism involving AQP1, which is localized to both the apical and basolateral domains [39]. Secretin, a gastrointestinal hormone secreted by S cells of the duodenum [45], promotes the movement of intracellular vesicles containing AQP1 to the apical plasma membrane, enhancing osmotic water permeability, a process essential to ductal bile secretion [39]. Furthermore, when vesicles are isolated from the apical and basolateral membranes of bile duct-ligated (BDL) rats treated with secretin, the apical vesicles became enriched in AQP1, while the basolateral vesicles express stable levels of AQP4 [46]. Thus, these observations suggest that AQP1 is regulated and mediates apical water flow, whereas AQP4 is constitutively expressed and mediates the basolateral movement of water [46]. In cholangiocytes isolated from the PCK rat, an animal model of autosomal recessive polycystic kidney disease (ARPKD), AQP1 is overexpressed at the basolateral membrane and may contribute to the expansion of cysts via influx of fluid [47].

Bicarbonate Secretion Another important function of cholangiocytes is biliary transport of HCO_3^-, which maintains bile alkalinity, preventing protonation of bile salts that would otherwise induce bile duct injury. In human and rat cholangiocytes, HCO_3^- secretion occurs mainly through the Na^+-independent Cl^-/HCO_3^- exchanger, AE2, and related apical Cl^- channels [48]. Biliary secretion of HCO_3^- initially requires modulation of intracellular levels of HCO_3^- in cholangiocytes. There are two mechanisms by which the intracellular level of HCO_3^- is regulated: (i) via direct loading from the basolateral membrane mediated by the Na^+/HCO_3^- cotransporter or (ii) via carbonic anhydrase-mediated generation of

HCO_3^- and H^+ from hydration of CO_2 with water [34]. The basolateral influx of HCO_3^- is mediated by the Na^+/HCO_3^- cotransporter in rats [1] and the Na^+-dependent Cl^-/HCO_3^- anion exchanger in humans [49]. Biliary secretion of HCO_3^- also involves the generation in the lumen of a negative potential, requiring activation of Cl^- channels and subsequent release of Cl^- ions [34]. It is well known that bile ducts express Ca^{2+}-dependent Cl^- channels [50]. HCO_3^- biliary secretion is influenced by at least three hormones, namely, acetylcholine, somatostatin, and gastrin [51]. Acetylcholine and muscarinic M3 subtype receptor interaction induce an increase in intracellular Ca^{2+} and activation of the Cl^-/HCO_3^- ion exchanger AE2. Somatostatin inhibits secretin-stimulated intracellular cAMP synthesis through a somatostatin receptor interaction [52, 53]. In addition, gastrin synthesis, generated by gastric antral G cells, decreases secretin-stimulated cAMP levels through both the downregulation of cyclic adenylate cyclase and decreased expression of secretin receptors [54].

Intracellular Signaling Cholangiocytes express a number of receptors through which autocrine and paracrine signaling pathways are modulated. Secretin receptors (SR)s are typical G protein-coupled receptors expressed on the basolateral domain of intrahepatic rodent and human large cholangiocytes [55]. In large intrahepatic cholangiocytes, cAMP levels increase upon secretin stimulation [56]. This activation induces phosphorylation of protein kinase A (PKA), which in turn promotes the opening of the apically located Cl^- channel (CFTR), resulting in Cl^- secretion into bile. This process further activates Cl^-/HCO_3^- exchange via AE2 resulting in HCO_3^- secretion into bile [21, 57]. BDL of rats induces hypercholeresis via secretin-mediated activation of SRs [58] in a mechanism that involves an increased number of secretin receptors per cell [59]. Importantly, studies by Glaser et al. [56] demonstrated that in SR knockout mice, the proliferation of large cholangiocytes is reduced during BDL compared to wild-type BDL mice. In addition, decreased levels of both basal- and secretin-stimulated cAMP as well as reduced phosphorylation of the extracellular signal-regulated protein kinases 1 and 2 (ERK1/2) were observed in large cholangiocytes from SR knockout BDL mice compared to large cholangiocytes from wild-type BDL mice. In vitro experiments showed that secretin increased the proliferation of cholangiocytes via cAMP/PKA/ERK1/2 signaling [56].

Cholangiocytes also express the G protein-coupled bile acid receptor, TGR5 (GPBAR-1, M-Bar, or GPR131). TGR5 is a transmembrane receptor linked to cAMP signaling expressed in a variety of human and rodent tissues that is encoded by a gene located on chromosome 1C3 in mouse and 2q35 in humans [60]. In cholangiocytes, TGR5 is found in multiple intracellular locations, including primary cilia on the apical domain, on the non-ciliary portion of the apical membrane, and on the inner and outer membrane of the cholangiocyte nucleus [61]. TGR5 is a major receptor for bile acid signaling in cholangiocytes, and its activation affects intracellular cAMP via coupling to $G\alpha_s$ or $G\alpha_i$ proteins subsequently triggering downstream signaling events [62]. A role for TGR5 in the development of gallstones was proposed by Keitel et al. In vitro experiments from the same study also showed that TGR5 stimulates the CFTR-dependent release of biliary Cl^- [63]. As mentioned above, primary cilia are key organelles involved in intracellular signaling and, as such, influence the response to TGR5 cholangiocyte activation. For example, in cholangiocytes, experimentally devoid of primary cilia, stimulation by TGR5 agonists enhanced cAMP activation via $G\alpha_i$, partially inhibiting ERK signaling, which results in reduced cholangiocyte proliferation [61]. Interestingly, the reverse outcomes were noted when ciliated cholangiocytes were challenged with the same TGR5 agonists [61]. Masyuk et al. demonstrated that primary cilia act as mechanosensors, responding to luminal fluid flow by alterations in intracellular Ca^{2+} and cAMP. The ciliary proteins involved in this transduction of mechanical stimuli include polycystin-1, a cell surface receptor, and polycystin-2, a Ca^{2+} channel [14]. Primary cilia also express the transient receptor potential 4 (TRPV4) protein, a Ca^{2+} permeable, nonselective cation channel, through which they can detect changes in osmolarity [15]. Gradilone et al. demonstrated that hypotonicity induces a rise in intracellular Ca^{2+} via TRPV4 activation in rat cholangiocytes. Furthermore, in vivo stimulation of cholangiocyte TRPV4 by intrabiliary saline increased adenosine triphosphate (ATP) production, HCO_3^- release, and thereby bile movement [15]. The role of cholangiocyte primary cilia as chemosensors has also been demonstrated. Primary cilia on rat cholangiocytes express the purinergic receptors, $P2Y_{12}$ and $P2Y_{13}$, that respond to changes in cAPM induced by adenosine diphosphate (ADP) and ATP-γS (nonhydrolyzed analog of ATP), two known agonists of $P2Y_{12}$ receptors. Moreover, suramin, an inhibitor of P2Y receptors, can prevent the ADP-dependent decrease of cAMP [16].

Cholangiocyte signaling also can occur in response to receptor-mediated recognition of microbial-derived molecules. Receptors involved include Toll-like receptors (TLRs), nucleotide oligomerization domain proteins [3], and purinoceptors [64]. TLRs, a family of conserved receptor proteins critical for pathogen recognition, are present on the apical membranes of cholangiocytes where they are well positioned to detect pathogenic molecules in bile notably pathogen-associated molecular patterns (PAMPs), as well as adaptor proteins such as myeloid differentiation protein 88 (MyD88) and intracellular kinases [65]. Human cholangiocytes express TLRs 1–10, MD-2, MyD88, and downstream effectors of the TLR pathway [66]. The responses triggered by activation of TLRs in cholangiocytes are described later in this chapter.

Communication Between Cells Cholangiocytes can communicate with each other and with other cells via the release of soluble molecules as well as by secreted extracellular vesicles (ECVs). ECVs are nano-vesicles secreted by various types of benign and malignant cells. Exosomes, a subset of ECVs 30–150 nm in diameter, are membrane-enclosed vesicles present in biological fluids in vivo that shuttle molecules from donor cells to proximal or distant target cells [18]. Exosomes are generated through the invagination of early endosomes, subsequently producing intraluminal vesicles (ILVs) that contain multiple molecules (e.g., proteins, RNA, etc.) that typically result in the formation of multivesicular bodies (MVBs). The dynamic MVB pathways can lead to either: (i) plasma membrane fusion followed by release of ILVs into the extracellular milieu (now termed exosomes) or (ii) lysosomal fusion resulting in degradation [18]. Liver epithelia, including hepatocytes and cholangiocytes, can release exosomes in culture and in vivo, consistent with an important role for exosomes in intercellular communication and signaling. The mechanisms by which exosomes may initiate signaling pathways in target cells remain poorly defined but include: (a) binding to specific membrane receptors to induce intracellular signaling processes; (b) fusion of the exosome with the target cell membrane followed by release of its encapsulated content; and (c) endocytosis of the entire exosome following convex-like membrane bending of the target cell plasma membrane [67].

Cholangiocytes secrete exosomes into the bile duct lumen [18]. Studies using cultured cholangiocytes show that exosomes isolated from bile induce ERK1/2 activation that is dependent on the presence of primary cilia and that can influence ERK1/2-mediated cholangiocyte proliferation and miRNA expression [18]. In addition, it has also been reported that cholangiocytes infected by the protozoan parasite, *Cryptosporidium parvum* (*C. parvum*), secrete increased numbers of apically derived exosomes that contain antimicrobial peptides, suggesting a role for cholangiocyte-derived exosomes in response to biliary infection [68].

Basolaterally released exosomes derived from intestinal epithelia as well as from cholangiocytes have also been described; however, their physiological relevance remains unclear [18, 69].

Cholangiocyte Plasticity

Cholangiocytes have the ability to adapt and respond to changes in their microenvironment. For instance, upon injury cholangiocytes become reactive, actively producing and secreting molecules that stimulate immune and wound-healing responses. Furthermore, as a mechanism to prevent malignancy, cholangiocytes undergo a state of senescence in which their proliferative capacity is shut down. Under certain circumstances, however, this mechanism can be bypassed, and cholangiocytes adopt a malignant phenotype characterized by hyperproliferation with a marked production of pro-inflammatory cytokines.

Cholangiocyte Reactivity Exposure of cholangiocytes to chemicals, microbes, and microbial products can induce cholangiocyte activation [3]. Activated cholangiocytes are characterized by: (i) increased resistance to apoptosis, allowing benign proliferative expansion of cholangiocytes; (ii) increased production and release of cytokines and chemokines that attract immune cells, amplifying the pro-inflammatory response already initiated; (iii) decreased expression of epithelial markers and acquisition of mesenchymal features; and (iv) overproduction and secretion of profibrotic molecules (Table 7.1) (Fig. 7.1) [5]. Reactive cholangiocytes, for example, secrete PDFG-BB, which induces the production of hedgehog (Hh) ligands by myofibroblasts and cholangiocytes. Importantly, activation of the Hh pathway appears necessary for activated cholangiocytes to maintain the reactive phenotype [5].

In an in vitro model of *C. parvum* infection of cholangiocytes, Chen et al. demonstrated that cholangiocytes respond and defend against this parasite by inducing activation of the nuclear factor kappa B (NF-kB) pathway via TLR-2, TLR-4, and subsequent production of IL-8 and human beta defensin 2 (HBD-2). Both TLRs and HBD-2 are key players of the innate immune system against pathogens [66]. Cholangiocytes can also be exposed to enteric bacterial-derived products via the enterohepatic circulation [70]. For instance, cholangiocytes in patients with primary sclerosing cholangitis (PSC) may be exposed to lipopolysaccharide (LPS), the bioactive part of gram-negative bacteria [71]. Recognition of LPS by cholangiocytes via TLR-4/MyD88 stimulates the NF-kB and N-Ras/ERK pathways. TLR-induced N-Ras activation requires transactivation of the epidermal growth factor receptor (EGFR) and the ADAM metallopeptidase domain 17 (TACE). Stimulation of the N-Ras/ERK pathway and NF-kB activation promote IL-6 expression, a known pro-inflammatory cytokine and mitogen, activating cholangiocyte proliferation [70, 72]. Several other molecules such as hormones, BAs, neuropeptides, and an increase in bile duct pressure are known to induce cholangiocyte proliferation [73].

Bile duct proliferation is another mechanism of response/defense of cholangiocytes upon injury. Acute injury of the biliary tree induces proliferation of large cholangiocytes to maintain internal stability within the bile ducts [3], whereas chronic injury triggers replication of both small and large cholangiocytes [3]. Acute and chronic biliary damage promotes regeneration and repair which modulates bile duct morphogenesis. Fabris et al. demonstrated that in human livers with bile duct injury, reactive bile ducts display features similar to what occurs during the early phase of bile duct morphogenesis [74].

Senescent Cholangiocytes Cellular senescence is an irreversible state in which cells, arrested in the G1 phase of the cell cycle, can no longer replicate. Cellular senescence is a characteristic of aging and is present in a variety of disorders, e.g., atherosclerosis, osteoarthritis, and chronic obstructive pulmonary disease [75]. It occurs as a result of genotoxic stimulation and constitutes a mechanism to prevent cancer growth as it halts proliferation of injured cells [6]. There are two major, but not mutually exclusive, tumor suppressor pathways that tightly control cellular senescence: the p53 and the $p16^{INK4a}$/pRB pathways. As mentioned earlier in this chapter, senescent cells may transition to a highly pro-inflammatory phenotype known as the senescence-associated secretory phenotype (SASP) [6]. This term was first proposed by Coppé et al. while studying an array of factors that human pre-senescent and senescent fibroblasts secrete [6]. Fibroblasts undergoing SASP secrete abundant levels of pro-inflammatory cytokines and immuno-attractant chemokines (IL-6, IL-7, IL-8, monocyte chemoattractant protein-2 [MCP-2], and macrophage inflammatory protein-3 alpha), growth regulatory molecules (growth-regulated oncogene, hepatocyte growth factor, and insulin-like growth factor-binding proteins [IGFBPs]), membrane/transmembrane receptors (intracellular adhesion molecules, urokinase receptor, and tumor necrosis factor [TNF] receptors), and survival mediators (osteoprotegerin and fibroblast growth factor) compared to pre-senescent fibroblasts [6].

Senescent cholangiocytes have been reported in different types of liver injury and have been implicated in the pathogenesis of various diseases. Indeed, a positive correlation between cholangiocyte senescence and the degree of rejection in acute liver allograft rejection has been reported [76]. Cholangiocyte senescence has been also associated with the progression of chronic liver diseases such as primary biliary cirrhosis, chronic viral hepatitis, and nonalcoholic steatohepatitis [77]. Further studies from the same group showed an association between fibrosis and inflammation in nonalcoholic fatty liver disease. Furthermore, the number of senescent cholangiocytes increased as the fibrosis progressed. Interestingly, the expression of MCP-1, a SASP secretory factor and chemoattractant of hepatic stellate cells (HSCs) and inflammatory cells, was also upregulated in bile ducts in the late stages of the disease. Coculture experiments also showed increase migration of HSCs toward senescent cholangiocytes. The authors concluded that senescent cholangiocytes most likely produce MCP-1 for the recruitment of HSCs to the sites of injury [78].

Recent studies have demonstrated that cellular senescence may play a key role in the pathogenesis of PSC [75]. Immunofluorescence of human PSC liver sections showed that cholangiocytes are not proliferative and express the senescent markers $p16^{INK4A}$ and γH2A.x, suggesting that cholangiocytes in PSC exhibit increased senescence [75]. Moreover, PSC cholangiocytes produce abundant levels of SASP factors, particularly IL-6, IL-8, plasminogen activator inhibitor-1, and MCP-1 compared to normal and disease control cholangiocytes (Table 7.1) (Fig. 7.1) [75]. As mentioned, SASP components engage in intercellular communication to induce pro-inflammatory and senescent phenotypes in target cells. Importantly, we recapitulated these findings in an in vitro model of stress-induced cholangiocyte senescence. In this same model, we found that cholangiocyte senescence is driven by the N-Ras pathway. Moreover, cholangiocytes isolated from livers of patients with PSC cholangiocytes secrete 23 and 46 times more IL-6 and IL-8, respectively, compared to normal cholangiocytes [79]. At the morphological level, PSC cholangiocytes display an enlarged shape with marked cytoskeletal filamentous proteins [79]. These cells also showed decreased tight junction integrity, evaluated by the low expression level of the tight junction marker ZO-1 [79].

Transformed Cholangiocytes Neoplastic transformation of cholangiocytes results in the development of cholangiocarcinoma (CCA) [80]. While the molecular mechanisms responsible for the malignant transformation of cholangiocytes and its progression to CCA are still unclear, CCA frequently occurs within bile ducts plagued by chronic inflammation [7].

Aberrant expression of the tyrosine kinase receptor ErbB-2/Neu and prostaglandin endoperoxide synthase cyclooxygenase-2 (COX-2) in biliary epithelia has been implicated in the development and progression of CCA (Table 7.1) (Fig. 7.1). Immunohistochemistry of human bile ducts has demonstrated that both COX-2 and ErbB-2 are several times fold upregulated in PSC and CCA patients compared to normal subjects. There was also a positive correlation between tumor differentiation and the overexpression of COX-2 and ErbB-2 with peak expression of both proteins observed in well-differentiated tumors [81].

In pathological conditions, chronic inflammation promotes oxidative stress via production of abnormal levels of reactive oxygen and nitrogen species. Reactive nitrogen species are generated from nitric oxide (NO). NO is a signaling molecule that at physiological concentrations inhibits inflammation and prevents platelet aggregation and integrin-dependent adhesion. NO is overproduced in a variety of pathological conditions and at high levels can promote carcinogenesis via inhibition of apoptosis, induction of DNA damage, and angiogenesis [82]. Jaiswal et al. demonstrated via immunohistochemistry cholangiocyte DNA damage and de novo production of the inducible nitric oxide synthase (iNOs) in cholangiocytes of patients with PSC [83]. Further studies revealed that iNOs induces malignant transformation of cholangiocytes and CCA progression [84]. The mechanism involves iNOs-dependent production of NO by PSC cholangiocytes. [84]. NO activates the Notch-1 signaling pathway leading to resistance of TRAIL-mediated apoptosis [84].

IL-6 is one of the pro-inflammatory cytokines that is abundantly expressed during chronic bile duct inflammation [7]. It is normally produced by various liver cell types and is particularly secreted at high levels by senescent cholangiocytes in patients with PSC [7, 79]. Several lines of evidence have shown that IL-6 potently stimulates normal cholangiocyte proliferation via autocrine and paracrine mechanisms [72, 73, 85, 86]. The role of IL-6 signaling in liver tumorigenesis and liver cancer progression has also been documented both in vivo and in vitro [87, 88]. Abrogation of the IL-6 signaling pathway by an antihuman IL-6 neutralizing antibody inhibits proliferation of the CCA line KMCH-1 [85]. Furthermore, stimulation of KMCH-1 cells with the pro-inflammatory cytokines IL1-β and TNF-α leads to an upregulation in IL-6 secretion [85]. In vitro and in vivo evidence suggests that IL-6 dysregulation is implicated in cholangiocyte malignant transformation and aggravation of CCA. Meng et al. showed that IL-6 promotes survival of human cell lines from intrahepatic, extrahepatic, and gallbladder tumors via increased expression of the myeloid cell leukemia protein-1, which in turn inhibited apoptosis and decreased sensitivity to chemotherapy [7].

Summary

In this chapter we have selectively summarized the latest literature regarding the biology of normal cholangiocytes. In addition, we present a model of cholangiocyte plasticity that includes the normal functions of cholangiocytes as well as their responses upon injury, focusing on the induction of senescence, the subsequent development of SASP, and ultimately cholangiocyte malignant transformation. The signaling pathways in which injured cholangiocytes communicate are also reviewed. The mechanisms that regulate the responses of cholangiocytes in each stage are not fully understood, and whether cholangiocytes can revert from one stage to another still remains to be elucidated. Understanding what regulates the plasticity of cholangiocytes during disease may lead to finding novel therapeutic targets that could trigger the resolution of the activated, senescent, and SASP phases.

References

1. Strazzabosco M, Fabris L. Functional anatomy of normal bile ducts. Anat Rec (Hoboken). 2008;291:653–60.
2. Syal G, Fausther M, Dranoff JA. Advances in cholangiocyte immunobiology. Am J Physiol Gastrointest Liver Physiol. 2012;303:G1077–86.
3. O'Hara SP, Tabibian JH, Splinter PL, LaRusso NF. The dynamic biliary epithelia: molecules, pathways, and disease. J Hepatol. 2013;58:1–16.
4. Milani S, Hermann H, Schuppan D, Stein H, Surrenti C. Transforming growth factors 1 and Are differentially expressed in fibrotic liver disease. Am J Pathol. 1991;139:1221–9.
5. Omenetti A, Diehl AM. Hedgehog signaling in cholangiocytes. Curr Opin Gastroenterol. 2011;27: 268–75.
6. Coppé JP, Patil CK, Rodier F, Sun Y, Muñoz DP, Goldstein J, et al. Senescence-associated secretory phenotypes reveal cell-nonautonomous functions of oncogenic RAS and the p53 tumor suppressor. PLoS Biol. 2008;6:2853–68.
7. Meng F, Yamagiwa Y, Ueno Y, Patel T. Overexpression of Interleukin-6 enhances cell survival and transformed cell growth in human malignant cholangiocytes. J Hepatol. 2006;44:1055–65.
8. Tabibian JH, Masyuk AL, Masyuk TV, O'Hara SP, LaRusso NF. Physiology of cholangiocytes. Compr Physiol. 2013;3:1–49.
9. Alpini G, Roberts S, Kuntz SM, Ueno Y, Gubba S, Podila PV, et al. Morphological, molecular, and functional heterogeneity of cholangiocytes from normal Rat liver. Gastroenterology. 1996;110:1636–43.
10. Tietz P, Levine S, Holman R, Fretham C, LaRusso NF. Characterization of apical and basolateral plasma membrane domains derived from cultured Rat cholangiocytes. Anal Biochem. 1997;254:192–9.

11. Huang BQ, Masyuk TV, Muff MA, Tietz PS, Masyuk AI, Larusso NF. Isolation and characterization of cholangiocyte primary cilia. Am J Physiol Gastrointest Liver Physiol. 2006;291:G500–9.
12. Gradilone SA, Lorenzo Pisarellob MJ, LaRussob NF. Primary Cilia in Tumor Biology: The primary cilium as a therapeutic target in cholangiocarcinoma. Curr Drug Targets. 2015. [Epub ahead of print.]
13. Satir P, Pedersen LB, Christensen ST. The primary cilium at a glance. J Cell Sci. 2010;123:499–503.
14. Masyuk AI, Masyuk TV, LaRusso NF. Physiology of cholangiocytes. In: Johnson LR, editor. Physiology of the gastrointestinal tract. 4th ed. Academic Press; Canada, 2006. p. 1505–33.
15. Gradilone SA, Masyuk AI, Splinter PL, Banales JM, Huang BQ, Tietz PS, et al. Cholangiocyte cilia express TRPV4 and detect changes in luminal tonicity inducing bicarbonate secretion. Proc Natl Acad Sci U S A. 2007;104:19138–43.
16. Masyuk AI, Gradilone SA, Banales JM, Huang BQ, Masyuk TV, Lee SO, et al. Cholangiocyte primary cilia are chemosensory organelles that detect biliary nucleotides via P2Y12 purinergic receptors. Am J Physiol Gastrointest Liver Physiol. 2008;295: G725–34.
17. Masyuk AI, Masyuk TV, LaRusso NF. Cholangiocyte primary cilia in liver health and disease. Dev Dyn. 2008;237:2007–12.
18. Masyuk AI, Huang BQ, Ward CJ, Gradilone SA, Banales JM, Masyuk TV, et al. Biliary exosomes influence cholangiocyte regulatory mechanisms and proliferation through interaction with primary cilia. Am J Physiol Gastrointest Liver Physiol. 2010;299: G990–9.
19. Marzioni M, Glaser SS, Francis H, Phinizy JL, LeSage G, Alpini G. Functional heterogeneity of cholangiocytes. Semin Liver Dis. 2002;22:227–40.
20. LeSage GD, Glaser SS, Marucci L, Benedetti A, Phinizy JL, Rodgers R, et al. Acute carbon tetrachloride feeding induces damage of large but not small cholangiocytes from BDL rat liver. Am J Physiol. 1999;276:G1289–301.
21. Afroze S, Meng F, Jensen K, McDaniel K, Rahal K, Onori P, et al. The physiological roles of secretin and its receptor. Ann Transl Med. 2013;1(3):1–14.
22. LeSage GD, Benedetti A, Glaser S, Marucci L, Tretjak Z, Caligiuri A, et al. Acute carbon tetrachloride feeding selectively damages large, but not small, cholangiocytes from normal rat liver. Hepatology [Research Support, Non-US Gov't Research Support, US Gov't, Non-PHS]. 1999;29(2):307–19.
23. Sell S. Comparison of liver progenitor cells in human atypical ductular reactions with those seen in experimental models of liver injury. Hepatology. 1998;27: 317–31.
24. Thiese ND, Saxena R, Portmann BC, Thung SN, Yee H, Chiriboga L, et al. The canals of hering and hepatic stem cells in humans. Hepatology. 1999;30:1425–33.
25. Sell S. Heterogeneity and plasticity of hepatocyte lineage cells. Hepatology. 2001;33:738–50.
26. Boyer JL. Bile formation and secretion. Compr Physiol. 2013;3:1035–78.
27. Farina A, Dumonceau JM, Lescuyer P. Proteomic analysis of human bile and potential applications for cancer diagnosis. Expert Rev Proteomics. 2009;6: 285–301.
28. Masyuk AI, Masyuk TV, LaRusso NF. Physiology of cholangiocytes. In: Johnson LR, editor. Physiology of the gastrointestinal tract. 5th ed. Elsevier; 2012. p. 1531–57.
29. Trauner M, Boyer JL. Bile salt transporters: molecular characterization, function, and regulation. Physiol Rev. Bethesda, MD, 2003;83:633–71.
30. Feranchak AP, Doctor RB, Troetsch M, Brookman K, Johnson SM, Fitz JG. Calcium-dependent regulation of secretion in biliary epithelial cells: the role of apamin-sensitive SK channels. Gastroenterology. 2004;127:903–13.
31. Fitz JG, Basavappa S, McGill J, Melhus O, Cohn JA. Regulation of membrane chloride currents in rat bile duct epithelial cells. J Clin Invest. 1993;91:319–28.
32. McGill JM, Basavappa S, Gettys TW, Fitz JG. Secretin activates Cl- channels in bile duct epithelial cells through a cAMP-dependent mechanism. Am J Physiol. 1994; 266:G731–6.
33. Singh SK, Mennone A, Gigliozzi A, Fraioli F, Boyer JL. Cl(−)-dependent secretory mechanisms in isolated rat bile duct epithelial units. Am J Physiol Gastrointest Liver Physiol. 2001;281:G438–46.
34. Banales JM, Prieto J, Medina JF. Cholangiocyte anion exchange and biliary bicarbonate excretion. World J Gastroenterol. 2006;12:3496–511.
35. Alpini G, Glaser SS, Rodgers R, Phinizy JL, Robertson WE, Lasater J, et al. Functional expression of the apical Na+–dependent bile acid transporter in large but not small rat cholangiocytes. Gastroenterology. 1997;113(5):1734–40.
36. Lazaridis KN, Tietz P, Wu T, Kip S, Dawson PA, LaRusso NF. Alternative splicing of the rat sodium/bile acid transporter changes its cellular localization and transport properties. Proc Natl Acad Sci U S A. 2000;97:11092–7.
37. Alpini G, Glaser S, Alvaro D, Ueno Y, Marzioni M, Francis H, et al. Bile acid depletion and repletion regulate cholangiocyte growth and secretion by a phosphatidylinositol 3-kinase-dependent pathway in rats. Gastroenterology. 2002;123:1226–37.
38. Ballatori N, Truong AT. Glutathione as a primary osmotic driving force in hepatic bile formation. Am J Physiol. 1992;263:G617–24.
39. Cova E, Gong A, Marinelli RA, LaRusso NF. Water movement across rat bile duct units is transcellular and channel-mediated. Hepatology. 2001;34:456–63.
40. Day R, Kitchen P, Owen DS, Bland C, Marshall L, Conner AC. Human aquaporins: regulators of transcellular water flow. Biochim Biophys Acta. 1840;2014:1492–506.
41. Ishibashi K. Aquaporin superfamily with unusual npa boxes: S-aquaporins (superfamily, sip-like and subcellular-aquaporins). Cell Mol Biol (Noisy-le-Grand). 2006;52(7):20–7.

42. Agre P, King LS, Yasui M, Guggino WB, Ottersen OP, Fujiyoshi Y. Aquaporin water channels--from atomic structure to clinical medicine. J Physiol. 2002;542: 3–16.
43. Yeung CH, Callies C, Rojek A, Nielsen S, Cooper TG. Aquaporin isoforms involved in physiological volume regulation of murine spermatozoa. Biol Reprod. 2009;80:350–7.
44. Masyuk AI, LaRusso NF. Aquaporins in the hepatobiliary system. Hepatology. 2006;43:S75–81.
45. Gossen D, Poloczek P, Svoboda M, Christophe J. Molecular architecture of secretin receptors: the specific covalent labelling of a 51 kDa peptide after cross-linking of [125I]iodosecretin to intact rat pancreatic acini. FEBS Lett. 1989;243:205–8.
46. Marinelli RA, Pham LD, Tietz PS, LaRusso NF. Expression of aquaporin-4 water channels in rat cholangiocytes. Hepatology. 2000;31:1313–7.
47. Banales JM, Masyuk TV, Bogert PS, Huang BQ, Gradilone SA, Lee SO, et al. Hepatic cystogenesis is associated with abnormal expression and location of ion transporters and water channels in an animal model of autosomal recessive polycystic kidney disease. Am J Pathol. 2008;173:1637–46.
48. Beuers U, Maroni L, Elferink RO. The biliary HCO(3)(−) umbrella: experimental evidence revisited. Curr Opin Gastroenterol. 2012;28:253–7.
49. Strazzabosco M, Joplin R, Zsembery A, Wallace L, Spirli C, Fabris L. Na(+)-dependent and -independent Cl-/HCO-3 exchange mediate cellular HCO3- transport in cultured human intrahepatic bile duct cells. Hepatology. 1997;25:976–85.
50. Jung J, Lee MG. Role of calcium signaling in epithelial bicarbonate secretion. Cell Calcium. 2014;55: 376–84.
51. Hirata K, Nathanson MH. Bile duct epithelia regulate biliary bicarbonate excretion in normal rat liver. Gastroenterology. 2001;121:396–406.
52. Tietz PS, Alpini G, Pham LD, Larusso NF. Somatostatin inhibits secretin-induced ductal hypercholeresis and exocytosis by cholangiocytes. Am J Physiol. 1995;269:G110–8.
53. Hogan MC, Masyuk TV, Page L, Holmes 3rd DR, Li X, Bergstralh EJ, et al. Somatostatin analog therapy for severe polycystic liver disease: results after 2 years. Nephrol Dial Transplant. 2012;27:3532–9.
54. Glaser SS, Rodgers RE, Phinizy JL, Robertson WE, Lasater J, Caligiuri A, et al. Gastrin inhibits secretin-induced ductal secretion by interaction with specific receptors on rat cholangiocytes. Am J Physiol. 1997;273:G1061–70.
55. Glaser SS, Gaudio E, Rao A, Pierce LM, Onori P, Franchitto A, et al. Morphological and functional heterogeneity of the mouse intrahepatic biliary epithelium. Lab Invest. 2009;89:456–69.
56. Glaser S, Lam IP, Franchitto A, Gaudio E, Onori P, Chow BK, et al. Knockout of secretin receptor reduces large cholangiocyte hyperplasia in mice with extrahepatic cholestasis induced by bile duct ligation. Hepatology. 2010;52:204–14.
57. Feranchak AP, Sokol RJ. Cholangiocyte biology and cystic fibrosis liver disease. Semin Liver Dis. 2001;21:471–88.
58. Alpini G, Ulrich CD, Phillips JO, Pham LD, Miller LJ, LaRusso NF. Upregulation of secretin receptor gene expression in rat cholangiocytes after bile duct ligation. Am J Physiol. 1994;266:G922–8.
59. Tietz PS, Hadac EM, Miller LJ, LaRusso NF. Upregulation of secretin receptors on cholangiocytes after bile duct ligation. Regul Pept. 2001;97:1–6.
60. Thomas C, Pellicciari R, Pruzanski M, Auwerx J, Schoonjans K. Targeting bile-acid signalling for metabolic diseases. Nat Rev Drug Discov. 2008;7:678–93.
61. Masyuk AI, Huang BQ, Radtke BN, Gajdos GB, Splinter PL, Masyuk TV, et al. Ciliary subcellular localization of TGR5 determines the cholangiocyte functional response to bile acid signaling. Am J Physiol Gastrointest Liver Physiol. 2013;304:G1013–24.
62. Reich M, Deutschmann K, Sommerfeld A, Klindt C, Kluge S, Kubitz R, et al. TGR5 is essential for bile acid-dependent cholangiocyte proliferation in vivo and in vitro. Gut. 2015.
63. Keitel V, Cupisti K, Ullmer C, Knoefel WT, Kubitz R, Häussinger D. The membrane-bound bile acid receptor TGR5 is localized in the epithelium of human gallbladders. Hepatology. 2009;50:861–70.
64. Burnstock G, Vaughn B, Robson SC. Purinergic signalling in the liver in health and disease. Purinergic Signal. 2014;10:51–70.
65. Rachmilewitz D, Katakura K, Karmeli F, Hayashi T, Reinus C, Rudensky B, et al. Toll-like receptor 9 signaling mediates the anti-inflammatory effects of probiotics in murine experimental colitis. Gastroenterology. 2004;126:520–8.
66. Chen XM, O'Hara SP, Nelson JB, Splinter PL, Small AJ, Tietz PS. Multiple TLRs are expressed in human cholangiocytes and mediate host epithelial defense responses to Cryptosporidium parvum via activation of NF-kappaB. J Immunol. 2005;175:7447–56.
67. Mathivanan S, Ji H, Simpson RJ. Exosomes: extracellular organelles important in intercellular communication. J Proteomics. 2010;73:1907–20.
68. Hu G, Gong AY, Roth AL, Huang BQ, Ward HD, Zhu G, et al. Release of luminal exosomes contributes to TLR4-mediated epithelial antimicrobial defense. PLoS Pathog. 2013;9(4), e1003261.
69. Bu HF, Wang X, Tang Y, Koti V, Tan XD. Toll-like receptor 2-mediated peptidoglycan uptake by immature intestinal epithelial cells from apical side and exosome-associated transcellular transcytosis. J Cell Physiol. 2010;222:658–68.
70. Trussoni CE, Tabibian JH, Splinter PL, O'Hara SP. Lipopolysaccharide (LPS)-induced biliary epithelial cell NRas activation requires Epidermal Growth Factor Receptor (EGFR). PLoS One. 2015;10:1–15.
71. Sasatomi K, Noguchi K, Sakisaka S, Sata M, Tanikawa K. Abnormal accumulation of endotoxin in biliary epithelial cells in primary biliary cirrhosis and primary sclerosing cholangitis. J Hepatol. 1998;29: 409–16.

72. O'Hara SP, Splinter PL, Trussoni CE, Gajdos GB, Lineswala PN, LaRusso NF. Cholangiocyte N-Ras protein mediates lipopolysaccharide-induced interleukin 6 secretion and proliferation. J Biol Chem. 2011;286:30352–60.
73. Park J, Gores GJ, Patel T. Lipopolysaccharide induces cholangiocyte proliferation via an interleukin-6-mediated activation of p44/p42 mitogen-activated protein kinase. Hepatology. 1999;29:1037–43.
74. Fabris L, Strazzabosco M, Crosby HA, Ballardini G, Hubscher SG, Kelly DA, et al. Characterization and isolation of ductular cells coexpressing neural cell adhesion molecule and Bcl-2 from primary cholangiopathies and ductal plate malformations. Am J Pathol. 2000;156:1599–611.
75. Tabibian JH, O'Hara SP, Splinter PL, Trussoni CE, LaRusso NF. Cholangiocyte senescence by Way of N-Ras activation is a characteristic of primary sclerosing cholangitis. Hepatology. 2014;6:2263–75.
76. Brain JG, Robertson H, Thompson E, Humphreys EH, Gardner A, Booth TA, et al. Biliary epithelial senescence and plasticity in acute cellular rejection. Am J Transplant. 2013;13:1688–702.
77. Sasaki M, Ikeda H, Yamaguchi J, Miyakoshi M, Sato Y, Nakamuna Y. Bile ductular cells undergoing cellular senescence increase in chronic liver diseases along with fibrous progression. Am J Clin Pathol. 2010;133: 212–23.
78. Chiba M, Sasaki M, Kitamura S, Ikeda H, Sato Y, Nakanuma Y. Participation of bile ductular cells in the pathological progression of non-alcoholic fatty liver disease. J Clin Pathol. 2011;64:564–70.
79. Tabibian JH, Trussoni CE, O'Hara SP, Splinter PL, Heimbach JK, LaRusso NF. Characterization of cultured cholangiocytes isolated from livers of patients with primary sclerosing cholangitis. Lab Invest. 2014;94:1126–33.
80. Lazaridis KN, LaRusso NF. The cholangiopathies. Mayo Clin Proc. 2015;90:791–800.
81. Endo K, Yoon BI, Pairojkul C, Demetris AJ, Sirica AE. ERBB-2 overexpression and cyclooxygenase-2 Up-regulation in human cholangiocarcinoma and risk conditions. Hepatology. 2002;36:439–50.
82. Aktan F. iNOS-mediated nitric oxide production and its regulation. Life Sci. 2004;75:639–53.
83. Jaiswal M, LaRusso NF, Shapiro RA, Billiar TR, Gores GJ. Nitric oxide-mediated inhibition of DNA repair potentiates oxidative DNA damage in cholangiocytes. Gastroenterology. 2001;120:190–9.
84. Ishimura N, Bronk SF, Gores GJ. Inducible nitric oxide synthase Up-regulates notch-1 in mouse cholangiocytes: implications for carcinogenesis. Gastroenterology. 2005;128:1354–68.
85. Park J, Gores GJ, Patel T. Inhibition of interleukin 6-mediated mitogen-activated protein kinase activation attenuates growth of a cholangiocarcinoma cell line. Hepatology. 1999;30:1128–33.
86. Xiao Y, Wang J, Yan W, Zhou Y, Chen Y, Zhou K, et al. Dysregulated miR-124 and miR-200 expression contribute to cholangiocyte proliferation in the cholestatic liver by targeting IL- 6/STAT3 signalling. J Hepatol. 2015;62:889–96.
87. Maione D, Di Carlo E, Li W, Musiani P, Modesti A, Peters M, et al. Coexpression of IL-6 and soluble IL-6R causes nodular regenerative hyperplasia and adenomas of the liver. EMBO J. 1998;5588–97.
88. Wan S, Zhao E, Kryczek I, Vatan L, Sadovskaya A, Ludema G, et al. Tumor-associated macrophages produce interleukin 6 and signal via STAT3 to promote expansion of human hepatocellular carcinoma stem cells. Gastroenterology. 2014;6:1393–404.
89. Fabris L, Strazzabosco M. Epithelial–mesenchymal interactions in biliary diseases. Semin Liver Dis. 2011;31:11–32.
90. Li ZR, Wei JL, Li ZZ. Mucins 1-shRNA inhibit the proliferation and HIF-1alpha protein expression on human cholangiocarcinoma cells. Cell Biol Int. 2013;37:121–5.
91. Ohtani N, Yamakoshi K, Takahashi A, Hara E. The p16INK4a-RB pathway: molecular link between cellular senescence and tumor suppression. J Med Invest. 2004;51:146–53.

Genetics of Primary Sclerosing Cholangitis

8

Tom Hemming Karlsen and Gideon M. Hirschfield

Introduction

For a disease such as primary sclerosing cholangitis (PSC) that presently lacks effective treatment, in part because of an absent overarching disease understanding, there is anticipated value in utilising genetic screening technologies to identify rare and common biologic pathways relevant to this chronic inflammatory biliary disease and its associated complications. From a genetic perspective, the phenotypic presentation of PSC shows important overlap with other diseases. The degree of co-morbidity with inflammatory bowel disease (IBD) is considerable but shows an important geographic variation. In Northern Europe and the United States, up to 60–70 % of the patients with PSC also have a clinical diagnosis of IBD; notably this may not be equal between sexes. In Southern Europe and Asia, this fraction is lower (in the range of 30–50 %). A large number of patients (approximately 25 %) also have autoimmune co-morbidities outside of the gut-liver axis, e.g. in the form of autoimmune thyroid disease, type 1 disease and rheumatoid arthritis. Furthermore, the high lifetime risk of bile duct and gallbladder cancer (up to 15 %) poses additional challenges for clinical management and currently comprises the cause of death in up to half of the patients.

The considerable complexity and phenotypic heterogeneity has led to a speculation that PSC might comprise a 'mixed bag' of hitherto undefined conditions and hence existing challenges in delineating the aetiology and pathogenesis. Geographic variability of the clinical co-morbidities supports such concepts, yet for the major subgroup of patients who have PSC in the context of IBD, a common pathophysiological basis likely exists. Even in Japan [1], where IBD frequency for PSC patients overall is reported as around 30 %, young-onset adult patients (20–40 years of age), who tend to progress towards liver transplantation, exhibit similar IBD frequencies as in Europe (almost 60 %) and thus likely represent a similar subset as observed in Western

T.H. Karlsen (✉)
Norwegian PSC Research Center,
Division of Cancer Medicine,
Surgery and Transplantation,
Department of Transplantation Medicine,
Oslo University Hospital Rikshospitalet,
Pb 4950 Nydalen, Oslo N-0424, Norway

Section of Gastroenterology, Division of Cancer Medicine, Surgery and Transplantation, Department of Transplantation Medicine, Oslo University Hospital Rikshospitalet, Oslo, Norway

Institute of Clinical Medicine, Faculty of Medicine, University of Oslo, Oslo, Norway

Research Institute of Internal Medicine,
Division of Cancer Medicine, Surgery
and Transplantation, Oslo University Hospital,
Oslo, Norway
e-mail: t.h.karlsen@medisin.uio.no

G.M. Hirschfield
Centre for Liver Research, NIHR Birmingham Liver Biomedical Research Unit, University of Birmingham, Birmingham B15 2TT, UK

L.M. Forman (ed.), *Primary Sclerosing Cholangitis*, DOI 10.1007/978 3 319 40908-5_8 countries [2]. The fraction of IBD patients represented by this entity has been estimated in the range of 2.5–4.5 %. However, long-term cholangiographic follow-up of patients with IBD points towards a higher prevalence of sclerosing cholangitis at 7.5 % [3]. Notwithstanding individual patient variation, PSC appears epidemiologically associated with particular clinical features of IBD (pancolitis, right-sided colitis, rectal sparing, ileitis and increased risk of colorectal cancer) as compared to ulcerative colitis (UC) and Crohn's disease.

In this chapter, we aim to review the genetic efforts in PSC in the perspective set by that of genetic studies in liver disease in general. An emphasis will be put on the relationship between the genetics of PSC and those of other inflammatory conditions, in particular pertaining to the molecular demarcation of PSC-IBD from other forms of IBD. The genetic basis of these reflections is given in Tables 8.1 and 8.2.

GWAS and Liver Disease Genetics

The first successful GWAS was published in 2005 [4], and the following decade saw a flourishing and widespread application of the successful study design, leading to the identification of more than 1,000 risk loci in a variety of human complex traits, in more than 2,000 original publications. A GWAS is in simple terms a case-control association analysis, comparing the frequencies of genetic variants spread throughout the genome between two groups, patients and healthy controls: a GWAS is a scientific experiment, requiring a clear hypothesis and a well-defined phenotype and appropriate interpretation. The impact of any genetic association, wherein at multiple loci the allele frequency differs between cases and controls, must reflect the study design, as well as the population studied. Hence disease risk and disease severity, for example, are distinct questions answered in different ways. Risk loci (susceptibility loci) are determined as chromosomal regions (sometimes within single genes, susceptibility genes) where there is a statistically significant difference in the occurrence of particular variants observed in the patients (Fig. 8.1). Notably it may not be possible to always confidently assign a gene to an identified

Table 8.1 Genome-wide significant ($P \leq 5 \times 10^{-8}$) risk loci in primary sclerosing cholangitis

Chromosome	Plausible risk gene	Study
1	*MMEL1*, *TNFRSF14*	Folseraas et al. (2012) [56]
2	*BCL2L11*	Melum et al. (2011) [59]
2	*CD28*, *CTLA4*	Liu et al. (2013) [27]
2	*CCL20*	Ellinghaus et al. (2016) [45]
2	*GPR35*	Ellinghaus et al. (2013) [60]
3	*MST1*	Melum et al. (2011) [59]
4	*NFKB1*	Ellinghaus et al. (2016) [45]
4	*IL2*, *IL21*	Liu et al. (2013) [27]
6	*BACH2*	Liu et al. (2013) [27]
6	The HLA complex	Karlsen et al. (2010) [32]
10	*IL2RA*	Srivastava et al. (2012) [61]
11	*SIK2*	Liu et al. (2013) [27]
12	*HDAC7*	Liu et al. (2013) [27]
12	*RFX4*, *RIC8B*	Ellinghaus et al. (2016) [45]
12	*SH2B3*, *ATXN2*	Liu et al. (2013) [27]
16	*CLEC16A*, *SOCS1*	Ellinghaus et al. (2016) [45]
18	*TCF4*	Ellinghaus et al. (2013)
18	*CD226*	Liu et al. (2013) [27]
19	*PRKD2*, *STRN4*	Liu et al. (2013) [27]
21	*PSMG1*	Liu et al. (2013) [27]

The risk gene annotation at each locus is based on circumstantial evidence, and no conclusive reports exist linking a PSC-associated genetic variant to distinct disease mechanisms. Such studies are urgently needed and often hampered by limited genetic insight of the risk loci (i.e. often there are more than one gene at associated loci)

Table 8.2 Primary sclerosing cholangitis susceptibility loci identified by two independent analytical assessments but not reaching the formal genome-wide significance threshold ($P \leq 5 \times 10^{-8}$)

	Liu et al. (2013) [27]		Ellinghaus et al. (2016) [45]	
Chromosome	Lead SNP	Gene	Lead SNP	Gene
2	rs12479056	*PUS10, REL*	rs7608910	*PUS10*
2	rs11676348	*TGR5, ARPC2, CXCR1/2*	rs11676348	*CXCR2*
8	rs10956390 rs13255292 rs2977035	*PVT1, MIRs 1204-1208*	rs2042011	*RN7SKP226*
10	rs7923837	*HHEX*	rs2497318	*EIF2S2P3*
10	rs10883371	*NKX2-3*	rs10748781	*NKX2-3*
11	rs694739	*PRDX5*	rs559928	*NA*
16	rs7404095	*PRKCB*	rs7404095	*PRKCB*
18	rs2847297	*PTPN2*	rs12968719	*PTPN2*
19	rs601338	*FUT2*	rs679574	*FUT2*
21	rs11203203	*UBASH3A*	rs1893592	*UBASH3A*

SNP, single nucleotide polymorphism (a genetic marker used in genome-wide association studies). The risk gene annotation at each susceptibility loci is done by circumstantial evidence and not causal or conclusive factors; hence, they differ on some instances between the two studies

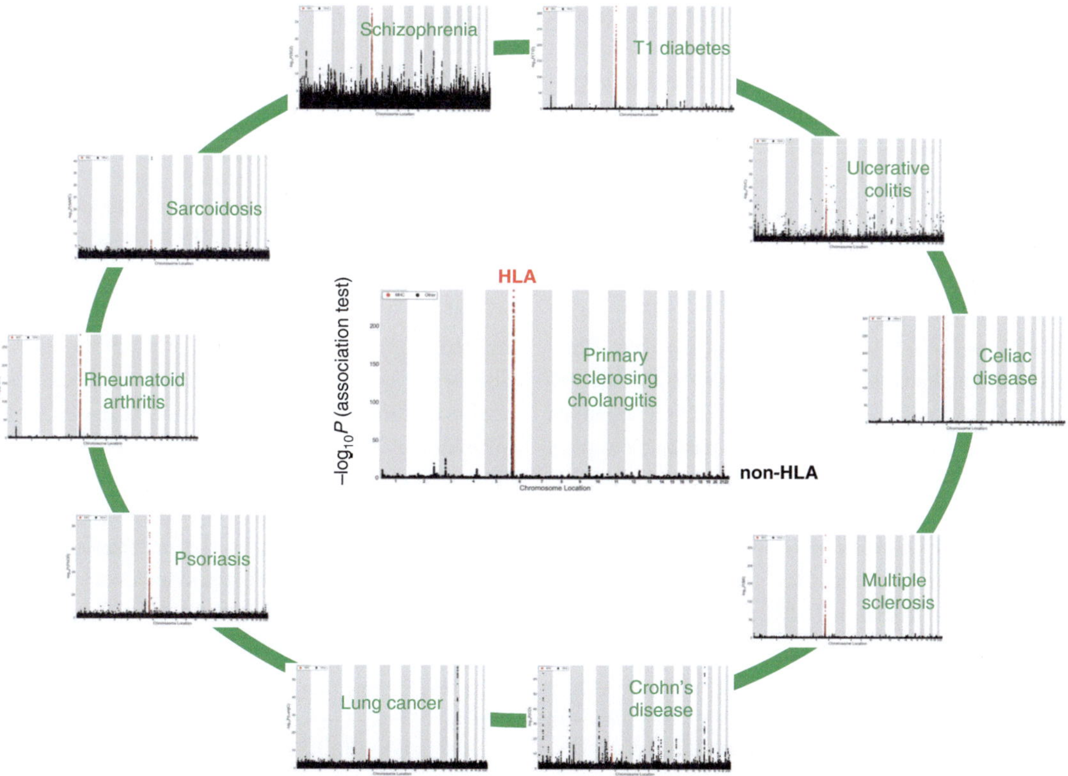

Fig. 8.1 The importance of HLA associations in PSC and other autoimmune diseases. The figure shows a selection of the so-called Manhattan plots in genome-wide association studies. The *X* axis of the plots shows the chromosome and position and the *Y* axis the significance level of association testing at each position. The purpose of showing the figure, with primary sclerosing cholangitis as the centre plot, is to highlight the immense predominance of the HLA associations at chromosome 6 (plotted in *red*). Similar HLA associations can be seen to a variable extent in a multitude of other diseases, most strongly in prototypical autoimmune diseases. The non-HLA associations are plotted in *black* (Further information on individual gene studies can be found at https://www.ebi.ac.uk/gwas/)

risk locus, and caution is therefore needed in making immediate biological interpretation of findings, not least because of the complexity of genetic interactions now recognised across the genome. Equally readers should be very sceptical of any study in the current era that adopts outdated single gene/variant analyses, unless it is apparent that appropriate validation cohorts are included in such candidate gene studies.

Given the high number of genetic variants tested (typically now around 1,000,000), statistical significance thresholds are stringently set by convention at $P \leq 5 \times 10^{-8}$ (so-called genome-wide significance) to avoid false-positive findings (type 1 errors), and generally external validation of findings is sought as well. Inherent to the study design (association analysis), variants detected at risk loci must have a relatively high frequency to be detectable (i.e. they are 'common', typically with a frequency above 1–5 % in the general population), and being common they generally also exert a relatively low impact on disease risk (odds ratio typically below 1.5) [5]. The latter fact also implies that large collections of cases and controls have been required for the study design to be useful, preferably thousands, and the networks organised to recruit patients for DNA collection have promoted a collaborative, international working environment which should be considered a beneficial 'side effect' of GWAS [6]. For rare diseases like PSC, the statistical stringency and the low effect size of implied variants inevitably lead to false negatives (type 2 statistical errors), and this has to be kept in mind as a limitation of the data herein reviewed.

During the 1990s, liver disease genetics was dedicated to Mendelian traits, starting with the identification of genes for hyperbilirubinemias and Wilson's disease [7–12] and a strong subsequent focus on cholestasis and hemochromatosis [13–23]. The interpretation of the gene findings in these studies has greatly influenced the thinking of susceptibility genes also in non-Mendelian (i.e. complex) diseases like PSC. This is important to be aware of, since the genetics as determined by GWAS represent fundamentally different mechanisms of causality. In Mendelian diseases, there is an approximately 1:1 relationship between genetic aberrations and disease traits (the genetic

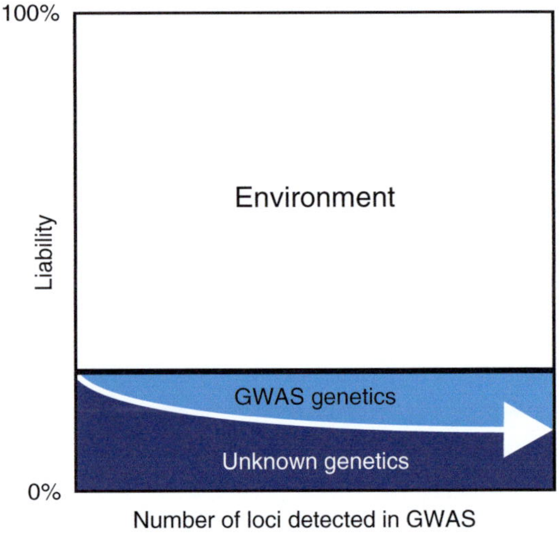

Fig. 8.2 Relative impact of genetic versus non-genetic factors in PSC. Genetic studies emphasise that the genetic contribution to overall primary sclerosing cholangitis (PSC) liability is low and that interacting and co-occurring environmental factors (*white*) are likely important. Outcomes of genome-wide association studies (GWAS; *light blue*) may aid in the identification of such factors, since the common variants have been exposed to the historical environment. Despite an increasing number of reported risk loci (at present 16), a fraction of the heritable contribution to PSC pathogenesis is not detectable by GWAS due to limitations of the study design (*dark blue*) (Reprinted with permission from Ref. [24])

variants 'cause disease' frequently as mutations are structurally damaging to protein function). This being said, given the time taken to mechanistically understand even Mendelian diseases, it is relevant to reflect that disease penetrance and clinical phenotype are often not so easily explained by a single mutation-single effect model, even for diseases as classic monogenic as hemochromatosis and Wilson's disease.

For GWAS findings, contextual factors (environment, gene-gene interactions, etc.) nevertheless play a considerably greater role than in Mendelian genetics (Fig. 8.2), making it inappropriate to assume susceptibility genes as causal (the disease-associated genetic variants in GWAS 'do not cause disease'). This distinction between Mendelian genetics and 'GWAS genetics' is underlined by the fact that the overall contribution of genetics to complex traits like PSC is limited [24]. GWAS outcomes, even by mathematical extrapolations, are

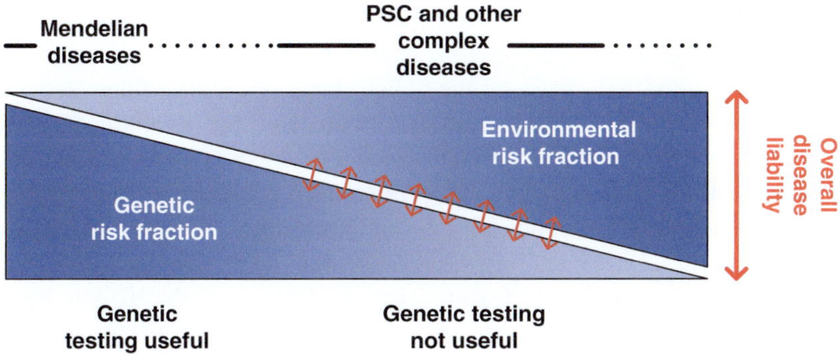

Fig. 8.3 Distinguishing Mendelian from complex liver affections. For complex phenotypes, the contribution from genetics to overall disease liability is limited (typically less than 50 %). In addition, only a fraction (for primary sclerosing cholangitis [PSC] less than 10 %) of the genetic susceptibility is known. In both Mendelian and complex disease manifestations, the gene findings serve as clues to the underlying pathophysiology. However, only for the case of Mendelian manifestations of liver affections do genetic findings have clinically useful predictive power (Reprinted with permission from Ref. [43])

likely to represent a minor fraction (probably less than one third) of the susceptibility to complex traits [25, 26], and PSC so far makes up less than 10 % of the overall disease liability [27].

The relative importance of genetic influences in PSC is also evident in studies of heritability. There are no formal twin studies as for many other diseases, but registry data from Sweden makes a hazard ratio estimate of 11.1 in siblings of PSC patients (complicated by the lack of an ICD10 code for precise case identification) [28]. Such an estimate places PSC at the same degree of heritability as in most other complex autoimmune and immune-mediated conditions. In these diseases, heritability estimates mostly range near a relative sibling risk of ~10 on most instances. Notably, this number is very low compared to Mendelian conditions where relative sibling risk (depending on the penetrance of involved genetic variants) ranges from several hundreds to several thousands [29], further underlining how our thinking on the outcomes of genetic studies in complex diseases like PSC must be different from that of monogenic traits (Fig. 8.3).

The HLA Association in PSC

As can be seen in Fig. 8.1, the genetic findings on chromosome 6 in PSC are several orders of magnitude stronger than those found in any other region. Throughout the rest of the genome, a number of weaker and less significant associations can be found. The important point about this overall genetic architecture in PSC is the fact that it resembles the genetic architecture of prototypical autoimmune diseases, e.g. type 1 diabetes, rheumatoid arthritis and multiple sclerosis. Prior to the genetic studies, it had been questioned whether PSC could be an autoimmune disease, particularly given the strong male predominance (two thirds of the patients are male) and lack of efficacy of immunosuppressive therapy. However, autoimmune diseases with a male predominance do exist (e.g. ankylosing spondylitis), and alongside other features observed (autoantibodies [30] and clonality of T cell receptors [31]), genetics clearly positions PSC as an inherently autoimmune condition, albeit one perhaps because of its biliary localisation that does not respond to classical immunosuppression. In many aspects, this global observation is one of the major outcomes of the genetic studies. The model contrasts that of other models of PSC development (e.g. toxic bile acid injury, gut leakage of bacterial components due to IBD [32]) whilst is compatible with models involving the cross-homing or cross-reactivity of lymphocytes between the bowel and the liver [33, 34].

The region involved in the chromosome 6 associations in PSC is called the human leucocyte antigen (HLA) complex or more generally the major histocompatibility complex (MHC).

This genetic region plays a critical role in immune function and spans approximately 250 protein coding genes over 7.6 million base pairs on the short arm of chromosome 6 [35]. Genetic variants in the region contribute almost without exception to risk of autoimmune and immune-mediated conditions, including infections [36]. For most conditions, the HLA class I and II genes appear to play primary roles, a point which suggests that the adaptive immune system is involved in disease development. The HLA class I molecules present endogenously (intracellular) antigens to CD8+ T cells (HLA-peptide-T cell receptor [TCR] interaction), whereas the CD4+ TCR recognises exogenously (extracellular) antigens presented by HLA class II molecules. A typical HLA class I variant binds between 2,000 and 10,000 different peptides, and more than 2,000 different peptides are estimated to bind an HLA class II variant. Within this spectrum of peptides, triggers of the adaptive immune response in HLA-associated diseases are likely to reside, as critically exemplified by celiac disease (Fig. 8.1) [37, 38]. Non-HLA genes within the HLA complex also likely contribute to the overall impact of the region onto autoimmune disease development [39–41].

The identities of peptide triggers in PSC and the majority of other autoimmune conditions remain unknown; intriguingly this is in contrast to primary biliary cholangitis, where greater insight exists as a result of a characteristic serologic abnormality and anti-mitochondrial antibodies. The relationship between gluten in celiac disease and the genetic HLA DQB1-association also serves as a model to illustrate how disease-related genetic variation in the HLA complex is likely to contain information of relevance to such triggers. In PSC, circumstantial evidence points in the direction of *HLA-DRB1* serving a similar role [42]. However, a complex association picture exists [40], with strong *HLA-B* associations also imminent. Interpretation of these findings is confounded by the allele nomenclature of the HLA variants, which is very complex because of the various methodologies that have been employed in describing HLA variation over the last 30–40 years. For this reason, elaborate descriptions of allelic associations serve currently little practical purpose and can be assessed elsewhere by the interested reader [43]. Furthermore, the evolutionary history of the region has led to complex rearrangements and relationships between genetic variants in different populations [36]. All these aspects jointly make the dissection and interpretation of the genetic findings in the HLA in PSC exceedingly difficult. However, when overcome, insights obtained from PSC-related HLA variants are likely to point towards critical antigenic triggers, potentially even causal ones.

Non-HLA Associations in PSC

Almost without exception, non-HLA genetic variants enhancing the risk of autoimmune and immune-mediated conditions appear in more than one disease. PSC is no exception, and the 19 non-HLA associations that have been identified at the time of writing all appear in related conditions. The phenomenon (genetically denominated 'pleiotropy') follows an apparently random pattern, meaning there is a collection of different risk genes that can predispose individuals to a variety of autoimmune conditions (Fig. 8.4) [44].

More recently, we have been able to describe this poorly understood pattern of genetic overlap in greater detail, suggesting more generally the existence of a 'hidden' molecular taxonomy that differs from the traditional classification of disease by organ or system [45]. A key outcome of these analyses is that despite the profound pleiotropy, clear demarcations of the genetic risk for the individual conditions exist. Most importantly, the analysis supports the clinical notions of PSC-IBD being a distinct condition, contrasting a model wherein biliary injury is a mere complication of classical ulcerative colitis and Crohn's disease. This is important, since genetic outcomes thus contrast two existing theories of PSC development: that of a primary alteration of biliary homeostasis ('toxic bile hypothesis') and that of a causal relationship between the bowel disease and biliary disease ('leaky gut' hypothesis). This does not mean

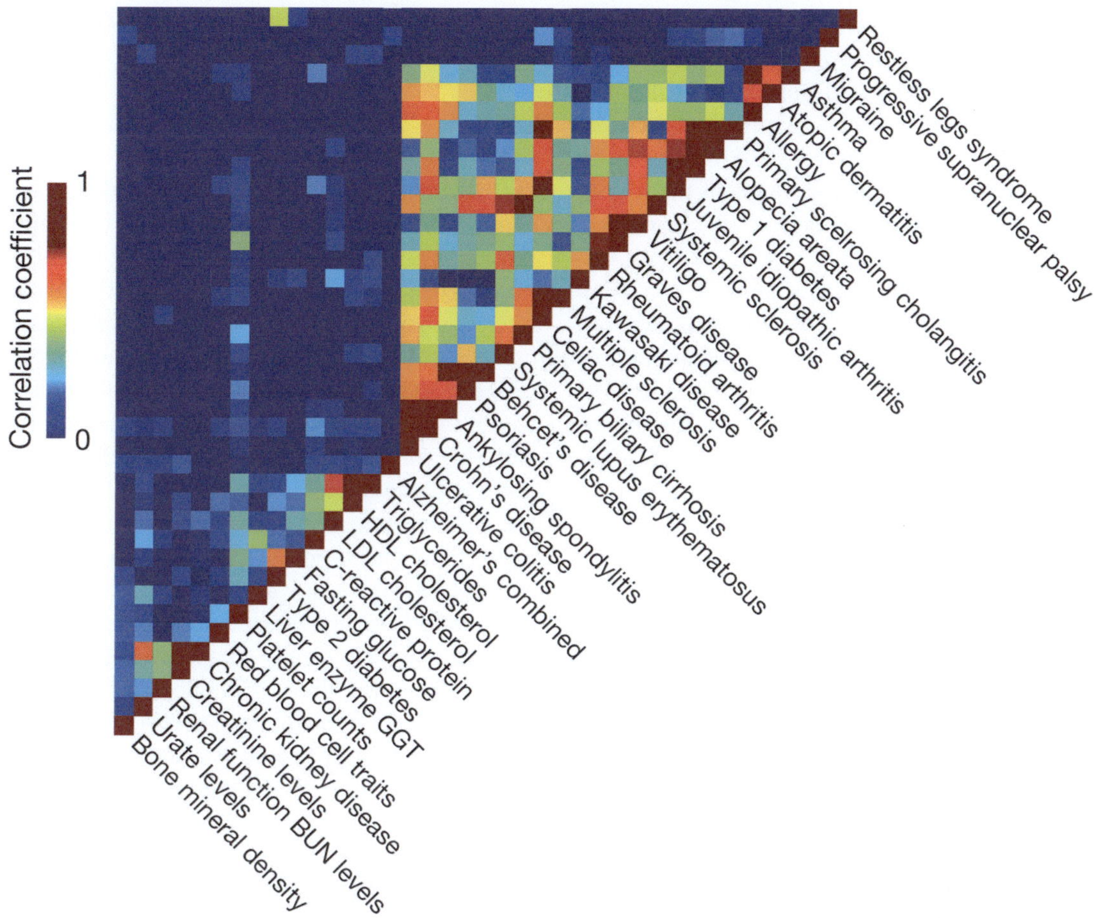

Fig. 8.4 Genetic relationship between PSC and other autoimmune conditions. The colour scale indicates correlation between phenotypes (*red* = high, *blue* = low) according to genetic findings published at https://www.ebi.ac.uk/gwas/. As shown, genetics of PSC cluster together with other autoimmune and immune-mediated diseases (Reprinted with permission from reference [44])

that such mechanisms are not of relevance to the chain of events leading to biliary injury but rather places autoimmune-like mechanisms presumably upstream. Clinically, this is compatible with the inconsistent timing of relationship between presentation of bowel disease and biliary disease in PSC-IBD (bowel disease presenting after biliary disease in a substantial fraction of patients and on some instances even only after liver transplantation [46]). Genetically, there is no evidence for primary disturbances of biliary homeostasis as per the known functions of detected susceptibility genes; only modifier effects have been so far reported in a single-centre patient series [47].

In popular terms, there are several ways to describe this pattern of genetic overlap for the non-HLA risk loci in PSC. Most notably, there is a mixture of IBD susceptibility loci and susceptibility loci involving in prototypical autoimmune conditions like type 1 diabetes, multiple sclerosis and rheumatoid arthritis [44]. Of note, out of the 163 established risk loci in ulcerative colitis and Crohn's disease [48], still only 11 demonstrate equally robust association in PSC, despite substantial statistical power in recent assessments [27, 45]. Some of the PSC risk loci do not show associations in IBD (e.g. *PRKD2* and *BCL2L11*) and contribute, together with the difference in HLA associations [49], to the demarcation of

PSC and PSC-IBD versus ulcerative colitis and Crohn's disease. From a clinical perspective, the overlap between risk loci in PSC and suggestive associations detected in autoimmune hepatitis (i.e. *SH2B3*, *MMEL1/TNFRSF14*, *CTLA4/CD28* and *BACH2*) [50] may help explain the clinical co-morbidity observed for the two conditions (slightly less than 10 % of the PSC patients showing features of autoimmune hepatitis [51]). In line with the rarity of patients with overlap between PSC and primary biliary cholangitis in the clinic, there is remarkably little overlap between the genetics of the two conditions, exceptions occurring though at *SH2B3* and *MMEL1/TNFRSF14*.

Another simplistic way of clustering the non-HLA risk genes is that of a demarcation between genes likely to involve in T cell development and function and those with other or less apparent biological functions. Belonging to the first group of genes are likely *CTLA4/CD28*, *IL2/IL21*, *IL2RA*, *MMEL1/TNFRSF14*, *CCL20*, *SIK2*, *HCDAC7*, *CD226* and potentially also *PRKD2*. Belonging to the second group of genes are likely *BCL2L11*, *GPR35*, *MST1*, *BACH2*, *TCF4*, *PSMG1* and *CLEC16A/SOSC1*. The demarcation holds some logic in substantiating the strong suggestions from the HLA associations of PSC being a T cell-mediated autoimmune disease, however making the critical assumption that currently published literature is relevant. This is a fundamental issue in the interpretation of genetic findings in hypothesis-free genetic studies, since published literature from pre hoc experiments do not account either for the disease relationship of genes in question nor their potentially different roles in different tissues (e.g. immune cells versus biliary epithelial cells). To a large extent, this phenomenon ('literature bias') also makes pathophysiological interpretations of gene findings speculative. In the opinion of the authors, excessive elaboration on the potential roles of single susceptibility genes in PSC pathogenesis in the absence of disease-specific data should be avoided and is herein not done. The interested reader can obtain further insight by published review articles that provide further details on the subject [52, 53].

Practical Implications of Novel Gene Associations

The field of PSC genetics is coming to a plateau, and even application of whole genome sequencing may not greatly add to our knowledge (in contrast to studies that focus on highly clinically described cohorts and patient subgroups, which might prove powerful). At the time of writing, the International PSC Study Group (www.ipscsg.org) has collected DNA from almost 5,000 PSC patients and is wrapping up the final studies based on this material. With 20 robust risk loci and an additional 10 for which sufficient evidence exists to conclude them relevant (Tables 8.1 and 8.2), it is timely to pause and ask what are the practical implications of these discoveries. For patients there are many needs; they are devoid of therapies effectively influencing disease progression, there is no means for predicting disease behaviour or the risk of cholangiocarcinoma, and they experience symptoms related to liver (pruritus, pain and fatigue) and colonic diseases significantly affecting their quality of life. There have been great expectations to genetics for potentially providing developments to meet these needs; however, it is increasingly clear that outcomes may need considerable further processing before clinical utility can be reached.

One tempting opportunity is considering whether risk genes represent novel drug targets. Particularly for targets where there are potential drugs already available, it is an intriguing possibility that such drugs may show beneficial effects in PSC (so-called drug repurposing), but careful use of such analogies is needed because risk of disease initiation is not equivalent to biological pathways to liver injury and repair. Although IL2RA-targeted therapy like basiliximab and daclizumab is perhaps unlikely to enter clinical practice in hepatology outside of current indications related to liver transplantation, they serve logical examples of therapeutics for which considerations in PSC could be made. Clinical trials for anti-CCL20 are underway in IBD (https://clinicaltrials.gov/ct2/show/NCT01984047) and could also serve a candidate example.

On a related note, there has also been the example of IL12/IL23 signalling in primary biliary cholangitis versus potential applicability of ustekinumab [54]. Whereas for genetic reasons, drugs targeting these signalling pathways might be a rational approach in primary biliary cholangitis, there was insufficient clinical efficacy as evaluated by crude markers of cholestasis for ustekinumab, and a clinical trial have has not shown any efficacy [55]. The reasons for this are unknown, but likely an individual risk gene cannot be taken out of its overall host genetic make-up and disease setting for direct therapeutic exploitation, as well as recognition that in evaluating new therapies patient heterogeneity at the time of recruitment can be relevant. This is furthermore particularly relevant to the cholestatic liver diseases wherein the response to immune-mediated injury, bile duct damage and cholestasis is inherently very powerful and has frequently deleterious biological effects, potentially more impactful than the initiating liver injury. Hence, the susceptibility genes are clues to important biological affections that only upon careful work-up of disease-specific mechanisms could lead to insights of relevance to therapy. Furthermore, and importantly, the elephant in the susceptibility room, environmental co-variables (Fig. 8.2), is likely to interact with the genetic factors. As long as these are unknown, the appreciation of risk gene biology will remain incomplete.

The field of 'personalised medicine', 'stratified medicine' or 'precision medicine' is under rapid development. Various definitions are found in the literature, but in essence personalised medicine means preventive, diagnostic, therapeutic or follow-up means adapted to an individual biological setting. There have been important accomplishments in the fields of oncology (druggable and prognostic mutations), Mendelian disease (where whole-genome sequencing has reduced the fraction of undeterminable aetiology), pharmacogenomics and to some extent also microbiology (resistance tracking). For complex diseases like PSC, a clinical role of high-throughput technologies remains undefined. Although enthusiasm is considerable, proof of concept for how to transform the increasing wealth of genetic insights from GWAS into tailored management for the individual patient is not yet clear. The large and poorly understood overlap in genetic susceptibility between different autoimmune diseases leads to low specificity. As shown in Fig. 8.2, the low contribution of currently identified risk genes to overall PSC liability (about 5–10%) [45] and hence pathophysiology also means diagnostic, and stratifying utility of risk variants is low. Further delineation of the underlying biological abnormities represented by gene findings may lead to marker phenomena better suited for the purpose, but unless family history suggests a Mendelian PSC variant (familial clustering), gene testing and gene profiling in patients with PSC should so far be avoided.

Overall, the greatest practical utility of current insights in PSC genetics comes for the research laboratory. The gene findings shown in Tables 8.1 and 8.2 serve as a basis for pathophysiological research that is likely more relevant to the human disease setting than model systems so far employed. In pursuing the individual risk genes, researchers use a variety of tools, including mouse models, cell cultures and other laboratory methods. Notably, in a complex disease setting where multiple genetic and environmental factors are required for disease development, none of these modelling experiments is likely to provide comprehensive insights. Rather, they are biological studies, providing biological pieces to a puzzle, where biology revealed most likely holds relevance for PSC given a basis in human data. This is important to acknowledge and as elaborated previously contrasts the paradigm of Mendelian diseases in which murine model systems are more likely to closer reflect the full features of human disease.

How to incorporate environmental factors in the follow-up experiments of the genetic studies remains to be clarified. Some of the risk genes, like *FUT2* [56], show distinct relationships with environmental co-variables (on this instance gut microbial community composition [57]). The HLA associations in this regard also serve a prototypical example. For other risk genes, there is less apparent a role for gene-environment interactions. What is clear from this perspective is that studies on these co-variables are now needed. As for the gut microbiota and dietary exposures, there are obvious therapeutic prospects. In case series and clinical trials with antibiotic treatment in PSC [58], some improvement in alkaline phosphatase has been seen. This should not be interpreted as clinical efficacy without further substantiation. Rather the findings add to the genetics pointing in the direction of gut-derived antigenic and other influences and serve as proof of concept that alterations in this domain might become of benefit for patients.

Conclusions

Genetic studies have positioned PSC as a complex autoimmune disease in which environmental factors play a significant role in driving disease development. The 30 susceptibility genes discussed in the present article all show associations in other autoimmune and immune-mediated conditions. Importantly, however, they clearly demarcate PSC and PSC-IBD from classical ulcerative colitis and Crohn's disease. The clinical utility of this pool of risk genes is so far not established and needs extension in ethnically diverse populations, and further work is needed to establish the underlying pathophysiological implications as well as the environmental cofactors. Larger-scale efforts identifying, if present, genetic markers of clinical course, response to treatment and clinical outcomes are now as worthy as initial genetic risk studies, and it is likely that as important as evolving genetic technologies is the curation of highly phenotyped cohorts for study. With the expectation that genomic data can be aligned to other 'omics', it is reasonable to be optimistic that the outcomes are providing increasingly clear directions for further PSC research. Ultimate patient benefit is therefore a strong expectation.

Acknowledgements We are grateful to the authors of reference 43 for allowing reprinting of Fig. 8.4.

We thank Xiaojun Jiang for the help in assembling Tables 8.1 and 8.2.

References

1. Tanaka A, Tazuma S, Okazaki K, et al. Nationwide survey for primary sclerosing cholangitis and IgG4-related sclerosing cholangitis in Japan. J Hepatobiliary Pancreat Sci. 2014;21:43–50.
2. Tanaka A, Tazuma S, Okazaki K, et al. Clinical profiles of patients with primary sclerosing cholangitis in the elderly. J Hepatobiliary Pancreat Sci. 2015;22:230–6.
3. Lunder AK, et al. Prevalence of Sclerosing Cholangitis, Detected by Magnetic Resonance Cholangiography, in Patients with Long-term Inflammatory Bowel Disease. Gastroenterology In press (doi: 10.1053/j.gastro.2016.06.021).
4. Klein RJ, Zeiss C, Chew EY, et al. Complement factor H polymorphism in age-related macular degeneration. Science. 2005;308:385–9.
5. Hindorff LA, Sethupathy P, Junkins HA, et al. Potential etiologic and functional implications of genome-wide association loci for human diseases and traits. Proc Natl Acad Sci U S A. 2009;106:9362–7.
6. Bulik-Sullivan BK, Sullivan PF. The authorship network of genome-wide association studies. Nat Genet. 2012;44:113.
7. Koiwai O, Nishizawa M, Hasada K, et al. Gilbert's syndrome is caused by a heterozygous missense mutation in the gene for bilirubin UDP-glucuronosyltransferase. Hum Mol Genet. 1995;4:1183–6.
8. Bosma PJ, Chowdhury JR, Huang TJ, et al. Mechanisms of inherited deficiencies of multiple UDP-glucuronosyltransferase isoforms in two patients with Crigler-Najjar syndrome, type I. FASEB J. 1992;6:2859–63.
9. Moghrabi N, Clarke DJ, Boxer M, et al. Identification of an A-to-G missense mutation in exon 2 of the UGT1 gene complex that causes Crigler-Najjar syndrome type 2. Genomics. 1993;18:171–3.
10. Petrukhin K, Fischer SG, Pirastu M, et al. Mapping, cloning and genetic characterization of the region containing the Wilson disease gene. Nat Genet. 1993;5:338–43.
11. Bull PC, Thomas GR, Rommens JM, et al. The Wilson disease gene is a putative copper transporting P-type ATPase similar to the Menkes gene. Nat Genet. 1993;5:327–37.
12. Paulusma CC, Kool M, Bosma PJ, et al. A mutation in the human canalicular multispecific organic anion transporter gene causes the Dubin-Johnson syndrome. Hepatology. 1997;25:1539–42.
13. Papanikolaou G, Samuels ME, Ludwig EH, et al. Mutations in HFE2 cause iron overload in chromosome 1q-linked juvenile hemochromatosis. Nat Genet. 2004;36:77–82.
14. Roetto A, Papanikolaou G, Politou M, et al. Mutant antimicrobial peptide hepcidin is associated with severe juvenile hemochromatosis. Nat Genet. 2003;33:21–2.

15. Njajou OT, Vaessen N, Joosse M, et al. A mutation in SLC11A3 is associated with autosomal dominant hemochromatosis. Nat Genet. 2001;28:213–4.
16. Montosi G, Donovan A, Totaro A, et al. Autosomal-dominant hemochromatosis is associated with a mutation in the ferroportin (SLC11A3) gene. J Clin Invest. 2001;108:619–23.
17. Strautnieks SS, Bull LN, Knisely AS, et al. A gene encoding a liver-specific ABC transporter is mutated in progressive familial intrahepatic cholestasis. Nat Genet. 1998;20:233–8.
18. Bull LN, van Eijk MJ, Pawlikowska L, et al. A gene encoding a P-type ATPase mutated in two forms of hereditary cholestasis. Nat Genet. 1998;18:219–24.
19. McDaniell R, Warthen DM, Sanchez-Lara PA, et al. NOTCH2 mutations cause Alagille syndrome, a heterogeneous disorder of the notch signaling pathway. Am J Hum Genet. 2006;79:169–73.
20. Feder JN, Gnirke A, Thomas W, et al. A novel MHC class I-like gene is mutated in patients with hereditary haemochromatosis. Nat Genet. 1996;13:399–408.
21. Kamath BM, Bauer RC, Loomes KM, et al. NOTCH2 mutations in Alagille syndrome. J Med Genet. 2012;49:138–44.
22. de Vree JM, Jacquemin E, Sturm E, et al. Mutations in the MDR3 gene cause progressive familial intrahepatic cholestasis. Proc Natl Acad Sci U S A. 1998;95:282–7.
23. Girelli D, Bozzini C, Roetto A, et al. Clinical and pathologic findings in hemochromatosis type 3 due to a novel mutation in transferrin receptor 2 gene. Gastroenterology. 2002;122:1295–302.
24. Henriksen EKK, Melum E, Karlsen TH. Update on primary sclerosing cholangitis genetics. Curr Opin Gastroenterol. 2014;30(3):310–9.
25. Stahl EA, Wegmann D, Trynka G, et al. Bayesian inference analyses of the polygenic architecture of rheumatoid arthritis. Nat Genet. 2012;44:483–9.
26. Wood AR, Esko T, Yang J, et al. Defining the role of common variation in the genomic and biological architecture of adult human height. Nat Genet. 2014;46:1173–86.
27. Liu JZ, Hov JR, Folseraas T, et al. Dense genotyping of immune-related disease regions identifies nine new risk loci for primary sclerosing cholangitis. Nat Genet. 2013;45:670–5.
28. Bergquist A, Montgomery SM, Bahmanyar S, et al. Increased risk of primary sclerosing cholangitis and ulcerative colitis in first-degree relatives of patients with primary sclerosing cholangitis. Clin Gastroenterol Hepatol. 2008;6:939–43.
29. Donaldson PT. Genetics of liver disease: immunogenetics and disease pathogenesis. Gut. 2004;53:599–608.
30. Hov JR, Boberg KM, Karlsen TH. Autoantibodies in primary sclerosing cholangitis. World J Gastroenterol. 2008;14:3781–91.
31. Liaskou E, Henriksen EK, Holm K, et al. High-throughput T-cell receptor sequencing across chronic liver diseases reveals distinct disease-associated repertoires. Hepatology. 2016;63(5):1608–19.
32. Karlsen TH, Schrumpf E, Boberg KM. Update on primary sclerosing cholangitis. Dig Liver Dis. 2010;42: 390–400.
33. Grant AJ, Lalor PF, Salmi M, et al. Homing of mucosal lymphocytes to the liver in the pathogenesis of hepatic complications of inflammatory bowel disease. Lancet. 2002;359:150–7.
34. Das KM. Immunopathogenesis of primary sclerosing cholangitis: possible role of a shared colonic and biliary epithelial antigen. J Gastroenterol Hepatol. 2004;19:S290–4.
35. Horton R, Wilming L, Rand V, et al. Gene map of the extended human MHC. Nat Rev Genet. 2004;5: 889–99.
36. Traherne JA. Human MHC, architecture and evolution: implications for disease association studies. Int J Immunogenet. 2008;35:179–92.
37. Molberg O, McAdam SN, Korner R, et al. Tissue transglutaminase selectively modifies gliadin peptides that are recognized by gut-derived T cells in celiac disease. Nat Med. 1998;4:713–7.
38. Sollid LM, Markussen G, Ek J, et al. Evidence for a primary association of celiac disease to a particular HLA-DQ alpha/beta heterodimer. J Exp Med. 1989;169:345–50.
39. Goyette P, Boucher G, Mallon D, et al. High-density mapping of the MHC identifies a shared role for HLA-DRB1*01:03 in inflammatory bowel diseases and heterozygous advantage in ulcerative colitis. Nat Genet. 2015;47:172–9.
40. Naess S, Lie BA, Melum E, et al. Refinement of the MHC risk map in a scandinavian primary sclerosing cholangitis population. PLoS One. 2014;9, e114486.
41. Lie BA, Thorsby E. Several genes in the extended human MHC contribute to predisposition to autoimmune diseases. Curr Opin Immunol. 2005;17: 526–31.
42. Hov JR, Kosmoliaptsis V, Traherne JA, et al. Electrostatic modifications of the human leukocyte antigen-DR P9 peptide-binding pocket and susceptibility to primary sclerosing cholangitis. Hepatology. 2011;53:1967–76.
43. Mells GF, Kaser A, Karlsen TH. Novel insights into autoimmune liver diseases provided by genome-wide association studies. J Autoimmun. 2013;46:41–54.
44. Farh KK, Marson A, Zhu J, et al. Genetic and epigenetic fine mapping of causal autoimmune disease variants. Nature. 2015;518:337–43.
45. Ellinghaus D, Jostins L, Spain SL, et al. Analysis of five chronic inflammatory diseases identifies 27 new associations and highlights disease-specific patterns at shared loci. Nat Genet. 2016;48(5):510–8.
46. Riley TR, Schoen RE, Lee RG, et al. A case series of transplant recipients who despite immunosuppression developed inflammatory bowel disease. Am J Gastroenterol. 1997;92:279–82.
47. Karlsen TH, Lie BA, Frey Froslie K, et al. Polymorphisms in the steroid and xenobiotic receptor gene influence survival in primary sclerosing cholangitis. Gastroenterology. 2006;131:781–7.

48. Jostins L, Ripke S, Weersma RK, et al. Host-microbe interactions have shaped the genetic architecture of inflammatory bowel disease. Nature. 2012;491: 119–24.
49. Karlsen TH, Boberg KM, Vatn M, et al. Different HLA class II associations in ulcerative colitis patients with and without primary sclerosing cholangitis. Genes Immun. 2007;8:275–8.
50. Hirschfield GM, Karlsen TH. Genetic risks link autoimmune hepatitis to other autoimmune liver disease. Gastroenterology. 2014;147:270–3.
51. Kaya M, Angulo P, Lindor KD. Overlap of autoimmune hepatitis and primary sclerosing cholangitis: an evaluation of a modified scoring system. J Hepatol. 2000;33:537–42.
52. Karlsen TH, Lammert F, Thompson RJ. Genetics of liver disease: from pathophysiology to clinical practice. J Hepatol. 2015;62:S6–14.
53. Folseraas T, Liaskou E, Anderson CA, et al. Genetics in PSC: what do the "risk genes" teach Us? Clin Rev Allergy Immunol. 2015;48(2–3): 154–64.
54. Hirschfield GM, Liu X, Xu C, et al. Primary biliary cirrhosis associated with HLA, IL12A, and IL12RB2 variants. N Engl J Med. 2009;360:2544–55.
55. Hirschfield GM, Gershwin ME, Strauss R, et al. PURIFI Study Group: Ustekinumab for patients with primary biliary cholangitis who have an inadequate response to ursodeoxycholic acid: A proof-of-concept study. Hepatology. 2016;64(1):189–99.
56. Folseraas T, Melum E, Rausch P, et al. Extended analysis of a genome-wide association study in primary sclerosing cholangitis detects multiple novel risk loci. J Hepatol. 2012;57(2):366–75.
57. Rausch P, Rehman A, Kunzel S, et al. Colonic mucosa-associated microbiota is influenced by an interaction of Crohn disease and FUT2 (Secretor) genotype. Proc Natl Acad Sci U S A. 2011;108:19030–5.
58. Tabibian JH, Talwalkar JA, Lindor KD. Role of the microbiota and antibiotics in primary sclerosing cholangitis. Biomed Res Int. 2013;2013:389537.
59. Melum E, Franke A, Schramm C, et al. Genome-wide association analysis in primary sclerosing cholangitis identifies two non-HLA susceptibility loci. Nat Genet. 2011;43(1):17–9. doi: 10.1038/ng.728. Epub 2010 Dec 12.
60. Ellinghaus D, Folseraas T, Holm K, et al. Genome-wide association analysis in primary sclerosing cholangitis and ulcerative colitis identifies risk loci at GPR35 and TCF4. Hepatology. 2013;58(3):1074–83. doi: 10.1002/hep.25977. Epub 2013 Jan 17.
61. Srivastava B, Mells GF, Cordell HJ, et al. Fine mapping and replication of genetic risk loci in primary sclerosing cholangitis. Scand J Gastroenterol. 2012;47(7):820–6. doi: 10.3109/00365521.2012.682090. Epub 2012 May 4.

Immunology of Primary Sclerosing Cholangitis

9

John M. Vierling

Abbreviations

aa	Amino acid
Ags	Antigens
AID	Autoimmune disease
APCs	Antigen-presenting cells
AutoAbs	Autoantibodies
AutoAg	Autoantigen
BSEP	Bile salt export protein
C'	Complement
CCL	Chemokine ligand for CC chemokine receptors
CCR5Δ32	Chemokine receptor 5 with 32 base pair deletion
CD	Crohn's disease
CFTR	Cystic fibrosis transmembrane conductance regulator
CpG	Bacterial dinucleotide PAMP
CTL	Cytotoxic T lymphocyte
CTLA4	Cytotoxic T lymphocyte antigen-4
DCs	Dendritic cells
ERCP	Endoscopic retrograde cholangiopancreatography
FISH	Fluorescence in situ hybridization
GALT	Gut-associated lymphoid tissue
HLA	Human leukocyte antigen complex (designation for human MHC)
IBD	Inflammatory bowel disease
ICAM-1	Intercellular adhesion molecule-1 (CD54)
IFNγ	Interferon gamma
IL	Interleukin
IMID	Immune-mediated inflammatory disease
LPS	Lipopolysaccharide
MADCAM-1	Mucosal vascular addressin cell adhesion molecule-1
Mdr2	Multidrug resistance gene product 2, the mouse homolog of human MDR3
MDR3	Multidrug resistance gene product 3, a human bile transporter
MHC	Major histocompatibility complex
MMPs	Matrix metalloproteinases
NK cell	Natural killer cell
NKT	Natural killer T cell
NSDC	Nonsuppurative destructive cholangitis
OLT	Orthotopic liver transplantation
PAMPs	Pathogen-associated molecular patterns
pANCAs	Perinuclear antineutrophil cytoplasmic antibodies
pANNAs	Peripheral antineutrophil nuclear antibodies
PBMC	Peripheral blood mononuclear cells
PDGF	Platelet-derived growth factor
PRRs	Pattern recognition receptors

J.M. Vierling, MD, FACP, FAASLD
Division of Abdominal Transplantation, Departments of Medicine and Surgery, Baylor College of Medicine, Baylor-St. Luke's Medical Center, Houston, TX, USA
e-mail: vierling@bcm.edu

L.M. Forman (ed.), *Primary Sclerosing Cholangitis*, DOI 10.1007/978-3-319-40908-5_9

PSC	Primary sclerosing cholangitis
TCRs	T cell receptors for peptide antigens
TGFβ	Transforming growth factor-beta
Th	T helper
TLRs	Toll-like receptors
TNFα	Tumor necrosis factor-alpha
Treg	Regulatory CD4 T cell
UC	Ulcerative colitis
VAP-1	Vascular adhesion protein-1
VCAM-1	Vascular cell adhesion molecule-1
Vβ	Variable region of β-chain of TCR

Introduction

Primary sclerosing cholangitis (PSC) is a rare, chronic, progressive hepatobiliary disease of undefined etiology that affects macroscopic intrahepatic and/or extrahepatic bile ducts in the majority and microscopic proximal bile ducts in a minority (<10 %) [1, 2]. PSC is associated with inflammatory bowel disease (IBD) of the colon in >75 % of cases; ulcerative colitis (UC) of a distinctive phenotype afflicts the majority and Crohn's disease (CD) the minority [3]. In PSC, peribiliary inflammation results in progressive circumferential fibrosis causing biliary strictures. Currently, PSC is classified as an "atypical" autoimmune disease (AID) because several features of PSC differ from those of a classical AID (Table 9.1) [4].

A form of secondary sclerosing cholangitis associated with elevations of serum IgG4 and/or IgG4-secreting B and plasma cells may mimic PSC [5]. Retrospective studies indicate that approximately 10 % of patients diagnosed with PSC instead may have IgG4 cholangiopathy [6]. IgG4 cholangiopathy can be distinguished by a prior history of pancreatitis, stricturing of both intrahepatic and extrahepatic bile ducts, propensity for jaundice, and the use of recently developed techniques [7].

Multiple immunological features suggest involvement of innate and adaptive immune responses in immunopathogenesis, including susceptibility and resistance associations with HLA haplotypes and autoantibodies (autoAbs), and evidence that gut-primed T effector T cells mediate peribiliary, fibrosing inflammation [4, 8]. The homing and retention of these gut-primed T cells are facilitated by the activated cholangiocytes that

Table 9.1 Comparison of characteristic features of classical autoimmune diseases and primary sclerosing cholangitis

Features	Classical AID	PSC
Autoantigen(s)	Yes	Possibly
Autoantibody	Yes, pathogenetic	Yes, biomarker
Age	Children and adults	Children and adults
Gender predilection	Female > male	Male > female
Genetic factors	HLA, non-HLA	HLA, non-HLA
Tissue- or organ-specific disease	Yes	Yes
Inflammatory cells	Autoreactive T cells	Gut-primed T cells, NK, NKT, macrophages, γδ T cells
Environmental factors	Yes	Yes
Associated AIDs	Yes	Yes
Response to immunosuppression	Yes	No
Examples	SLE Myasthenia gravis Graves' disease Pernicious anemia Type 1 diabetes AIH PBC	

Abbreviations: *AID* autoimmune disease, *HLA* human major histocompatibility complex, *NK* natural killer cells, *NKT* natural killer T cells, *SLE* systemic lupus erythematosus, *AIH* autoimmune hepatitis, *PBC* primary biliary cholangitis express ligands and receptors and secretion of inflammatory cytokines and chemokines [9]. Thus, the cholangiocytes are not passive targets of the immune response but participate in the immunopathogenesis of PSC [4].

The goal of this chapter is to provide a progress report on the immunology of PSC. Emphasis is placed on immunological findings advancing our understanding of the immunopathogenesis of PSC.

Biliary Anatomic Features and PSC

The branching network of bile ducts is lined by cholangiocytes with tight junctions that retain bile within the duct lumens (Fig. 9.1) [10, 11]. Each bile duct is accompanied by a branch of the hepatic artery of equal caliber that gives rise to a peribiliary capillary plexus surrounding each duct. Lymphatic channels adjacent to the peribiliary capillaries drain lymph formed in the space of Disse that contains cytokines and other constituents produced in the hepatic lobules. The portal venous blood from the small bowel and colon contains pathogen-associated molecular patterns (PAMPs) from the cell walls and unmethylated DNA of gut bacteria and fungi, metabolites produced by the gut microbiota, and viable microbial pathogens when the gut mucosal barrier is breached. PSC markedly alters these homeostatic anatomic relationships.

Pathology of PSC

The histopathology of PSC is unique among primary biliary tract diseases (Fig. 9.2) [12]. Lymphoplasmacytic infiltrates of the portal tracts localize to the peribiliary space, where they promote peribiliary fibrosis without apoptotic destruction of the cholangiocytes. The density of portal inflammation is scant, especially when compared to either autoimmune hepatitis (AIH) or primary biliary cholangitis (PBC). A key feature distinguishing PSC from PBC is the absence of effector cell-mediated apoptosis of cholangiocytes in PSC [13].

Progressive fibrosis leads to concentric, circumferential laminations around intact intrahe-

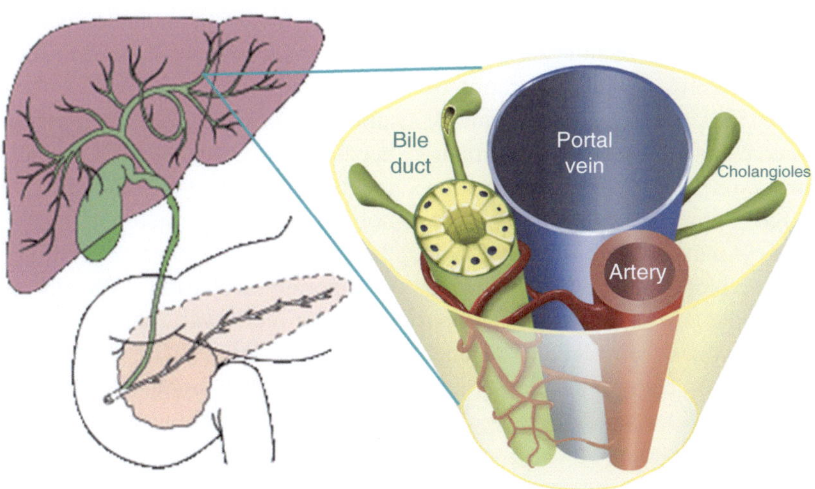

Fig. 9.1 Biliary anatomic features involved in primary sclerosing cholangitis. An intralobular bile duct receives the bile secreted by hepatocytes through cholangioles at the periphery of the portal tract. Each intrahepatic bile duct is accompanied by a branch of the hepatic artery of equal caliber. The arteries supply a peribiliary capillary plexus surrounding each duct, while lymphatic channels lie adjacent to the peribiliary capillaries and drain lymph formed in the space of Disse that contains cytokines and other constituents produced in the hepatic lobules. The portal venous blood from the small bowel and colon contains pathogen-associated molecular patterns (PAMPs) from the cell walls and unmethylated DNA of gut bacteria and fungi, metabolites produced by the gut microbiota, and viable microbial pathogens when the gut mucosal barrier is breached

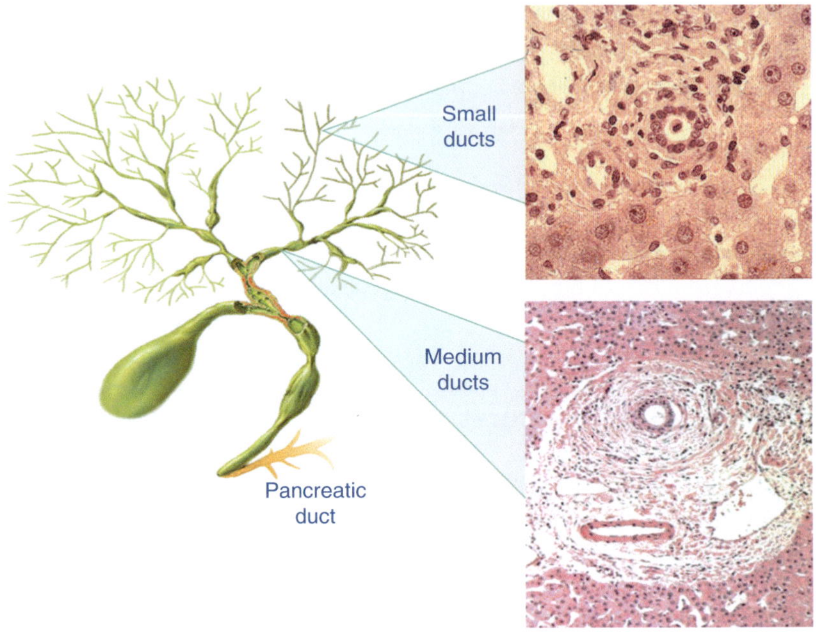

Fig. 9.2 Histopathology of small duct and medium duct primary sclerosing cholangitis. The histopathology of PSC includes the small duct variant and the fibrous inflammatory lesions of medium-caliber intrahepatic ducts. Compared to either AIH or PBC, the inflammatory infiltrates in PBC are sparse. Periductal, concentric fibrosis of the medium-caliber intralobular bile ducts pushes the peribiliary capillary plexi away from the basement membranes of the bile ducts

patic bile ducts, referred to as "onion skin" fibrosis, that displace the peribiliary capillary plexi, creating a physical and spatial barrier to oxygenation and maintenance of the cholehepatic countercurrent circulation between the bile duct and artery [14]. Thus, the pathogenesis of stricturing, circumferential peribiliary fibrosis also involves relative arterial or capillary ischemia. Stimuli of periductal fibrosis include secretion of chemokines and cytokines by innate immune cells and activated cholangiocytes and the inflammatory and fibrotic response to toxic bile leaking between injured cholangiocytes [4, 15]. Proinflammatory cytokines and/or microbial molecules in lymph or blood induce cholangiocyte expression of chemokine receptors and secretion of chemokines and cytokines involved in the chemoattraction of effector cells to the peribiliary space and promotion of fibrogenesis [4, 16].

Innate and Adaptive Immunity

Innate Immunity

Innate immunity provides immediate reactions against microbial pathogens and cells altered by stress, infection, or neoplasia [17, 18]. Innate immune responses are mediated by macrophages (including Kupffer cells), dendritic cells (DCs), natural killer (NK), and NKT cells. Macrophages and DCs constitutively express pattern recognition receptors (PRRs) for invariant microbial molecules, collectively called PAMPs, and for CD14 and activated complement (C') molecules. Toll-like receptors (TLRs) are the most prominent PRRs, expressed on innate immune cells and epithelial cells, including cholangiocytes and hepatocytes. Since PAMPs are molecular fragments of microbes, innate immune responses do not require viable microbes. PAMPs relevant to the immunopathogenesis of PSC [11, 19] include (1) lipopolysaccharide (LPS, aka endotoxin), the signature cell wall component of all Gram-negative bacteria; (2) lipoteichoic acid, the signature cell wall component of Gram-positive bacteria; (3) peptidoglycans, essential cell wall components of all bacteria; and (4) unmethylated, bacterial CpG dinucleotide motifs. Class I chain-related MICA and MICB genes encode ligands expressed by cells damaged by stress, infection, or neoplasia that bind to NKG2D receptors on NK cells, NKT cells, macrophages, and $\gamma\delta$T cells causing target cell lysis. In addition, MICA ligands also costimulate CD8 CTLs through their NKG2D receptors.

Innate Immunity in PSC

Intense, unregulated innate immune responses are involved in PSC immunopathogenesis [4, 20]. The cholangiocytes of PSC patients express normal amounts of TLR4 and nucleotide-binding oligomerization domain-containing protein (NOD)-like receptor family pyrin domain-containing 3 (NLRP3) but excessive TLR9 [21]. TLR9 expression correlated with fibrosis stages and greater risk for orthotopic liver transplantation (OLT). Cholangiocytes activated by TLRs, proinflammatory cytokines, and interferon-γ (IFNγ) produce cytokines and chemokines involved in the peribiliary localization of specific inflammatory cells and peribiliary fibrogenesis (Fig. 9.3, discussed below) [4, 9, 22].

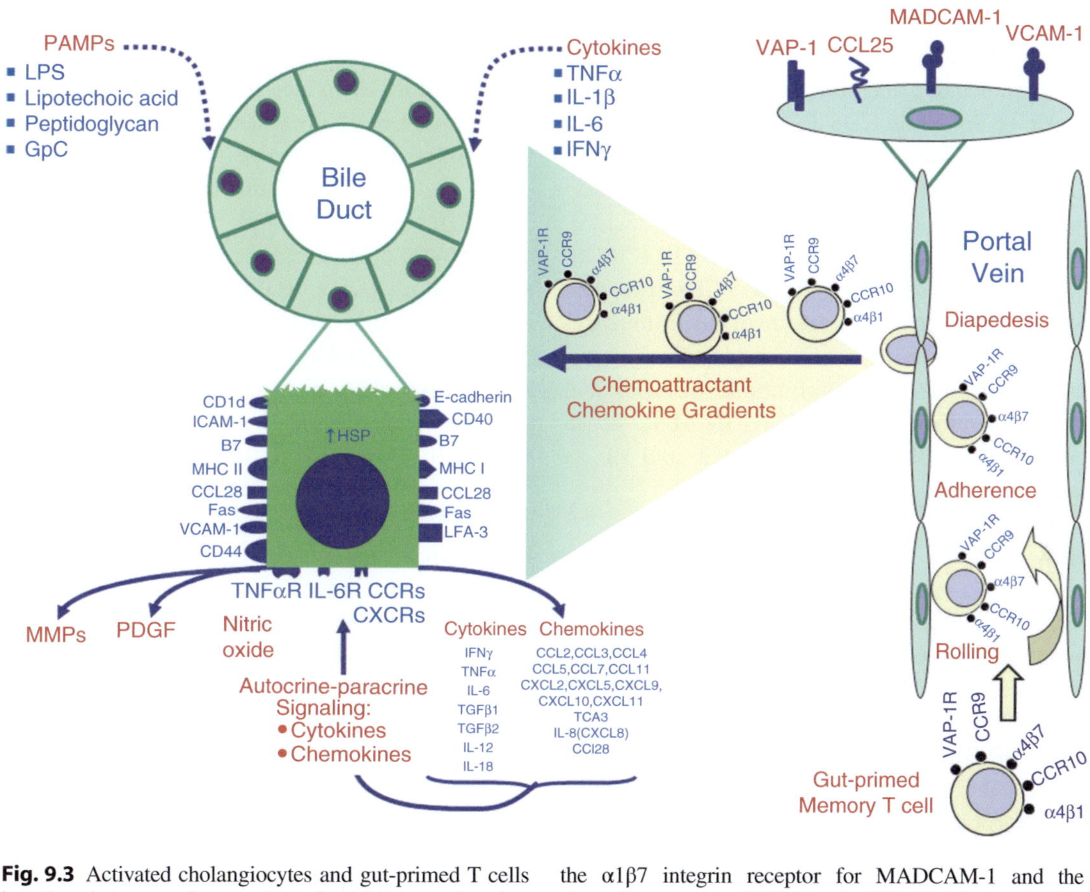

Fig. 9.3 Activated cholangiocytes and gut-primed T cells in the immunopathogenesis of primary sclerosing cholangitis. Cholangiocytes are activated by PAMPs and by proinflammatory cytokines TNFα, IL-1β, IL-6, and IFNγ. Activated gene expression leads to cholangiocyte production of multiple immunological ligands and receptors, chemokines, cytokines, MMPs, PDGF, NO, and aberrant class II HLA. In PSC, cholangiocytes secrete the chemokine CCL25, the ligand for CCR9 on gut-primed T cells. Portal endothelial cells in PSC livers express VAP-1, whose amine oxidase function in the presence of proinflammatory cytokines, especially TNFα, results in aberrant expression of MADCAM-1 and display of CCL25. This permits adhesion and diapedesis of gut-primed memory T cells bearing the α1β7 integrin receptor for MADCAM-1 and the chemokine receptor CCR9 for the CCL25. After transendothelial migration, gut-primed memory T cells migrate along the gradients of chemokines secreted by activated cholangiocytes to congregate in the peribiliary space. The chemokine CCL28 facilitates peribiliary recruitment of T cells bearing its chemokine receptor, CCR10, while VCAM-1 on the cell surface of cholangiocytes acts as ligand for the T cell integrin receptor α1β4. This postulated scheme does not require the presence of gut Ag(s) that originally primed the T cells in the GALT. The absence of cholangiocyte expression of the priming gut Ag(s) may explain the observation that peribiliary T cells do not cause apoptosis of cholangiocytes in PSC

Adaptive Immunity

Adaptive immunity involves delayed immune responses of T cell receptors (TCRs) to processed peptide antigens (Ags, potentially including autoAgs) presented within Ag-binding grooves of class I and II major histocompatibility complex molecules (MHC, designated HLA in humans) expressed by professional antigen-presenting cells (APCs) [23, 24]. Professional APCs include DCs of the innate immune system and activated B cells. CD4 T cell TCRs react with processed exogenous Ags presented by class II MHC molecules and stimulate Ag-specific CD4 T cell TCRs, while CD8 TCRs are stimulated by endogenous (including viral) Ags presented by class I MHC molecules. MHC binding of specific peptide Ags is genetically determined [25, 26]. The non-polymorphic MHC class I-like molecule, CD-1, presents lipid Ags to TCRs expressed by γδT cells. γδT cells are involved in mucosal immunity, surveillance of neoplastic changes, and protection from autoimmune diseases and microbial infections [27]. Class III MHC genes encode TNFα/β; C' factors C4, C2, and Bf; as well as heat shock proteins [25, 26].

HLA

HLA genes are inherited from each parent to form haplotype pairs [25, 26]. Class I HLA, expressed by HLA-A, HLA-B, and HLA-Cw loci, presents peptide Ags to TCRs of cytotoxic CD8 T cells. Class II HLA, expressed by HLA-DR, HLA-DQ, and HLA-DP loci, presents processed peptide Ags to TCRs of CD4 T cells. Polymorphic HLA class I and II Ag-binding grooves determine whether binding and presentation of specific peptide Ags occur, thus conferring susceptibility or resistance to development of a disease like PSC. The class III locus encodes polymorphic immune response proteins, including TNFα/β, complement (C') factors, and heat shock proteins.

Effector T Cells and Cytokines

Ag activation of CD4 T helper (Th) cells triggers exclusive pathways of differentiation that generate Ag-specific Th1, Th2, Th17, Th9, and T follicular helper (Tfh) cells and T regulatory (Treg) subsets [28]. A milieu containing IL-12, IL-18, and INFγ favors CD4 differentiation into Th1 cells that secrete the signature cytokines of Th1 cells: IL-2, INFγ, and TNFα/β. Th1 cytokines provide help for proliferation and differentiation of CD8 T cells, also called cytotoxic T lymphocytes (CTLs), and activate macrophages. Th1 cytokines also induce B cell secretion of C'-fixing IgG2a. In contrast, a milieu containing IL-4 favors CD4 differentiation into Th2 that secretes the signature cytokine profile of Th2 cells, IL, and activates eosinophils and mast cells. The signature cytokines of CD4 Th1 inhibit the proliferation of Th2 cells and vice versa, creating a dynamic balance between Th1 and Th2 subsets within inflammatory infiltrates. Transforming growth factor-beta (TGFβ), IL-6, IL-21, IL-23, and retinoic acid receptor-related orphan receptors γ and α (RORγ, RORα) promote generation of Th17 cells that can become either protective or pathogenic. Both Th1 IFNγ and Th2 IL-4 inhibit Th17 differentiation. Pathogenic Th17 cells are induced by IL-23 and IL-1β to secrete IL-17A, IL-17F, IL-21, and IL-22. In autoimmunity, Th17 effector cells intensify and perpetuate tissue inflammation. Th9 cells have not been evaluated in PSC; however, several functions indicate that they may be relevant to immunopathogenesis [29]. For example, secretion of IL-9 increases gut permeability, activates mast cells, and increases leukocyte recruitment. Th9 cells also secrete IL-21, which promotes IFNγ production by NK cells and CD8 T cells, and IL-3, which enhances DC survival. Tfh cells localize within B cell follicles in lymph nodes and Peyer's patches, where they promote selection and survival of B cell clones by expression of CD40 ligand and secretion of IL-4 and IL-21 [30].

CD4 Treg cells mediate Ag-specific suppression of T cell responses by local secretion of IL-10 and transforming growth factor-beta (TGFβ) [28]. The protective Th17 subset of Treg17 cells is induced by IL-6 and TGFβ.

Adaptive Immunity in PSC

Recent studies have focused on the role and functions of Tregs in PSC. Genome-wide association studies (GWAS) identified single nucleotide polymorphisms (SNPs) that could affect Treg cells, which led to studies of circulating and hepatic quantities of $CD4^{+}$-$CD25^{high}$-$FOXP3^{+}$-$CD127^{low}$ Tregs [31]. Tregs were significantly decreased in the blood and liver, and their suppressor function was reduced. Reduced Tregs in the blood significantly correlated with homozygosity for the major allele of the SNP rs10905718 in the IL-2RA gene. These findings provide a genetic basis for immune dysregulation caused by reduced Treg numbers in PSC. Another study of Tregs in peripheral blood mononuclear cells (PBMC) of patients with concurrent PSC and UC showed higher frequencies of Tregs compared to those in patients with UC alone [32].

Among the autoAbs associated with PSC is an IgA anti-cholangiocyte Ab, which occurs at high frequency and is correlated with more rapid progression to death or OLT compared to PSC patients without this autoAb [33]. The signature cytokine of Th17 cells, IL-17A, promotes hepatic inflammation and fibrosis [34]. To investigate Th17 immune responses to pathogens in PSC, hepatic bile obtained using endoscopic retrograde cholangiopancreatography (ERCP) was cultured, and liver biopsies were stained using 16sRNA fluorescence in situ hybridization (FISH) [34]. The bile grew multiple bacterial and fungal species and FISH detected microbes in 12 of 13 (92 %) of portal tracts. Stimulation PBMC with microbes cultured from the bile generated high frequencies of Th17 cells, especially in response to *Candida albicans*. Th17 cells expressing IL-17A were detected in the peribiliary space, indicating a pathogenic role in the generation of fibrosing inflammation.

Transendothelial Leukocyte Trafficking into Tissues

Activated, circulating leukocytes enter tissues by a multistep process of transendothelial migration [8, 9, 16]. Cellular injury or stress causes secretion of chemokines that are taken up by endothelial cells and displayed on their luminal surfaces along with adhesion molecules. As circulating, activated leukocytes expressing chemokine receptors and counter-receptors for adhesion molecules encounter activated endothelial cells, their leukocyte selectin receptors cause them to roll along the endothelium. Rolling ceases when firm leukocyte adhesion occurs due to binding of leukocyte chemokine receptors to chemokines displayed by endothelial cells and leukocyte integrin adhesion molecules to endothelial cellular adhesion molecules. This initiates diapedesis of leukocytes through endothelial tight junctions and basement membranes into the tissue, where they are chemoattracted along the chemokine gradient toward the source of chemokine secretion. Thus, both chemokines and adhesion molecules expressed on the endothelium determine the composition of inflammatory infiltrates entering the tissue from the blood. As discussed below, this process appears to play a key role in the immunopathogenesis of PSC [8, 9, 16].

Progress Toward an Understanding of Immunopathogenesis

Genetics

Genome-Wide Association Studies (GWAS)

Genetic susceptibility to PSC was assessed in a GWAS of 443,816 single nucleotide polymorphisms (SNPs) in 285 Norwegian PSC patients and 298 healthy controls [35]. Detected associations were reassessed in independent case-control panels in 766 PSC patients and 2,935 controls from Scandinavia, Belgium, the Netherlands, and Germany. The strongest associations were near the HLA-B locus (rs3099844, OR –4.8, 95 % CI 3.6–6.5, $p=2.6 \times 10^{-26}$, and rs2844559, OR 4.7, 95 % CI 3.5–6.4, $p=4.2 \times 10^{-26}$). Non-HLA rs9524260 on chromosome 13q31 was significantly associated with three of four groups. This locus encodes glycan 6, and inhibition of glycan 6 in a cholangiocyte cell line resulted in upregulation of proinflammatory markers.

Subsequent dense genotyping of 130,422 SNPs in immune-related disease regions was performed in 3,789 PSC patients of European ancestry and compared with 2,079 controls [36]. In addition to confirming three significant non-HLA associations, nine new non-HLA associations were detected. Six of the nine were more strongly associated with PSC than with comorbid IBD. These studies have expanded the genetic risk map of PSC, providing a better understanding of the relationship of PSC and other immune-mediated diseases.

Fucosyltransferase 2 (FUT2)

FUT2 introduces fucose into glycoproteins and glycolipids. FUT2 activity influences interactions between the host and microbes [37]. The nonsense mutation G428A and missense mutation A385T are the principal variants that cause 20 % of people to be FUT2 "nonsecretors," incapable of secreting fucose-containing Ags and lacking epithelial cell fucosylation. GWAS indicated that inactivating FUT2 variants were associated with PSC, Crohn's disease, and biochemical markers of biliary injury [37]. The microbiome of nonsecretors was characterized by reduced bifidobacteria, increased *Firmicutes*, and decreased *Proteobacteria* and *Actinobacteria*. The bacterial content of the bile also differed from that of secretors. Lack of fucosylated glycans on the surface of cholangiocytes is potentially deleterious because it would interrupt the glycocalyx required for the protective biliary bicarbonate umbrella that shields cholangiocytes from hydrophobic bile salt toxicity.

HLA and Susceptibility to PSC

PSC susceptibility is most strongly associated with four distinct HLA haplotypes (Table 9.2) [35, 38–41]. The highest susceptibility is conferred by homozygosity for MICA*008 (OR 5.01), suggesting that this allele is closely linked to a true susceptibility allele [42]. The MICA*008 allele contains the MICA5.1 microsatellite allele, which explains the microsatellite's significant association with PSC. It is possible that the NKG2D ligand produced by the MICA*008 allele might explain the increased numbers of NK and γδT cells in PSC livers [43, 44]. The MICB microsatellite allele MICB24 is also significantly associated with PSC. Of note, PSC associations with both MICA5.1 and MICB24 microsatellites are observed exclusively with the HLA-B8-DR3 haplotype [45].

Table 9.2 Immunogenetic associations of PSC with HLA and non-HLA alleles

Susceptibility haplotypes	*Odds ratio*
B8-MICA*008-TNFA*2-DRB3*0101-DRB1*0301-DQA1*0501 DQB1*0201	2.69
DRB3*0101-DRB1*1301-DQA1*0103-DQB1*0603	3.80
MICA*008-DRB5*0101-DRB1*1501-DQA1*0102-DQB1*0602	1.52
(MICA*008 homozygosity)	5.01
Resistance haplotypes	
DRB4*-DRB1*0401-DQA1*0301-DQB1*0302	0.26
DRB4*-DRB1*0701-DQA1*0201-DQB1*0303	0.15
MICA*002	0.12
Non-MHC associations	
ICAM-1	NA
MMP-1, MMP-3	NA
CTLA4	NA
CCR5Δ32 deletion	NA
CFTR	NA

The fact that the HLA-DR3 haplotype is absent from the other two HLA haplotypes associated with the second greatest susceptibility risk (OR 3.80) has been interpreted as evidence of linkage disequilibrium among HLA-B8, MICA*008, TNFα promoter (TNFA*2), and a yet unidentified susceptibility allele. Since DRB1 alleles are present in all three extended susceptibility HLA haplotypes, V or G at position 86 of the DRβ chain was analyzed. V86 was associated with susceptibility alleles DRB1*0301, DRB1*1301, and DRB1*1501 (OR 3.01), while G86 was associated with resistance alleles DRB1*0401 and DRB1*04 (OR 0.17). Modeling of susceptibility and resistance indicated that K87 and P55 in the DQB also could explain susceptibility (OR 2.78) or resistance (OR 0.28).

Of interest, one of the HLA susceptibility haplotypes contains the TNFA*2 allele (Table 9.2). Autoimmunity is associated with TNF-2 allele -308A [46], but a G-308A substitution in the TNFα promoter is linked with susceptibility only with the DRB3*0101 haplotype [47]. PSC susceptibility was not associated with the A to G polymorphism of Fas (encoded by the TNFSF6 gene) [48].

A single HLA susceptibility allele may exist in PSC, but it is more likely that PSC susceptibility is genetically complex, involving multiple HLA and non-HLA SNPs. Currently, PSC susceptibility can be explained for only 50 % of PSC cases on the basis of any allele, amino acid substitutions in the DRβ peptide, or homozygosity for MICA*008 [38]. This is independent of IBD, since UC is unassociated with these HLA haplotypes or MICA*008. Further investigations will require studies of SNPs identified in GWAS.

Susceptibility associations of HLA-DR3 and class III TNFA*2 and the G-308A substitution in the TNFα promoter may explain the association of PSC with AIDs [49]. HLA-DR3$^+$ leukocytes secrete significantly greater amounts of IL-2, IL-5, IL-12, and IFNγ than do HLA-DR3$^-$ leukocytes, before and after mitogen stimulation in vitro [50]. In contrast, HLA-DR3 haplotype does not influence secretion of anti-inflammatory Th2 cytokines IL-4 or IL-10. Susceptibility for PSC may reflect overproduction of TNFα and IFNγ. If high levels of these cytokines are obligatory for immunopathogenesis, it would be plausible that patients capable of generating similar levels of cytokines might develop PSC in the absence of HLA-DR3.

Non-MHC Genes and Susceptibility to PSC

Polymorphic non-HLA gene products involved in inflammation and immunoregulation may be biomarkers of progression and severity of PSC. No susceptibility associations have been identified for Nod2, IL-1, IL-1B, and IL-RN [19, 48]. CTLA4, a T cell receptor for costimulatory B7 ligands that downregulates T cell activation, is of great interest, since CTLA4 polymorphisms increase the risk of multiple organ-specific AIDs [51]. Susceptibility for PSC remains controversial, being present in one study and not in another [48]. The mutant chemokine receptor 5 with a deletion of 32 base pairs (CCR5Δ32) has reduced expression and function. Although initial results were controversial, a recent study showed that PSC susceptibility was significantly associated with CCR5Δ32 [52]. Fibrosis results from a dynamic imbalance between matrix metalloproteinases (MMPs) and inhibitors of metalloproteinases. The MMP-3 gene, encoding stromelysin, exhibits a promoter sequence polymorphism (5A or 6A repeat). A 5A allelic association was observed in one study but was not confirmed in another [53, 54]. The 5A allele was found more frequently in PSC patients with UC (60 %) than in PSC alone (45 %) [54]. The MMP-9 polymorphism R279Q was significantly associated with susceptibility [55]. No association was noted with MMP-1 promoter polymorphisms [54]. The TGFB1 gene encoding the profibrotic and immunosuppressive cytokine TGFβ was not associated with PSC [48]. The absence of the murine bile transporter, Mdr2 (Abcb4), caused regurgitation of toxic bile through leaky cholangiocyte tight junctions, resulting in PSC-like lesions. In contrast, PSC is characterized by normal bile acid transporter haplotypes for MDR3 (human homolog of murine Mdr2), ABCB4, and bile salt export protein (BSEP) ABCB11; thus, there is no evidence of a susceptibility association [56]. Of note, claudin-1 gene mutations compromise tight junctions and are associated with neonatal ichthyosis and sclerosing cholangitis [57]. PSC-like lesions in cystic fibrosis prompted testing for mutations in the cystic fibrosis transmembrane conductance regulator (CFTR). One report indicated an increased prevalence of CFTR mutations and defective nasal CFTR Cl^- channel function [58], but others failed to confirm these findings [59]. Induction of experimental colitis in cftr−/− knockout mice did cause PSC-like lesions, suggesting that CFTR mutations might contribute to pathogenesis of PSC in the presence of active IBD [60].

MHC Genes and Resistance to PSC

Three HLA haplotypes reduce the risk of PSC (Table 9.2). HLA-DR4 is the most protective; however, when PSC occurs in HLA-DR4-positive patients, they paradoxically have poorer prognosis and an increased risk of cholangiocarcinoma [61]. One copy of either the MICA*002 allele or its satellite allele MICA9 also confers significant resistance [42, 45]. Given the strong susceptibility risk of PSC bestowed by MICA*008, the resistance association with MICA*002 strongly suggests that MICA-encoded ligands for the NKG2D receptors of innate immune-responsive cells and CD8 CTLs are determinants of the immunopathogenesis of PSC. MICA allelic associations also imply involvement of innate immune effector cells and microbial PAMPs in immunopathogenesis.

Non-MHC Genes and Resistance to PSC

PSC patients have significantly lower frequencies for both ICAM-1 (CD54)-E469E homozygosity and its extended G241-E469/G241-E469 haplotype [62]. E469E homozygosity may protect against PSC by altering the adhesion required for transendothelial migration and target cell engagement. Resistance occurs with or without coexistent IBD.

Immunogenetics of Disease Progression and Complications of PSC

HLA and non-HLA alleles appear to be involved in PSC progression, severity, and complications. A study of HLA class II alleles in 265 PSC patients from five European countries reported that heterozygosity for the DRB1*03-DQA1*0501-DQB1*02 (HLA-DR3, HLA-DR2 extended haplotype) significantly increased the risk of death or liver transplantation (HR 1.63, 95 % CI 1.06–2.52) [63]. In the absence of HLA-DR3 and HLA-DR2, a HLA-DQ6 allele encoding DQB1*0603 or DQB1*0602 significantly reduced both risks (HR 0.57, 95 % CI 0.36–0.88). HLA-DR4 and HLA-DQ8 showed a nonsignificant trend for an increased risk of cholangiocarcinoma. The CCR5Δ32 genotype was more prevalent in advanced PSC (45 %) than in mild disease (21 %), suggesting that it promotes progression [52]. In MMP-3 gene encoding stromelysin, homozygosity for the 5A polymorphism was a significant risk for portal hypertension, indicative of a role in fibrogenesis [53].

Autoantibodies in PSC

Nuclear Envelope Autoantigens and Bacterial Mimicry

PSC is associated with a wide variety of autoAbs, many of which may be immunologic epiphenomena [64]. The most studied of the autoAbs in PSC are the atypical perinuclear antineutrophil cytoplasmic antibodies (pANCAs), which occur in ≤88 % of PSC patients, with or without UC [55, 65, 66]. In PSC, IBD, and AIH, pANCA autoAbs rarely react with the classical pANCA Ags: cytoplasmic actin, catalase, or enolase [67]. Instead, the atypical pANCAs in PSC react with nuclear envelope Ags in neutrophils rather than cytoplasmic Ags. This changed their designation to peripheral antineutrophil nuclear antibodies (pANNAs) [67].

Analyses of pANNA epitope specificity showed that 92 % of atypical pANNAs from patients with IBD or hepatobiliary diseases react with a 50 kDa myeloid-specific nuclear envelope protein [68] and subsequently identified a tubulin-beta isotype 5 [69]. Alpha and beta tubulins are highly conserved proteins that share 40 % aa sequence homology, undergo multiple posttranslational modifications, and have multiple isotypes [70]. pANNAs against tubulin-beta isotype 5 were not PSC specific, but also occurred in AIH [69]. Subsequent studies showed that pANNAs react with the highly conserved bacterial cell division protein FTsZ and that preabsorption of PSC sera with FTsZ abolished pANNA reactivity. This indicates molecular mimicry between bacterial FTsZ and nuclear Ags of human neutrophils [71]. Of note, pANNA titers do not decrease after transplantation or colectomy for UC [67]. pANNAs also may be correlated with biliary complications [72], intrahepatic rather than extrahepatic strictures [73], and cirrhosis at high titers [74]. Unfortunately, these studies were not powered sufficiently to reach firm conclusions.

Future studies of circulating and liver-infiltrating CD4 and CD8 T cell TCR reactions against tubulin-beta isotype 5 with appropriate healthy and diseased controls should clarify the importance of this autoAg/bacterial molecular mimic in PSC pathogenesis. Computer modeling of the binding affinities of putative autoAg(s) for HLA class II molecules associated with PSC susceptibility and resistance may help define their Ag specificities.

IgG ANCA in the bile is correlated significantly with PSC risk and formation of dominant strictures, but not with risk of death, OLT, or cholangiocarcinoma [75]. The frequency of pANCA is also significantly higher in UC than Crohn's disease [76]. Moreover, the combination of typical multi-Ag-specific ANCA, ANA, and SMA is 67 % sensitive for the diagnosis of PSC [76].

AutoAbs reacting with cholangiocytes have multiple consequences. The majority of PSC patients have serum IgA autoAbs that bind to cultured human cholangiocytes, while they are absent in the sera of healthy controls [33]. High titers correlated with total serum IgA levels and were clinically correlated with faster disease progression. IgG autoAbs in PSC sera also reacted against cultured human cholangiocytes and induced expression of TLR4 and TLR9 [77]. The addition of the LPS ligand for TLR4 and the CpG DNA ligand for TLR9 induced cholangiocytes to secrete copious amounts of proinflammatory cytokines, TNFα, Il-1β, and IL-6, along with IFNγ, TGFβ, and granulocyte-macrophage colony-stimulating factor. Bile ducts stained for TLR4 and TLR9 in biopsies of 58 % of PSC patients with IgG anti-cholangiocyte autoantibodies, indicating concordance between the in vitro observation and pathophysiology.

Induction of murine colitis by bacterial Ags and production of pANCA support the hypothesis that immune responses to bacterial Ags or other Ags cross-reactive with enteric Ags can induce pANNA in PSC [78, 79]. The fact that up to 81 % of PSC patients have antibodies against enterobacterial proteins also supports the hypothesis [65]. Bacterial/permeability-increasing protein (BPI), an endotoxin-binding neutrophil leukocyte-granular protein with antibacterial and antiendotoxin activity [80], is also an ANCA Ag in PSC, IBD, cystic fibrosis, and vasculitis [81]. Titers of BPI-ANCA correlate with inflammation and tissue damage, suggesting that BPI-ANCA might retard clearance of LPS, promoting inflammation and LPS stimulation of biliary TLR4 [77].

Cholangiocyte-Specific Autoantigens and CD44

Serum autoAbs reacting with human intrahepatic cholangiocytes from a healthy person were detected in 63 % of patients with PSC, 37 % with PBC, 16 % with AIH, and 8 % of healthy controls [82]. Western blotting showed that PSC patients exclusively had autoAbs reacting with a 40 kDa Ag. Anti-cholangiocyte antibodies from PSC and PBC patients, but not AIH patients, induced cholangiocyte secretion of proinflammatory IL-6, which stimulates cholangiocyte proliferation and inhibits apoptosis.

In PSC, but not PBC or AIH, both IgG and IgM autoAbs induced cholangiocyte expression of the CD44 cell adhesion receptor for the extracellular matrix ligand, hyaluronic acid, which also plays roles in cell proliferation, differentiation, presentation of cytokines, chemokines, and growth factors to their receptors, protease docking to cell membranes, and angiogenesis [83]. Blocking of the CD44v7 isoform on T cells and activated macrophages in an experimental murine model of IBD caused apoptosis of effector cells and clinical recovery [84]. Anti-CD44 reduced induction of experimental arthritis by collagen or proteoglycan PAMPs by preventing pathological interactions of synovial-like fibroblasts and cartilaginous matrix [85]. Thus, PSC-specific autoAbs against cholangiocyte autoAgs stimulate PSC-specific expression of CD44 isoforms potentially capable of reducing recruitment of effector leukocytes to the peribiliary space, suggesting the possibility of therapeutic inhibition of CD44 in PSC.

Nonspecific Autoantibodies

Multiple nonspecific autoAbs observed in PSC are likely epiphenomena related to chronic inflammation and immunogenetics favoring vigorous immune responses [64]. Frequencies of nonspecific autoAbs included antinuclear antibodies in 7–77 %, smooth muscle antibodies in 13–20 %, antimitochondrial antibodies in 0–9 %, anti-cardiologic antibodies in 4–66 %, anti-thyroperoxidase antibodies in 7–16 %, anti-thyroglobulin antibodies in 4 %, and anti-Ig rheumatoid factor in 15 %. AutoAbs against tropomycin found in either UC or PSC mediated antibody-dependent cellular cytotoxicity of cells expressing the HLA-DPw9 allele [86].

Immunological Epiphenomena

In addition to nonspecific autoAbs, multiple immunological abnormalities described in PSC also appear to be epiphenomena consistent with the concept that PSC is associated with disordered immunoregulation [55, 64, 66]. These abnormalities include evidence of:(1) Decreased proportions of peripheral blood T cells and CD8 T cells [87, 88](2) Increased proportions of circulating B cells [89](3) Decreased T suppressor cell function [90](4) Increased autologous mixed lymphocyte reactivity [91](5) C' activation with increased levels of C3b and C4d [92](6) Deposits of C3d on hepatic arteries, but not bile ducts [93] (7) Immune complexes in the blood and bile [94] (8) Diminished clearance of artificial immune complexes by Kupffer cells in vivo [95] and (9) Aberrant expression of blood group antigens on biliary and colonic epithelia [96]

Cholangiocytes in the Immunopathogenesis of PSC

Cholangiocytes as Immunological Targets in PSC

Ductopenia occurs in PSC; however, inflammatory-mediated apoptosis of cholangiocytes is absent in PSC [13]. In contrast, apoptosis is the hallmark of CD8 T cell-mediated nonsuppurative destructive cholangitis (NSDC) leading to ductopenia in PBC, chronic graft-versus-host disease (GVHD), and hepatic allograft rejection (HAR) [11]. The near absence of NSDC in PSC [97] is intriguing, since PSC cholangiocytes express an activated phenotype of increased class I HLA, aberrant class II HLA, and ICAM-1 that would facilitate recognition by Ag-specific CD8 CTLs. Portal infiltrates in PSC also differ from those in PBC by containing neutrophils, CD4 T >>CD8 T cells, macrophages, NK, and γδT cells [44, 87, 88, 98, 99]. Evidence of a paucity of peribiliary CD8 CTLs in the precirrhotic stages of PSC strongly argues against cholangiocytes as primary target cells [88].

Immunomodulatory Roles of Cholangiocytes

It is now clear that cholangiocytes, rather than being passive target cells or innocent bystanders, play a seminal role in determining the composition of peribiliary inflammatory infiltrates and likely participate in periductular fibrogenesis in PSC (Fig. 9.3) [4, 8, 11, 100, 101]. Activated cholangiocytes express TLR4 and TLR9 for the PAMP ligands LPS and unmethylated CpG DNA molecules, respectively. Cholangiocytes also have receptors for proinflammatory cytokines TNFα, IL-1β, IL-6, as well as IFNγ. These stimuli induce cholangiocyte expression of chemokine receptors and secretion of multiple chemokines, cytokines, matrix metalloproteinases, and growth factors that immunomodulate inflammation and fibrogenesis (Fig. 9.3). Cholangiocyte secretion of multiple chemokines in PSC (Fig. 9.3) dictates the composition of peribiliary inflammatory infiltrates containing innate immune cells and T cells bearing specific chemokine receptors, including a pathogenetic population of PSC-specific T cells primed in the gut (discussed below) [8, 102]. Secretions of profibrotic TGFβ by activated cholangiocytes, along with profibrogenic cytokines secreted by peribiliary inflammatory cells, are likely causes of the concentric layers of circumferential fibrosis characteristic of PSC.

Endothelial Cells and the Role of Arterial Ischemia in PSC

Direct injury of hepatic arteries or arterioles causes secondary ischemic sclerosing cholangitis [103–105]. While there is no evidence of an immunological attack against endothelial cells of hepatic arteries or peribiliary capillary plexi in PSC [14, 97], it is now clear that concentric layers of circumferential peribiliary fibrosis progressively push peribiliary capillary plexi away from the basement membranes of bile ducts [14]. An experimental mouse model [106] suggests that a microcirculatory barrier to diffusion of O_2 and nutrients and disruption of the cholehepatic circulation created by fibrous displacement of the peribiliary capillary plexi might explain the atrophic, senescent appearance of cholangiocytes in PSC. An unsubstantiated but correlative hypothesis postulated that biliary ischemia resulted from aberrant production of angiotensin II or endothelin by PSC cholangiocytes, leading to vasoconstriction of peribiliary capillary plexi and arterioles [107].

Emerging Role of Gut Microbiota

Gut microbiota play essential roles in health and disease. Published studies are limited but indicate that gut microbial profile in PSC is distinctly different than that in UC without PSC or healthy controls [108]. Specifically, PSC patients have significantly reduced bacterial diversity compared with healthy controls and a different microbial composition compared to either controls or patients with UC alone. Microbiota were similar for PSC patients, regardless of the presence or absence of IBD. Eleven of 12 microbial genera were reduced in PSC, while the *Veillonella* genus (anaerobic, Gram-negative cocci) was significantly increased compared with controls of patients with UC. Of potential importance, the *Veillonella* genus is associated with other chronic inflammatory and fibrotic conditions. A study of ileocecal biopsies confirmed the low microbial diversity in the gut microbiota of PSC patients and noted significantly lower abundance of uncultured *Clostridiales II* compared with controls or patients with UC [109]. As noted above, FUT2 nonsecretors have low abundance of fecal bifidobacteria, *Proteobacteria*, and *Actinobacteria* and an increase in *Firmicutes* [37]. Finally, a study of the microbiota of the bile showed *Helicobacter pylori* DNA in microdissected hilar bile ducts in 9 of 56 (16%) end-stage PSC patients, suggesting that bile reflux can carry *H. pylori* into the distal biliary tract from the duodenum [110]. Further studies of the microbiota should lead to an understanding of the gut-liver axis in health and disease [111].

Immunopathogenic Role of Gut-Primed T Cells, Aberrant Expression of Adhesion Molecules, Chemokines, and Cytokines

A series of elegant studies have brought the immunomodulatory roles of cholangiocytes and the portal venous and arterial endothelia to the forefront of studies of PSC immunopathogenesis [8, 102]. Collectively, these studies demonstrated that hepatic inflammatory infiltrates in PSC contain T cells primed by Ags in gut-associated lymphoid tissues (GALT). These studies also link the immunopathogenesis of PSC to that of IBD [101, 112–116]. Early studies of extraintestinal manifestations of IBD in the eye, skin, and synovial tissues showed that inflammation was mediated by gut-primed lymphocytes that had inappropriately migrated to these tissues [9]. A similar pathogenetic mechanism in PSC did not appear likely, since PSC can occur in the absence of active gut inflammation, may be present years before the onset of IBD, or may even begin after total colectomy for UC. This led to the hypothesis that PSC is mediated by memory T cells primed in the gut that migrated into the peribiliary space as a result of aberrant expression of gut-specific adhesion molecules and cholangiocyte secretion of gut-specific chemokines [114, 116, 117]. Ag-specific activation of naïve T cells by gut DCs in Peyer's patches and mesenteric lymph nodes produces a gut-specific T cell phenotype (Fig. 9.3) characterized by expression of $\alpha 4\beta 7$ and $\alpha 4\beta 1$ integrins and chemokine receptors CCR9 and CCR10 [118, 119]. Hepatic DCs are incapable of imprinting this gut-specific phenotype.

Normally, circulating memory T cells of this phenotype interact only with gut endothelial cells, due to exclusive endothelial expression of the gut addressin mucosal vascular address cell adhesion molecule-1 (MADCAM-1) and the chemokine ligand CCL25, which bind to gut-primed T cell $\alpha 4\beta 7$ and CCR9, respectively. Evidence that portal venous endothelial cells in PSC, but not other inflammatory liver diseases, aberrantly express MADCAM-1 and CCL25 provided a novel mechanism for the homing of gut-primed T cells into the portal tracts.

Further studies showed that the aberrant expression of MADCAM-1 on hepatic endothelial cells was caused by the physiologic interaction of natural dietary and microbial amines and vascular adhesion protein-1 (VAP-1) present on hepatic endothelial cells. VAP-1 functions as an adhesion molecule for the VAP-1 receptor (VAP-1R) and as an amine oxidase. The amine oxidase function of endothelial VAP-1 activates endothelial cell production of H_2O_2, which, in the presence of proinflammatory cytokines (e.g., TNFα), leads to activation of NFkB and ultimately aberrant expression of MADCAM-1 and CCL25 by portal venous endothelial cells. In accord with VAP-1 roles in adhesion and amine metabolism, the absence of hepatic endothelial VAP-1 in VAP-1$^{-/-}$ knockout mice significantly reduced both portal inflammation and fibrosis in murine models of hepatic injury [8]. As discussed above, PSC cholangiocytes activated by cytokines, PAMPs, or autoAbs also secrete the CCL25 chemokine required for transendothelial migration of gut-primed T cells into the portal tracts (Fig. 9.3). Cholangiocyte secretion of CCL25 explains migration of gut-primed CCR9-positive T cells along the concentration gradient to the peribiliary space.

Peribiliary localization and survival of gut-primed T cells also involve cholangiocyte expression of additional adhesion molecules and chemokines [8]. Cholangiocyte expressions of CCL28 and vascular cell adhesion molecule-1 (VCAM-1) appear to play critical roles for peribiliary recruitment of gut-primed T cells expressing the α4β1 integrin receptor for VCAM-1 and the CCL28 ligand for the chemokine receptor CCR10. Since cholangiocyte expression of CCL28 has been observed in other chronic inflammatory liver diseases, its role in chemoattraction of CCR10-positive T cells is nonspecific. However, stimulation of cholangiocyte TLR4 with LPS and the proinflammatory cytokine IL-1β, both shown to be present in PSC, induces secretion of CCL28, augmenting the α4β1 interaction of T cells with cholangiocyte VCAM-1. In contrast, neither TNFα nor IFNγ induces cholangiocyte secretion of CCL28. Thus, the innate immune response of the cholangiocytes to LPS in a proinflammatory cytokine milieu appears necessary for transendothelial migration and peribiliary recruitment of gut-primed T cells.

Gut-primed T cells appear to be activated by enteric Ags or Ags that cross-react with enterocytes. T cell lines propagated from the inflamed common bile ducts of two PSC patients expressed oligoclonal TCRs, indicating recruitment of T cells activated by a limited number of Ags [120]. Since TCR oligoclonality was unchanged in a second biopsy performed more than a year later, it appeared that extrahepatic T cells expressing oligoclonal TCRs were repopulating the periductal tissue, possibly from mesenteric lymph nodes or Peyer's patches. These T cells proliferated in response to human enterocytes and mediated enterocyte cytotoxicity, consistent with gut-specific Ag stimulation. T cells from other PSC livers also preferentially expressed Vβ3 TCR [121], which did not correlate with the histopathological stage of disease.

Other studies showed that liver-infiltrating lymphocytes in PSC contain T cells that proliferate poorly to mitogens, have intracytoplasmic IL-1β and TNFα, and secrete copious amounts of IL-1β and TNFα and lower levels of IL-2, IL-10, and IFNγ in vitro [122]. Neither hepatic T cells nor NK cells were cytotoxic in vitro. Anti-TNFα antibodies partially restored the proliferation and cytotoxicity of PSC liver-infiltrating lymphocytes, suggesting an immunopathogenic role for high portal tract concentrations of TNFα. The fact that Kupffer cells in PSC are threefold greater in number than in other liver diseases [123] may increase the amounts of IL-1β and TNFα in peribiliary lymphatics. Serum levels of the major profibrotic cytokine TGFβ are also significantly increased in PSC, presumably due to secretion by Kupffer cells, portal macrophages, and cholangiocytes chronically stimulated by proinflammatory cytokines [123].

It remains unknown whether transendothelial migration of gut-primed T cells into the portal tracts can be mediated solely by hepatic endothelial cells expressing VAP-1 and aberrantly expressing MADCAM-1 and CCL25 or also requires expression of the original priming Ag(s). The absence of gut-primed T cell-mediated cytolysis of cholangiocytes suggests that cholangiocyte HLA molecules do not express priming antigenic peptides [13]. Chronic portal and peribiliary inflammation may be intensified by Th17 cells, and expression of multiple cholangiocyte adhesion molecules and chemokines induced by PAMPs and proinflammatory cytokines likely determines the composition of portal inflammatory infiltrates in PSC [34]. This may explain the fact that only 20 % of portal inflammatory cells are gut-primed T cells [8]. However, the composition of the portal inflammatory infiltrates does not adequately explain why lesions of fibrous obliterative cholangitis associated with periductal concentric fibrosis occur only sporadically along the lengths of individual bile ducts and are absent in the small duct variant of PSC.

Key Unanswered Questions About PSC Immunopathogenesis

It remains unknown if circulating gut-primed, memory T cells provide immunological surveillance of both the liver and gut prior to initiation of PSC or only after hepatobiliary injury and proinflammatory cytokines facilitate VAP-1 induction of aberrant hepatic expression of MADCAM-1 and CCL25. Were livers of patients susceptible to PSC to express aberrant MADCAM-1 and CCL25 prior to the onset of PSC, it would suggest that the development of PSC requires a "second hit" such as cholangiocyte activation by PAMPs and proinflammatory IL-1β to induce VCAM-1 and secretion of CCL25 and CCL28 for recruitment and migration of gut-primed T cells to the peribiliary space.

Conversely, if VAP-1-mediated aberrant expression of hepatic endothelial MADCAM-1 and CCL25 were to occur only as an initial manifestation of overt PSC, then the etiopathogenesis of PSC would require a "multi-hit" hypothesis. Recurrence of PSC in transplanted liver allografts strongly suggests that aberrant expression of MADCAM-1 and CCL25 is not a primary expression of susceptibility but instead can be induced in a previously non-susceptible allograft. The role of the gut in posttransplant recurrence remains intriguing, since colectomy performed prior to or at the time of transplant protects against recurrence of PSC in UC patients. Colectomy performed later after transplant has no protective effect.

Animal studies support the key roles for PAMPs and proinflammatory cytokines in PSC immunopathogenesis [124]. PAMP-induced colitis with muramyl peptide [125] and *Escherichia coli* chemotactic peptide N-formyl L-leucine L-tyrosine (fMLT) [126] was complicated by PSC-likc hepatic lesions. In genetically susceptible rats, the PAMP peptidoglycan-polysaccharide produced by small bowel bacterial overgrowth in a surgically created blind loop caused PAMP production, portal inflammation, bile ductular proliferation, and strictures of both intra- and extrahepatic bile ducts [127, 128]. Injury was correlated significantly with TNFα production by Kupffer cells. Mutanolysin cleavage of peptidoglycan-polysaccharide, palmitate blockade of Kupffer cell phagocytosis, and pentoxifylline inhibition of TNFα secretion by Kupffer cells prevented hepatobiliary inflammation and biliary strictures. These data are in accord with evidence that PSC susceptibility is associated with the class III HLA TNFA*2 allele and that patients with extended HLA-DR3 haplotypes secrete excessive amounts of TNFα. PAMPs and proinflammatory cytokines appear to play seminal roles in the immunopathogenesis of PSC.

Bile Regurgitation into the Peribiliary Space and Consequences of Biliary Obstruction

Bile contains noxious constituents, including toxic hydrophobic bile acids, PAMPs, and glycoproteins. Regurgitation of the bile into the peribiliary space as a result of disruption of the tight junctions between cholangiocytes results in toxic bile injury and periductal concentric fibrosis in the Mdr2 (Abcb4)$^{-/-}$ knockout mouse model [15]. Regurgitation of the bile into the peribiliary space induces neutrophilic inflammation, followed by lymphocytic infiltration and production of both proinflammatory cytokines and profibrotic TGFβ. As observed in PSC, progressive laminations of periductal fibrous tissue displace peribiliary capillary plexi, and cholangiocytes became atrophic, presumably due to microcirculatory ischemia and nutrient deprivation. Biliary casts showed focal, macroscopic strictures and ectasias similar to those seen in PSC. However, PSC is not associated with abnormal haplotypes for MDR3, the human homolog of murine Mdr2.

Although the bile in the Mdr2 $(Abcb4)^{-/-}$ knockout mouse contains increased proportions of hydrophobic bile acids, it is important to note that the bile also contains other constituents with potential roles in immunopathogenesis. For example, fMLT, a chemotactic peptide of *Escherichia coli* in portal venous blood, is also secreted by hepatocytes into the bile [129]. CD66a, also known as biliary glycoprotein, is also present in the human bile [130]. As the human homolog of rat cell adhesion molecule, it is expressed by neutrophils, monocytes, ductular epithelia, endothelial cells, gut intraepithelial lymphocytes, and myoepithelial cells within infiltrative scars and sclerosing adenosis of the breast [131]. CD66a binds to E-selectin, galectin-3, and bacterial type 1 fimbriae and CD66b/66c and inhibits the cytotoxic function of gut intraepithelial lymphocytes [132]. Thus, several constituents of the bile may modulate inflammation and possibly fibrogenesis if they were regurgitated into the portal tracts.

Contribution of Biliary Obstruction to Pathogenesis

Obstruction of the biliary tract results in increased proximal intraluminal pressures, increasing the potential for bile regurgitation. Experimental obstruction results in increased LPS concentrations in portal tracts; innate immune activation of Kupffer cells and portal tract macrophages by LPS and/or other PAMPs; secretion of proinflammatory cytokines IL-1β, TNFα, IL-6, TGFα/β, and leukotrienes by macrophages; leaky cholangiocyte tight junctions; and regurgitation of the bile into the peribiliary space [133, 134]. Accumulation of LPS inhibits cholangiocyte HCO_3^- secretion (required for the protective biliary bicarbonate umbrella) and compromises cholehepatic cycling between cholangiocytes and displaced peribiliary capillaries that may prevent removal of noxious molecules from the peribiliary space. A peribiliary milieu of proinflammatory cytokines, chemokines, and LPS recruits and activates neutrophils, monocytes, and T cells. Biliary obstruction also induces ductular proliferation of cholangiocytes lining canals of Hering at the margin of the portal tracts [97]. Proliferating ductules secrete platelet-derived growth factor (PDGF) [133], a potent mitogen for activated stellate cells, that promotes results in projections of fibrous septa into the parenchyma and, ultimately, secondary biliary cirrhosis.

References

1. Williamson KD, Chapman RW. Primary sclerosing cholangitis. Dig Dis. 2014;32(4):438–45.
2. Hirschfield GM, Karlsen TH, Lindor KD, Adams DH. Primary sclerosing cholangitis. Lancet. 2013; 382(9904):1587–99.
3. de Vries AB, Janse M, Blokzijl H, Weersma RK. Distinctive inflammatory bowel disease phenotype in primary sclerosing cholangitis. World J Gastroenterol. 2015;21(6):1956–71.
4. O'Mahony CA, Vierling JM. Etiopathogenesis of primary sclerosing cholangitis. Semin Liver Dis. 2006;26(1):3–21.
5. Zen Y, Kawakami H, Kim JH. IgG4-related sclerosing cholangitis: all we need to know. J Gastroenterol. 2016;51(4):295–312.
6. Benito de Valle M, Muller T, Bjornsson E, Otten M, Volkmann M, Guckelberger O, et al. The impact of elevated serum IgG4 levels in patients with primary sclerosing cholangitis. Dig Liver Dis. 2014;46(10): 903–8.
7. Doorenspleet ME, Hubers LM, Culver EL, Maillette de Buy Wenniger LJ, Klarenbeek PL, Chapman RW, et al. IgG4+ B-cell receptor clones distinguish IgG4-related disease from primary sclerosing cholangitis and biliary/pancreatic malignancies. Hepatology. 2016;64(2):501–507.
8. Trivedi PJ, Adams DH. Mucosal immunity in liver autoimmunity: a comprehensive review. J Autoimmun. 2013;46:97–111.
9. Eksteen B, Miles AE, Grant AJ, Adams DH. Lymphocyte homing in the pathogenesis of extra-intestinal manifestations of inflammatory bowel disease. Clin Med (Lond). 2004;4(2):173–80.
10. Alpini G, McGill JM, Larusso NF. The pathobiology of biliary epithelia. Hepatology. 2002;35(5): 1256–68.
11. Vierling JM, Braun M, Wang H-M. Immunopathogenesis of vanishing bile duct syndromes. In: Alpini G, Alvaro D, Marzioni M, LeSage G, Larusso N, editors. The pathophysiology of biliary epithelia. Georgetown: Landes Bioscience; 2004. p. 330–56.
12. Scheuer PJ. Ludwig symposium on biliary disorders – part II. Pathologic features and evolution of primary biliary cirrhosis and primary sclerosing cholangitis. Mayo Clin Proc. 1998;73(2):179–83.

13. Kawata K, Kobayashi Y, Gershwin ME, Bowlus CL. The immunophysiology and apoptosis of biliary epithelial cells: primary biliary cirrhosis and primary sclerosing cholangitis. Clin Rev Allergy Immunol. 2012;43(3):230–41.
14. Washington K, Clavien PA, Killenberg P. Peribiliary vascular plexus in primary sclerosing cholangitis and primary biliary cirrhosis. Hum Pathol. 1997; 28(7):791–5.
15. Fickert P, Pollheimer MJ, Beuers U, Lackner C, Hirschfield G, Housset C, et al. Characterization of animal models for primary sclerosing cholangitis (PSC). J Hepatol. 2014;60(6):1290–303.
16. Borchers AT, Shimoda S, Bowlus C, Keen CL, Gershwin ME. Lymphocyte recruitment and homing to the liver in primary biliary cirrhosis and primary sclerosing cholangitis. Semin Immunopathol. 2009; 31(3):309–22.
17. Mathison J. Innate immunity. J Pediatr Gastroenterol Nutr. 2005;40 Suppl 1:S13–5.
18. Staros EB. Innate immunity: new approaches to understanding its clinical significance. Am J Clin Pathol. 2005;123(2):305–12.
19. Podolsky DK. Innate immunity, NOD-2 and primary sclerosing cholangitis. http://videocast.nih.gov/PastEvents.asp. NIDDK Research Workshop on Primary Sclerosing Cholangitis 2005.
20. Harada K, Nakanuma Y. Innate immunity in the pathogenesis of cholangiopathy: a recent update. Inflamm Allergy Drug Targets. 2012;11(6):478–83.
21. Matsushita H, Miyake Y, Takaki A, Yasunaka T, Koike K, Ikeda F, et al. TLR4, TLR9, and NLRP3 in biliary epithelial cells of primary sclerosing cholangitis: relationship with clinical characteristics. J Gastroenterol Hepatol. 2015;30(3):600–8.
22. Adams DH, Afford SC. The role of cholangiocytes in the development of chronic inflammatory liver. Front Biosci. 2002;7:e276–85.
23. Delves PJ, Roitt IM. The immune system. Second of two parts. N Engl J Med. 2000;343(2):108–17.
24. Delves PJ, Roitt IM. The immune system. First of two parts. N Engl J Med. 2000;343(1):37–49.
25. Klein J, Sato A. The HLA system. Second of two parts. N Engl J Med. 2000;343(11):782–6.
26. Klein J, Sato A. The HLA system. First of two parts. N Engl J Med. 2000;343(10):702–9.
27. Ulrichs T, Porcelli SA. CD1 proteins: targets of T cell recognition in innate and adaptive immunity. Rev Immunogenet. 2000;2(3):416–32.
28. Hirahara K, Nakayama T. CD4+ T-cell subsets in inflammatory diseases: beyond the Th1/Th2 paradigm. Int Immunol. 2016;28(4):163–71.
29. Kaplan MH, Hufford MM, Olson MR. The development and in vivo function of T helper 9 cells. Nat Rev Immunol. 2015;15(5):295–307.
30. Ivanova EA, Orekhov AN. T helper lymphocyte subsets and plasticity in autoimmunity and cancer: an overview. Biomed Res Int. 2015;2015:327470.
31. Sebode M, Peiseler M, Franke B, Schwinge D, Schoknecht T, Wortmann F, et al. Reduced FOXP3(+) regulatory T cells in patients with primary sclerosing cholangitis are associated with IL2RA gene polymorphisms. J Hepatol. 2014;60(5):1010–6.
32. Kekilli M, Tunc B, Beyazit Y, Kurt M, Onal IK, Ulker A, et al. Circulating CD4+CD25+ regulatory T cells in the pathobiology of ulcerative colitis and concurrent primary sclerosing cholangitis. Dig Dis Sci. 2013;58(5):1250–5.
33. Berglin L, Bjorkstrom NK, Bergquist A. Primary sclerosing cholangitis is associated with autoreactive IgA. Scand J Gastroenterol. 2013;48(6):719–28.
34. Katt J, Schwinge D, Schoknecht T, Quaas A, Sobottka I, Burandt E, et al. Increased T helper type 17 response to pathogen stimulation in patients with primary sclerosing cholangitis. Hepatology. 2013; 58(3):1084–93.
35. Karlsen TH, Franke A, Melum E, Kaser A, Hov JR, Balschun T, et al. Genome-wide association analysis in primary sclerosing cholangitis. Gastroenterology. 2010;138(3):1102–11.
36. Liu JZ, Hov JR, Folseraas T, Ellinghaus E, Rushbrook SM, Doncheva NT, et al. Dense genotyping of immune-related disease regions identifies nine new risk loci for primary sclerosing cholangitis. Nat Genet. 2013;45(6):670–5.
37. Maroni L, van de Graaf SF, Hohenester SD, Oude Elferink RP, Beuers U. Fucosyltransferase 2: a genetic risk factor for primary sclerosing cholangitis and Crohn's disease – a comprehensive review. Clin Rev Allergy Immunol. 2015;48(2–3):182–91.
38. Donaldson PT. Genetics of primary sclerosing cholangitis. http://videocast.nih.gov/PastEvents.asp. NIDDK Research Workshop on Primary Sclerosing Cholangitis 2005.
39. Donaldson PT. Genetics of autoimmune and viral liver diseases; understanding the issues. J Hepatol. 2004;41(2):327–32.
40. Donaldson PT. Genetics of liver disease: immunogenetics and disease pathogenesis. Gut. 2004;53(4): 599–608.
41. Webb GJ, Hirschfield GM. Genetics of autoimmune liver disease: a brief summary for clinicians. Dig Dis. 2014;32(5):e1–6.
42. Norris S, Kondeatis E, Collins R, Satsangi J, Clare M, Chapman R, et al. Mapping MHC-encoded susceptibility and resistance in primary sclerosing cholangitis: the role of MICA polymorphism. Gastroenterology. 2001;120(6):1475–82.
43. Hata K, Van Thiel DH, Herberman RB, Whiteside TL. Phenotypic and functional characteristics of lymphocytes isolated from liver biopsy specimens from patients with active liver disease. Hepatology. 1992;15(5):816–23.
44. Martins EB, Graham AK, Chapman RW, Fleming KA. Elevation of gamma delta T lymphocytes in peripheral blood and livers of patients with primary sclerosing cholangitis and other autoimmune liver diseases. Hepatology. 1996;23(5):988–93.
45. Wiencke K, Spurkland A, Schrumpf E, Boberg KM. Primary sclerosing cholangitis is associated to an

extended B8-DR3 haplotype including particular MICA and MICB alleles. Hepatology. 2001;34(4 Pt 1):625–30.
46. Abraham LJ, Kroeger KM. Impact of the −308 TNF promoter polymorphism on the transcriptional regulation of the TNF gene: relevance to disease. J Leukoc Biol. 1999;66(4):562–6.
47. Mitchell SA, Grove J, Spurkland A, Boberg KM, Fleming KA, Day CP, et al. Association of the tumour necrosis factor alpha −308 but not the interleukin 10–627 promoter polymorphism with genetic susceptibility to primary sclerosing cholangitis. Gut. 2001;49(2):288–94.
48. Donaldson PT, Norris S. Immunogenetics in PSC. Best Pract Res Clin Gastroenterol. 2001;15(4): 611–27.
49. Saarinen S, Olerup O, Broome U. Increased frequency of autoimmune diseases in patients with primary sclerosing cholangitis. Am J Gastroenterol. 2000;95(11):3195–9.
50. Lio D, Candore G, Romano GC, D'Anna C, Gervasi F, Di LG, et al. Modification of cytokine patterns in subjects bearing the HLA-B8, DR3 phenotype: implications for autoimmunity. Cytokines Cell Mol Ther. 1997;3(4):217–24.
51. Holmberg D, Cilio CM, Lundholm M, Motta V. CTLA-4 (CD152) and its involvement in autoimmune disease. Autoimmunity. 2005;38(3):225–33.
52. Eri R, Jonsson JR, Pandeya N, Purdie DM, Clouston AD, Martin N, et al. CCR5-Delta32 mutation is strongly associated with primary sclerosing cholangitis. Genes Immun. 2004;5(6):444–50.
53. Satsangi J, Chapman RW, Haldar N, Donaldson P, Mitchell S, Simmons J, et al. A functional polymorphism of the stromelysin gene (MMP-3) influences susceptibility to primary sclerosing cholangitis. Gastroenterology. 2001;121(1):124–30.
54. Wiencke K, Louka AS, Spurkland A, Vatn M, Schrumpf E, Boberg KM. Association of matrix metalloproteinase-1 and -3 promoter polymorphisms with clinical subsets of Norwegian primary sclerosing cholangitis patients. J Hepatol. 2004;41(2):209–14.
55. Worthington J, Cullen S, Chapman R. Immunopathogenesis of primary sclerosing cholangitis. Clin Rev Allergy Immunol. 2005;28(2):93–103.
56. Pauli-Magnus C, Kerb R, Fattinger K, Lang T, Anwald B, Kullak-Ublick GA, et al. BSEP and MDR3 haplotype structure in healthy Caucasians, primary biliary cirrhosis and primary sclerosing cholangitis. Hepatology. 2004;39(3):779–91.
57. Hadj-Rabia S, Baala L, Vabres P, Hamel-Teillac D, Jacquemin E, Fabre M, et al. Claudin-1 gene mutations in neonatal sclerosing cholangitis associated with ichthyosis: a tight junction disease. Gastroenterology. 2004;127(5):1386–90.
58. Sheth S, Shea JC, Bishop MD, Chopra S, Regan MM, Malmberg E, et al. Increased prevalence of CFTR mutations and variants and decreased chloride secretion in primary sclerosing cholangitis. Hum Genet. 2003;113(3):286–92.
59. Girodon E, Sternberg D, Chazouilleres O, Cazeneuve C, Huot D, Calmus Y, et al. Cystic fibrosis transmembrane conductance regulator (CFTR) gene defects in patients with primary sclerosing cholangitis. J Hepatol. 2002;37(2):192–7.
60. Blanco PG, Zaman MM, Junaidi O, Sheth S, Yantiss RK, Nasser IA, et al. Induction of colitis in cftr−/− mice results in bile duct injury. Am J Physiol Gastrointest Liver Physiol. 2004;287(2):G491–6.
61. Mehal WZ, Lo YM, Wordsworth BP, Neuberger JM, Hubscher SC, Fleming KA, et al. HLA DR4 is a marker for rapid disease progression in primary sclerosing cholangitis. Gastroenterology. 1994;106(1): 160–7.
62. Yang X, Cullen SN, Li JH, Chapman RW, Jewell DP. Susceptibility to primary sclerosing cholangitis is associated with polymorphisms of intercellular adhesion molecule-1. J Hepatol. 2004;40(3):375–9.
63. Boberg KM, Spurkland A, Rocca G, Egeland T, Saarinen S, Mitchell S, et al. The HLA-DR3, DQ2 heterozygous genotype is associated with an accelerated progression of primary sclerosing cholangitis. Scand J Gastroenterol. 2001;36(8):886–90.
64. Hov JR, Boberg KM, Karlsen TH. Autoantibodies in primary sclerosing cholangitis. World J Gastroenterol. 2008;14(24):3781–91.
65. Vierling JM. Aetiopathogenesis of primary sclerosing cholangitis. In: Manns MP, Chapman RW, Stiehl A, Wiesner RH, editors. Primary sclerosing cholangitis. London: Kluwer Academic Publishers; 1998. p. 37–45.
66. Vierling JM. Hepatobiliary complications in ulcerative colitis and Crohn's disease. In: Zakim D, Boyer TD, editors. Hepatology. 4th ed. Philadelphia: WB Saunders; 2002. p. 1221–72.
67. Terjung B, Worman HJ. Anti-neutrophil antibodies in primary sclerosing cholangitis. Best Pract Res Clin Gastroenterol. 2001;15(4):629–42.
68. Terjung B, Spengler U, Sauerbruch T, Worman HJ. "Atypical p-ANCA" in IBD and hepatobiliary disorders react with a 50-kilodalton nuclear envelope protein of neutrophils and myeloid cell lines. Gastroenterology. 2000;119(2):310–22.
69. Terjung B, Muennich M, Gottwein J, Soehne J, Worman HJ, Sauerbruch T, et al. Identification of myleloid-specific tubulin-beta isotype 5 as target antigen of antineutrophil cytoplasmic antibodies in autoimmune liver diseases. Hepatology. 2005;42:288A.
70. Tubulin-beta, isotype 5. http://www.ncbi.nlm.nih.gov/entrez/query.fcgi?CMD=search&DB=protein. 2005.
71. Terjung B, Sohne J, Lechtenberg B, Gottwein J, Muennich M, Herzog V, et al. p-ANCAs in autoimmune liver disorders recognise human beta-tubulin isotype 5 and cross-react with microbial protein FtsZ. Gut. 2010;59(6):808–16.
72. Pokorny CS, Norton ID, McCaughan GW, Selby WS. Anti-neutrophil cytoplasmic antibody: a prognostic indicator in primary sclerosing cholangitis. J Gastroenterol Hepatol. 1994;9(1):40–4.

73. Bansi DS, Bauducci M, Bergqvist A, Boberg K, Broome U, Chapman R, et al. Detection of antineutrophil cytoplasmic antibodies in primary sclerosing cholangitis: a comparison of the alkaline phosphatase and immunofluorescent techniques. Eur J Gastroenterol Hepatol. 1997;9(6):575–80.
74. Mulder AH, Horst G, Haagsma EB, Limburg PC, Kleibeuker JH, Kallenberg CG. Prevalence and characterization of neutrophil cytoplasmic antibodies in autoimmune liver diseases. Hepatology. 1993;17(3): 411–7.
75. Lenzen H, Weismuller TJ, Negm AA, Wlecke J, Loges S, Strassburg CP, et al. Antineutrophil cytoplasmic antibodies in bile are associated with disease activity in primary sclerosing cholangitis. Scand J Gastroenterol. 2013;48(10):1205–12.
76. Dobric S, Popovic D, Nikolic M, Andrejevic S, Spuran M, Bonaci-Nikolic B. Anti-neutrophil cytoplasmic antibodies (ANCA) specific for one or several antigens: useful markers for subtypes of ulcerative colitis and associated primary sclerosing cholangitis. Clin Chem Lab Med. 2012;50(3): 503–9.
77. Karrar A, Broome U, Sodergren T, Jaksch M, Bergquist A, Bjornstedt M, et al. Biliary epithelial cell antibodies link adaptive and innate immune responses in primary sclerosing cholangitis. Gastroenterology. 2007;132(4):1504–14.
78. Mizoguchi E, Mizoguchi A, Chiba C, Niles JL, Bhan AK. Antineutrophil cytoplasmic antibodies in T-cell receptor alpha-deficient mice with chronic colitis. Gastroenterology. 1997;113(6):1828–35.
79. Seibold F, Brandwein S, Simpson S, Terhorst C, Elson CO. pANCA represents a cross-reactivity to enteric bacterial antigens. J Clin Immunol. 1998;18(2):153–60.
80. Schultz H, Schinke S, Weiss J, Cerundolo V, Gross WL, Gadola S. BPI-ANCA in transporter associated with antigen presentation (TAP) deficiency: possible role in susceptibility to Gram-negative bacterial infections. Clin Exp Immunol. 2003;133(2):252–9.
81. Schultz H, Weiss J, Carroll SF, Gross WL. The endotoxin-binding bactericidal/permeability-increasing protein (BPI): a target antigen of autoantibodies. J Leukoc Biol. 2001;69(4):505–12.
82. Xu B, Broome U, Ericzon BG, Sumitran-Holgersson S. High frequency of autoantibodies in patients with primary sclerosing cholangitis that bind biliary epithelial cells and induce expression of CD44 and production of interleukin 6. Gut. 2002;51(1):120–7.
83. Nagano O, Saya H. Mechanism and biological significance of CD44 cleavage. Cancer Sci. 2004; 95(12):930–5.
84. Wittig BM, Stallmach A, Zeitz M, Gunthert U. Functional involvement of CD44 variant 7 in gut immune response. Pathobiology. 2002;70(3):184–9.
85. Naor D, Nedvetzki S. CD44 in rheumatoid arthritis. Arthritis Res Ther. 2003;5(3):105–15.
86. Sakamaki S, Takayanagi N, Yoshizaki N, Hayashi S, Takayama T, Kato J, et al. Autoantibodies against the specific epitope of human tropomyosin(s) detected by a peptide based enzyme immunoassay in sera of patients with ulcerative colitis show antibody dependent cell mediated cytotoxicity against HLA-DPw9 transfected L cells. Gut. 2000;47(2):236–41.
87. Si L, Whiteside TL, Schade RR, Starzl TE, Van Thiel DH. T-lymphocyte subsets in liver tissues of patients with primary biliary cirrhosis (PBC), patients with primary sclerosing cholangitis (PSC), and normal controls. J Clin Immunol. 1984;4(4):262–72.
88. Whiteside TL, Lasky S, Si L, Van Thiel DH. Immunologic analysis of mononuclear cells in liver tissues and blood of patients with primary sclerosing cholangitis. Hepatology. 1985;5(3):468–74.
89. Valenski WR, Herrod HG, Williams JW. In vitro evidence for B cell dysfunction in patients with chronic liver disease. J Clin Lab Immunol. 1989;28(4): 169–72.
90. Kilby AE, Krawitt EL, Albertini RJ, Chastenay BF, John A. Suppressor T-cell deficiency in primary sclerosing cholangitis. Case and family study. Dig Dis Sci. 1991;36(9):1213–6.
91. Lindor KD, Wiesner RH, Larusso NF, Homburger HA. Enhanced autoreactivity of T-lymphocytes in primary sclerosing cholangitis. Hepatology. 1987; 7(5):884–8.
92. Senaldi G, Donaldson PT, Magrin S, Farrant JM, Alexander GJ, Vergani D, et al. Activation of the complement system in primary sclerosing cholangitis. Gastroenterology. 1989;97(6):1430–4.
93. Garred P, Lyon H, Christoffersen P, Mollnes TE, Tranum-Jensen J. Deposition of C3, the terminal complement complex and vitronectin in primary biliary cirrhosis and primary sclerosing cholangitis. Liver. 1993;13(6):305–10.
94. Bodenheimer Jr HC, Larusso NF, Thayer Jr WR, Charland C, Staples PJ, Ludwig J. Elevated circulating immune complexes in primary sclerosing cholangitis. Hepatology. 1983;3(2):150–4.
95. Minuk GY, Angus M, Brickman CM, Lawley TJ, Frank MM, Hoofnagle JH, et al. Abnormal clearance of immune complexes from the circulation of patients with primary sclerosing cholangitis. Gastroenterology. 1985;88(1 Pt 1):166–70.
96. Bloom S, Heryet A, Fleming K, Chapman RW. Inappropriate expression of blood group antigens on biliary and colonic epithelia in primary sclerosing cholangitis. Gut. 1993;34(7):977–83.
97. Ludwig J. Histopathology of primary sclerosing cholangitis. In: Manns MP, Chapman RW, Stiehl A, Wiesner RH, editors. Primary sclerosing cholangitis. Boston: Kluwer Academic Publishers; 1998. p. 14–21.
98. Dienes HP, Lohse AW, Gerken G, Schirmacher P, Gallati H, Lohr HF, et al. Bile duct epithelia as target cells in primary biliary cirrhosis and primary sclerosing cholangitis. Virchows Arch. 1997;431(2): 119–24.
99. Ponsioen CY, Kuiper H, Ten Kate FJ, van Milligen de WM, van Deventer SJ, Tytgat GN.

Immunohistochemical analysis of inflammation in primary sclerosing cholangitis. Eur J Gastroenterol Hepatol. 1999;11(7):769–74.
100. Adams DH, Afford SC. The role of cholangiocytes in the development of chronic inflammatory liver disease. Front Biosci. 2002;7:e276–85, e276–e285.
101. Adams DH, Eksteen B, Grant A, Lalor PF, Miles A. Long-lived mucosal T cells drive hepatic inflammation in PSC. http://videocast.nih.gov/PastEvents.asp. NIDDK Research Workshop on Primary Sclerosing Cholangitis 2005.
102. Trivedi PJ, Adams DH. Gut-liver immunity. J Hepatol. 2016;64(5):1187–9.
103. Batts KP. Ischemic cholangitis. Mayo Clin Proc. 1998;73(4):380–5.
104. Beaussier M, Wendum D, Fouassier L, Rey C, Barbu V, Lasnier E, et al. Adaptative bile duct proliferative response in experimental bile duct ischemia. J Hepatol. 2005;42(2):257–65.
105. Benninger J, Grobholz R, Oeztuerk Y, Antoni CH, Hahn EG, Singer MV, et al. Sclerosing cholangitis following severe trauma: description of a remarkable disease entity with emphasis on possible pathophysiologic mechanisms. World J Gastroenterol. 2005; 11(27):4199–205.
106. Fickert P, Fuchsbichler A, Wagner M, Zollner G, Kaser A, Tilg H, et al. Regurgitation of bile acids from leaky bile ducts causes sclerosing cholangitis in Mdr2 (Abcb4) knockout mice. Gastroenterology. 2004;127(1):261–74.
107. Patel T. Aberrant local renin-angiotensin II responses in the pathogenesis of primary sclerosing cholangitis. Med Hypotheses. 2003;61(1):64–7.
108. Kummen M, Holm K, Anmarkrud JA, Nygard S, Vesterhus M, Hoivik ML, et al. The gut microbial profile in patients with primary sclerosing cholangitis is distinct from patients with ulcerative colitis without biliary disease and healthy controls. Gut. 2016. gutjnl-2015-310500 Published Online First: doi:10.1136/gutjnl-2015-310500.
109. Rossen NG, Fuentes S, Boonstra K, D'Haens GR, Heilig HG, Zoetendal EG, et al. The mucosa-associated microbiota of PSC patients is characterized by low diversity and low abundance of uncultured Clostridiales II. J Crohns Colitis. 2015;9(4):342–8.
110. Krasinskas AM, Yao Y, Randhawa P, Dore MP, Sepulveda AR. Helicobacter pylori may play a contributory role in the pathogenesis of primary sclerosing cholangitis. Dig Dis Sci. 2007;52(9):2265–70.
111. Eksteen B. The gut-liver axis in primary sclerosing cholangitis. Clin Liver Dis. 2016;20(1):1–14.
112. Viney JL, Jones S, Chiu HH, Lagrimas B, Renz ME, Presta LG, et al. Mucosal addressin cell adhesion molecule-1: a structural and functional analysis demarcates the integrin binding motif. J Immunol. 1996;157(6):2488–97.
113. Hillan KJ, Hagler KE, MacSween RN, Ryan AM, Renz ME, Chiu HH, et al. Expression of the mucosal vascular addressin, MAdCAM-1, in inflammatory liver disease. Liver. 1999;19(6):509–18.
114. Grant AJ, Lalor PF, Hubscher SG, Briskin M, Adams DH. MAdCAM-1 expressed in chronic inflammatory liver disease supports mucosal lymphocyte adhesion to hepatic endothelium (MAdCAM-1 in chronic inflammatory liver disease). Hepatology. 2001;33(5):1065–72.
115. Grant AJ, Goddard S, hmed-Choudhury J, Reynolds G, Jackson DG, Briskin M, et al. Hepatic expression of secondary lymphoid chemokine (CCL21) promotes the development of portal-associated lymphoid tissue in chronic inflammatory liver disease. Am J Pathol. 2002;160(4):1445–55.
116. Eksteen B, Grant AJ, Miles A, Curbishley SM, Lalor PF, Hubscher SG, et al. Hepatic endothelial CCL25 mediates the recruitment of CCR9+ gut-homing lymphocytes to the liver in primary sclerosing cholangitis. J Exp Med. 2004;200(11): 1511–7.
117. Grant AJ, Lalor PF, Salmi M, Jalkanen S, Adams DH. Homing of mucosal lymphocytes to the liver in the pathogenesis of hepatic complications of inflammatory bowel disease. Lancet. 2002;359(9301): 150–7.
118. Lalor PF, Edwards S, McNab G, Salmi M, Jalkanen S, Adams DH. Vascular adhesion protein-1 mediates adhesion and transmigration of lymphocytes on human hepatic endothelial cells. J Immunol. 2002; 169(2):983–92.
119. Mora JR, Bono MR, Manjunath N, Weninger W, Cavanagh LL, Rosemblatt M, et al. Selective imprinting of gut-homing T cells by Peyer's patch dendritic cells. Nature. 2003;424(6944):88–93.
120. Probert CS, Christ AD, Saubermann LJ, Turner JR, Chott A, Carr-Locke D, et al. Analysis of human common bile duct-associated T cells: evidence for oligoclonality, T cell clonal persistence, and epithelial cell recognition. J Immunol. 1997;158(4): 1941–8.
121. Broome U, Grunewald J, Scheynius A, Olerup O, Hultcrantz R. Preferential V beta3 usage by hepatic T lymphocytes in patients with primary sclerosing cholangitis. J Hepatol. 1997;26(3):527–34.
122. Bo X, Broome U, Remberger M, Sumitran-Holgersson S. Tumour necrosis factor alpha impairs function of liver derived T lymphocytes and natural killer cells in patients with primary sclerosing cholangitis. Gut. 2001;49(1):131–41.
123. Cameron RG, Blendis LM, Neuman MG. Accumulation of macrophages in primary sclerosing cholangitis. Clin Biochem. 2001;34(3):195–201.
124. Vierling JM. Animal models of primary sclerosing cholangitis. http://videocast.nih.gov/PastEvents.asp. NIDDK Research Workshop on Primary Sclerosing Cholangitis 2005.
125. Kuroe K, Haga Y, Funakoshi O, Mizuki I, Kanazawa K, Yoshida Y. Extraintestinal manifestations of granulomatous enterocolitis induced in rabbits by long-term submucosal administration of muramyl dipeptide emulsified with Freund's incomplete adjuvant. J Gastroenterol. 1996;31(2):199–206.

126. Yamada S, Ishii M, Liang LS, Yamamoto T, Toyota T. Small duct cholangitis induced by N-formyl L-methionine L-leucine L-tyrosine in rats. J Gastroenterol. 1994;29(5):631–6.
127. Lichtman SN, Keku J, Clark RL, Schwab JH, Sartor RB. Biliary tract disease in rats with experimental small bowel bacterial overgrowth. Hepatology. 1991;13(4):766–72.
128. Lichtman SN, Okoruwa EE, Keku J, Schwab JH, Sartor RB. Degradation of endogenous bacterial cell wall polymers by the muralytic enzyme mutanolysin prevents hepatobiliary injury in genetically susceptible rats with experimental intestinal bacterial overgrowth. J Clin Invest. 1992;90(4):1313–22.
129. Hobson CH, Butt TJ, Ferry DM, Hunter J, Chadwick VS, Broom MF. Enterohepatic circulation of bacterial chemotactic peptide in rats with experimental colitis. Gastroenterology. 1988;94(4):1006–13.
130. Watt SM, Fawcett J, Murdoch SJ, Teixeira AM, Gschmeissner SE, Hajibagheri NM, et al. CD66 identifies the biliary glycoprotein (BGP) adhesion molecule: cloning, expression, and adhesion functions of the BGPc splice variant. Blood. 1994;84(1):200–10.
131. Riethdorf L, Lisboa BW, Henkel U, Naumann M, Wagener C, Loning T. Differential expression of CD66a (BGP), a cell adhesion molecule of the carcinoembryonic antigen family, in benign, premalignant, and malignant lesions of the human mammary gland. J Histochem Cytochem. 1997;45(7):957–63.
132. Morales VM, Christ A, Watt SM, Kim HS, Johnson KW, Utku N, et al. Regulation of human intestinal intraepithelial lymphocyte cytolytic function by biliary glycoprotein (CD66a). J Immunol. 1999;163(3):1363–70.
133. Grappone C, Pinzani M, Parola M, Pellegrini G, Caligiuri A, DeFranco R, et al. Expression of platelet-derived growth factor in newly formed cholangiocytes during experimental biliary fibrosis in rats. J Hepatol. 1999;31(1):100–9.
134. Pinzani M. Liver fibrosis. Springer Semin Immunopathol. 1999;21(4):475–90.

Pruritus in Primary Sclerosing Cholangitis: New Insights into Cause and Treatment

10

Mark G. Swain

Introduction

Pruritus is a common complaint among patients with cholestatic liver diseases. Specifically, pruritus is a distinct and profound symptom associated with intrahepatic cholestasis of pregnancy (ICP) and benign recurrent intrahepatic cholestasis (BRIC). Moreover, pruritus is commonly encountered in patients with primary biliary cholangitis (PBC), affecting up to three-fourths of PBC patients to some degree [1]. In patients with PBC, itch can also be severe, significantly impairing patient quality of life (QOL) leading to depression, social withdrawal, and even suicidal ideation. In rare cases, severe itch can even be an indication for liver transplantation [1, 2].

In contrast, the prevalence and impact of pruritus in PSC patients are less well understood. The prevalence of pruritus in PSC patients at the time of diagnosis has been reported for a number of well-characterized patient cohorts. In Scandinavia, in a cohort of 305 patients with PSC, 30 % had pruritus at the time of their diagnosis [3]. However, in a cohort of PSC patients followed at the Mayo Clinic in Rochester, Minnesota [4], pruritus was almost twice as common at the time of diagnosis (59 %) compared to the frequency reported by Broome et al. [3]. This discrepancy likely reflects the specialized referral pattern for PSC patients seen at the Mayo Clinic. Moreover, among the Mayo patient cohort, 75 % of the patients who were symptomatic at diagnosis reported pruritus [4]. In another Scandinavian study, 65 PSC patients were provided with daily diaries and asked to report symptoms over a 3-year period [5]. A majority of patients (84 %) reported the occurrence of symptoms during this period, including pruritus, however these symptoms were typically intermittent and transient (lasting 1–2 days). In these patients, pruritus correlated closely with serum alkaline phosphatase levels [5]. Berquist et al. [6] examined a cohort of 246 PSC patients and divided them into those diagnosed before ($n = 185$) and after ($N = 61$) 1998. At the time of PSC diagnosis, 20 % of patients complained of pruritus. Interestingly, pruritus in these patients was significantly more common in women (28 %) than in men (16 %), a finding paralleling observations from PBC patients where women are more likely to be pruritic than men [7]. These observations are suggestive of hormonal regulation of pruritus in cholestasis and are consistent with the common clinical observation that pruritus in PBC patients often worsens around the time of menses. Perhaps not surprisingly, pruritus was reported in 25 % of patients diagnosed with PSC by endoscopic retrograde cholangiopancreatography (ERCP), compared to 5 % of patients diagnosed using magnetic resonance cholangiopancreatography (MRCP). The frequency of pruritus at the time of diagnosis

M.G. Swain, MD, MSc, FRCPC, FAASLD
Division of Gastroenterology and Hepatology, Department of Medicine, University of Calgary, Calgary, AB, Canada
e-mail: swain@ucalgary.ca

L.M. Forman (ed.), *Primary Sclerosing Cholangitis*, DOI 10.1007/978-3-319-40908-5_10

was similar in patients diagnosed before and after 1998 (22 % vs 15 %, respectively) [6].

In general, pruritus in cholestatic patients can have a profound effect on their health-related quality of life (HRQOL) [1, 2]. Similar findings of a pruritus-related detriment in HRQOL have been reported in patients with PSC. Gotthardt et al. administered HRQOL questionnaires to 113 PSC patients (SF-36 and Patient Health Questionnaire) and found that more frequent pruritus was associated with considerable reductions in HRQOL, as reflected by scores obtained in most of the QOL scales tested [8]. Moreover, pruritus was the most prominent factor affecting HRQOL and was associated with higher depression scores [8]. Similar findings were reported by Benito de Valle et al. in 182 patients with PSC [9]. Interestingly, in this group of patients, systemic symptoms such as pruritus were associated with lower HRQOL scores, whereas diseases severity was not [9].

The Pathophysiology of Itch

Pruritus is defined as an irritating skin sensation which leads to a desire to scratch. To better understand pruritus as it relates to cholestatic liver diseases, including PSC, it is important to appreciate the neural pathways that initiate and regulate itch. Pruritus may originate from diseases occurring within the CNS (e.g., stroke, tumors); however, more commonly pruritus has a peripheral origin that results from a pruritogen acting at the level of the skin to activate cutaneous "itch" nerve endings. Signals generated by activation of these cutaneous itch nerve endings are carried in unmyelinated C-fibers, through the dorsal root ganglion, to ultimately synapse with and activate spinal neurons within the dorsal horn of the spinal cord. Within the dorsal horn, itch-selective neurons carry the itch signal to the contralateral spinothalamic tract which relays the itch signal to the thalamus and ultimately to a number of itch-responsive areas of the brain [10]. An important role for the brain in regulating itch is routinely demonstrated by the observation that the itch sensation can be provoked in non-itchy people, simply by watching a person scratch an itch – a process termed "contagious itch" [11].

Much of our current understanding of itch comes from studies of *acute* itch induced by the application of a pruritogen. In contrast, pruritus associated with systemic disease, including cholestatic liver disease, is most commonly *chronic* in nature. The sensations of pain and itch are closely related but are distinct sensations subserved by separate nerve pathways [12]. Interestingly, painful stimuli (including scratching) often improves acute itch but is less effective in ameliorating chronic itch [13]. Based on relatively recent pioneering studies in models of acute itch, two types of peripheral C-fiber nerve pathways carrying itch signals from the skin to the spinal cord have been defined (Fig. 10.1):

(i) The *histaminergic itch pathway* involving mechanically insensitive C-fibers, as defined by Schmelz et al. [14].
(ii) The *non-histaminergic itch pathway* which is a histamine-independent pathway involving mechanically sensitive polymodal C-fibers, as originally described by Namer et al. [15].

Importantly, the histaminergic and non-histaminergic itch pathways activate distinct populations of dorsal horn spinothalamic tract neurons within the spine (Fig. 10.1) [16]. Therefore, the itch sensation can be driven by either of these two pathways, although it is generally believed that itch related to chronic systemic disease (e.g., cholestasis) *involves mainly the non-histaminergic itch pathway* [17], consistent with routine clinical observations that cholestasis-related itch is poorly relieved by antihistamines.

Four histamine receptors have been identified (H1R–H4R), with H1R being implicated as the major receptor involved in histamine-induced itch via activation of transient receptor potential cation channel V1 (TRPV1) [18]. In addition, H4R has been linked to chronic itch [19], although the pathways involved remain unclear. Cowage, a protein extract isolated from the legume *M. pruriens*, is commonly used experimentally to activate the non-histaminergic itch pathway. Cowage contains a cysteine protease

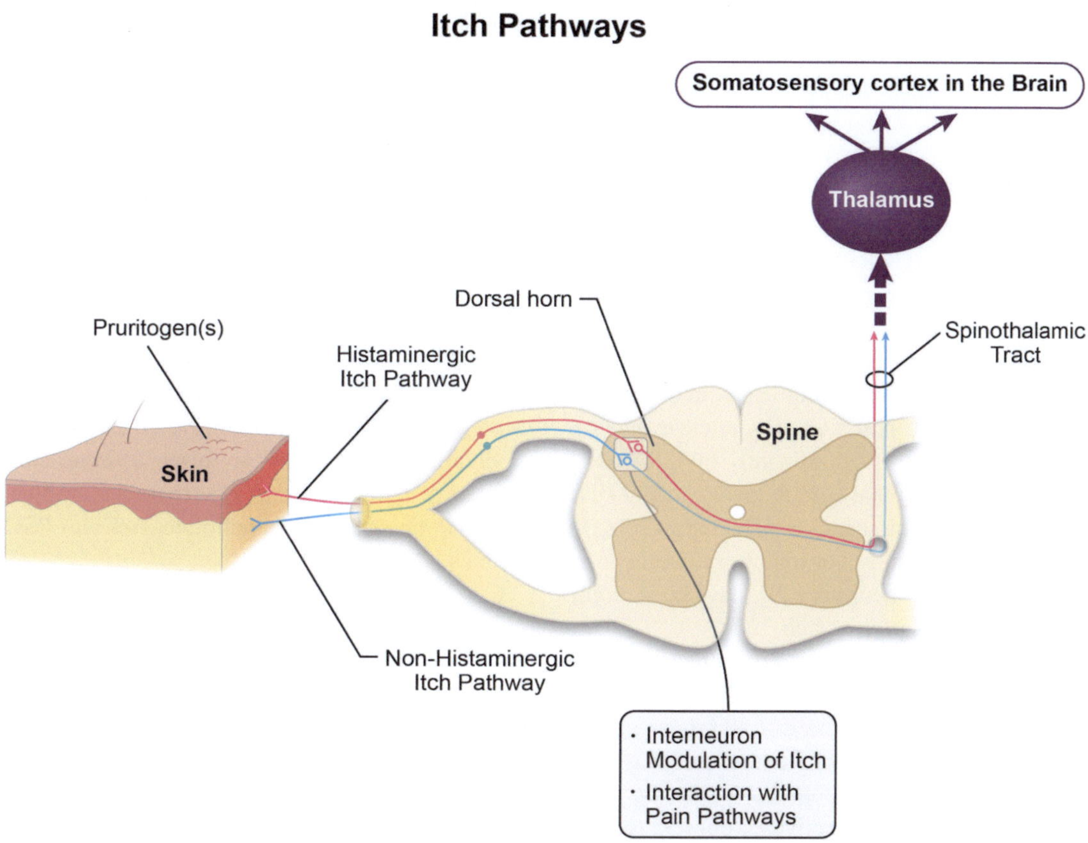

Fig. 10.1 Itch pathways. The two main peripheral itch pathways include the histaminergic pathway (*red line* stimulated by histamine) and the non-histaminergic pathway (*blue line* stimulated by a number of agents, including a protease contained in cowhage). The pruritogen present in cholestatic PSC patients is presumed to activate receptors located in the dermis of the skin to generate signals which are carried in polymodal C-fibers of the non-histaminergic itch pathway. These nerve fibers synapse with secondary neurons in the dorsal horn of the spinal cord where the itch signal can be modulated by input from neurotransmitters released from a variety of spinal interneurons and by interactions with pain pathways. Secondary afferent nerves carry the itch signal in the contralateral spinothalamic tract and synapse in the thalamus from which nerves project to a number of somatosensory areas within the brain

(mucunain) which activates protease-activated receptors 2 and 4 (PAR-2 and PAR-4) [20]. PAR-2 and PAR-4 have been implicated in the development of non-histaminergic itch [21], and PAR-2 specifically appears to be important in chronic itch [22, 23]. Interestingly, PAR-2 activation has been linked to transient receptor potential ankyrin 1 (TRPA1), a channel modulated by cold and cannabinoids [21, 24], with implications with regard to potential therapeutic approaches for treating itch. PAR-2 is co-expressed with TRPV1, and PAR-2 agonists increase afferent nerve signaling by sensitizing TRPV1 which in turn induces sensory nerve endings to become more responsive to other non-histaminergic pruritogens [25], an effect likely relevant in chronic itch syndromes.

At the level of the spinal cord, a close interplay between the histaminergic and non-histaminergic itch pathways appears to occur, through the activation of similar receptors (including G-protein-coupled receptors) and downstream messengers, as well as with pain-signaling pathways [17]. Both itch pathways activate phospholipase C and TRPV1 within the spinal dorsal root ganglion. Moreover, pain and itch pathways are in turn cross regulated through excitatory and inhibitory interneurons within the spinal cord that modulate the activity of each other. In addition, descending modulatory neural pathways from the brain also profoundly regulate both pain and itch pathways [17]. Within the dorsal horn of the spinal cord, a number of neurotransmitters and associated receptors have been implicated in the regulation of itch pathways. These include calcitonin gene-related peptide (CGRP), substance P, glutamate, gastrin-releasing peptide (GRP), glycine, and gamma-aminobutyric acid (GABA) [10, 17]. Gastrin-releasing peptide receptor (GRPR) activation has been strongly implicated in the generation of itch [26]; however, it is unclear whether GRPR is activated predominantly by GRP or by glutamate in the spinal cord to invoke itch [27]. In contrast, the neurotransmitters glycine and GABA [28], as well as a subset of inhibitory interneurons termed "Bhlhb5" neurons [29], have been implicated in the inhibition of itch.

Acute histaminergic and non-histaminergic itch pathway stimulation in healthy individuals results in neuronal signaling which is carried within specific spinal cord neural pathways and results in activation of neurons within the thalamus and subsequently activates numerous areas of the brain that are involved in the regulation of perception, emotion, motor control, pain regulation, attention, and motivation [10]. In contrast, this distinct representation of activation of different brain regions involved in acute itch processing induced by these two pathways is blurred in the context of diseases associated with chronic itch [30]. Interestingly, in uremic pruritus, increased PAR-2 expression in the skin, leading to chronic overstimulation of the PAR-2-mediated itch pathway, has been implicated in altered responses to acute activation of non-histaminergic itch pathways in these patients [30].

Summary

Chronic itch, as commonly experienced by PSC patients, likely involves non-histaminergic peripheral nerve pathways from the skin, where the pruritogen(s) in PSC is postulated to act, to the dorsal horn of the spinal cord where these nerves synapse with other neurons (Fig. 10.1). Pruritogenic stimuli carried in this pathway may in turn be significantly modulated in the spine by interactions with stimuli carried in the histaminergic and pain nerve pathways, from itch-modulating spinal interneurons involving a number of neurotransmitters and receptors and/or from descending inhibitory neural pathways from the brain. Therefore, itch is a very complex sensory response that is even more challenging to understand in the context of a chronic disease such as PSC, which in turn has its own complex pathophysiology. However, the multiple levels through which pruritogenic nerve stimuli can be modulated would seem to offer a significant number of potential targets for therapeutic interventions designed to ameliorate itch in PSC patients.

What Causes PSC Patients to Itch?

The peripheral and central pathways involved in the generation of cholestatic itch, and its regulation, are poorly understood. Moreover, a specific pruritogen(s) has not been identified in cholestatic patients; however, the accumulation or creation of the cholestasis-related pruritogen must in some way be related to an impairment of bile flow into the gut lumen as this is by definition a central component of the cholestatic syndrome. In addition, it is quite possible that different pruritogenic pathways may be primarily responsible for the generation of itch in different cholestatic syndromes (e.g., ICP, BRIC, PBC, PSC). Many studies have been published examining different therapeutic approaches to cholestatic itch. Unfortunately, no single effective therapy for all patients with cholestatic itch has been identified to date. However, these studies, when evaluated together, do provide insight into the pathophysiology of cholestatic itch and allow for the generation of novel hypotheses that can be tested which may lead to therapies that are more specific and effective for cholestatic patients in general and PSC patients specifically.

Cholestasis is associated with elevated circulating histamine levels [31], suggesting that mast cells are likely activated in cholestatic patients.

However, cholestatic itch is not associated clinically with a classical histamine-related wheal and flare reaction in the skin, and antihistamines are poorly effective in treating cholestatic itch [1, 2]. Mast cells are a rich source of histamine, but also secrete proteases (e.g., tryptase) which are strong activators of PAR-2 [32] which, as outlined earlier, plays an important role in modulating the activity of the non-histaminergic itch pathway. Therefore, it is plausible that mast cell stabilizers may be beneficial in treating cholestatic itch by decreasing mast cell release of PAR-2 activating proteases and warrants further study.

Bile acids have historically been most commonly implicated as the causative pruritogen in cholestasis. However, serum and skin bile acid levels correlate poorly with itch in cholestatic patients, and in PBC patients with advanced disease, pruritus often decreases or disappears completely despite the persistence of high serum bile acid levels [2]. Cholestyramine is widely used to treat cholestatic itch, presumably based on its ability to bind bile acids in the gut lumen [33]. However, the highly potent oral bile acid sequestrant colesevelam was not effective in treating cholestatic itch (including 14 patients with PSC) [34]. These findings suggest that the clinical efficacy of cholestyramine in treating cholestatic itch is likely distinct from its ability to bind bile acids and is consistent with cholestyramine potentially binding some other unknown pruritogen or pruritus-regulating substance in the gut lumen. Furthermore, obeticholic acid, a bile acid that is a strong farnesoid X receptor (FXR) agonist, induces itch but reduces levels of circulating bile acids in PBC patients [35]. Therefore, circulating bile acids do not appear to be primary mediators of cholestatic itch. Recently, a role for bile acids in cholestatic itch was supported by the finding that the TGR5 receptor, which is expressed in primary sensory neurons, can be activated by bile acids to induce itch through activation of TRPA1 channels [36, 37]. In contrast to the suggestion that bile acids are acting as pruritogens in cholestatic patients, another possibility is that altering the bile acid composition within the gut lumen, as part of the cholestatic syndrome or after treatment with obeticholic acid or cholestyramine, in turn alters the gut microbiota in such a way to either enhance or reduce specific bacterial species within the gut that facilitate or inhibit the generation of a pruritogenic substance. The concept that the pruritogen in cholestasis is secreted in the bile has led to other approaches to divert bile flow away from the gut, in an attempt to treat cholestatic itch. Nasobiliary drainage has been used in this regard and has been highly effective in treating refractory cholestatic itch in patients with BRIC and to a lesser extent in patients with PBC [38, 39]. However, it remains unclear whether nasobiliary drainage is an effective therapy for intractable itch associated with PSC.

The concept of a potential gut-derived pruritogen as a driver of cholestatic itch, which is created as a result of cholestasis-related changes in the gut microbiota, is supported by a number of other clinical observations. Specifically, rifampin is an antibiotic widely used to effectively treat cholestatic itch, including patients with PSC [40, 41]. Although the mechanism whereby rifampin alleviates cholestatic itch remains unknown, it is clear that rifampin has broad spectrum antimicrobial properties, and therefore ingestion of rifampin likely profoundly alters the gut microbiota [42]. Consistent with this possibility, treatment of PSC patients with high doses of the antibiotic metronidazole significantly decreased pruritus [43, 44]. The bile acid obeticholic acid is a powerful FXR agonist, and its administration to both cholestatic and non-cholestatic patients causes itch [35]. However, it is clear that FXR activation also strongly induces the production of a number of antimicrobial peptides [45], significantly altering the gut microbiome [46]. These FXR-mediated effects could potentially drive the gut microbial community to generate more pruritogenic substances. In contrast to the antipruritic effects of antibiotics, treatment of PSC patients with a probiotic mixture did not improve pruritus [47].

Lysophosphatidic acid (LPA) has recently been implicated as a potential mediator of cholestatic itch [48], and LPA is formed through the action of the enzyme autotaxin. Interestingly, LPA also stimulates basophils to release histamine, and this has recently been implicated in the development of itch in a patient with PSC [49]. Importantly, autotaxin activity in the serum is increased in cholestatic patients with pruritus and is decreased in cholestatic patients who have been effectively treated with antipruritic regimens, including nasobiliary drainage and rifampin [48, 50]. Indeed, Kremer et al. have suggested that the antipruritic effect of rifampin in cholestasis can be explained, at least in part, by rifampin-related activation of pregnane X receptor (PXR) which inhibits autotaxin expression at the transcriptional level [50]. However, other clinical observations do not support this hypothesis. Bezafibrate has been increasingly used as a treatment for patients with PBC, in part, due to its effects as a PXR agonist [51, 52]. However, bezafibrate has no effect on PBC-related pruritus [40, 52]. Moreover, autotaxin activity is highest and correlates most closely with itch in women with intrahepatic cholestasis of preagnancy (ICP); however, ursodeoxycholic acidhep (UDCA) therapy is highly effective in relieving itch in ICP patients but is without effect for itch in PBC and PSC patients [1, 2, 53, 54]. Moreover, LPA has a very short biological half-life and is highly lipophilic, and its receptors are located intracellularly making the case for a significant role for LPA in cholestatic itch challenging [2]. Interestingly, serum autotaxin activity is also often significantly increased clinically in a number of non-cholestatic clinical syndromes but is not associated with the development of itch [2].

Opioids have historically been closely linked to both pain and itch pathways, as administration of opioids (e.g., morphine) relieves pain but often induces itch. Endogenous opioids accumulate in the serum of cholestatic patients [55] and have been shown to modulate pain pathways in cholestasis by acting at peripheral opioid receptors located on cutaneous nerve endings [56]. Moreover, blockade of opioid receptors with naloxone, naltrexone, or nalmefene is clinically effective in treating some patients with cholestatic itch [40, 57–59]. However, the induction of an opioid withdrawal-type reaction in pruritic cholestatic patients treated with opioid receptor blockers suggests that endogenous opioids may be acting centrally, to modulate the perception of itch, and not peripherally to generate itch [57, 59].

Inflammatory mediators, including cytokines, can modulate pain and itch pathways. In particular, TNFα can activate nociceptive primary afferent nerve fibers [60], and topical application of TNFα to peripheral nerves causes mechanical hyperalgesia [61]. In addition, TNFα modulates spinal cord dorsal horn pain-related synaptic activity [62], and TNFα increases the expression of the TRPV1 receptor in the spinal dorsal root ganglia [63]. Inhibition of TNFα using etanercept reduces pain-related behaviors in a model of neuropathy [64]. A potential role for TNFα in modulating cholestatic itch is supported by a number of clinical observations. Circulating TNFα levels are increased in cholestatic patients, and treatment of profoundly pruritic cholestatic patients with MARS is associated with a significant reduction in serum TNFα levels [65]. In addition, thalidomide treatment (which inhibits TNFα production) decreased itch in PBC patients [66]. In contrast, treatment of PSC patients with pentoxifylline (also inhibits TNFα production) did not alter pruritus; however, the patients included in this study were not significantly pruritic at the start of treatment [67]. In another study, treatment of PSC patients with the TNFα inhibitor etanercept resulted in a reduction in pruritus [68]. Activated B cells produce significant amounts of TNFα [69], and we have shown that elimination of B cells with rituximab in PBC patients resulted in a significant improvement in pruritus, without altering serum indicators of cholestasis severity [70]. These observations suggest that targeting TNFα may be a novel approach to treat pruritus in PSC patients and may be linked to therapeutic approaches for inflammatory bowel disease (IBD) which commonly coexists in these patients.

The cutaneous itch signal is transmitted to secondary neurons within the spinal cord. These secondary neurons can be extensively modulated by input from excitatory and inhibitory interneurons (Fig. 10.1) and by descending inhibitory neural pathways from the brain [10, 17]. Itch signal processing and regulation within the spinal cord and brain therefore represent potential targets for therapeutic modulation of cholestatic itch. Cannabinoids are widely used clinically for their ability to modulate pain and decrease nausea, most likely by acting on receptors within the CNS. A pilot study in three cholestatic patients with treatment refractory itch, treated with the cannabinoid dronabinol, showed an improvement in itch [71]. Interestingly, histamine-induced itch is attenuated by a peripherally administered cannabinoid receptor agonist [72]. These findings suggest that cannabinoids may be beneficial in cholestatic itch by acting both peripherally and centrally. Serotonin also regulates itch, and a role for serotonin in cholestatic itch is supported by the well-documented clinical efficacy of the selective serotonin reuptake inhibitor (SSRI) sertraline in treating patients with cholestatic itch, including patients with PSC [73]. However, it remains unclear whether the clinical effect of sertraline in improving itch in these patients is due to the effects on serotonergic neurotransmission within the brain, spinal cord, or skin. One serotonin receptor in particular, the 5-HT3 receptor, has been examined as a potential driver of cholestatic itch. However, a number of studies have been performed using 5-HT3 antagonists in patients with cholestatic itch, but no significant beneficial effects could be consistently documented [40, 74].

Rational Approach to Treating Pruritus in PSC Patients

(i) *Defining the severity and impact of pruritus*: Evaluating patients in the clinic with regard to the severity of pruritus and its impact on their HRQOL (including physical, emotional, and social impacts) should be addressed at each visit. This evaluation can include simple to administer methods such as asking a patient to score their pruritus using a visual analog scale (VAS) [73, 75] or by asking the patient to rate their itch using a simple subjective-descriptive numerical scale, as previously described [67, 76].

(ii) *Dominant strictures and endoscopic therapies*: In PSC patients, the new onset or worsening of pruritus, especially when coupled with clinical deterioration of serum markers of cholestasis, suggests the possible development of a dominant stricture (benign or malignant) or a worsening of their overall disease. Dominant strictures occur commonly in PSC patients, occurring at a frequency ranging from 36 to 57 % over 10 years of follow-up [77]. Benign strictures can often be managed effectively endoscopically with an associated relief of, or improvement in, associated pruritus (Fig. 10.2).

(iii) *Medical management of pruritus in PSC patients*: As outlined earlier, since the specific cause of pruritus in PSC patients remains unknown, therapeutic approaches to treat itch in these patients must therefore remain somewhat empiric. However, in general, the therapeutic medical approach outlined in Fig. 10.2 is a useful framework for treating pruritic PSC patients and will be effective to satisfactorily ameliorate pruritus in the majority of these patients. Choosing a second-line therapy for treatment (Fig. 10.2) often comes down to personal preference, as there have been no head-to-head comparison studies of these therapies, and none of these treatments work in every pruritic patient. Therefore, therapy often needs to be individualized. In my own practice, I typically choose rifampin as my first choice, followed by sertraline and then naltrexone. For patients who are refractory to these first- and second-line therapies for pruritus, phototherapy, plasmapheresis, and/or albumin dialysis (MARS) can be considered; however, their potential utility is based on anecdotal experience and/or reports from small groups of cholestatic patients of with diseases of mixed etiology.

(iv) *Surgical management of pruritus in PSC patients*: In general, surgery has almost no role in the treatment of PSC-related pruritus. However, if pruritus is intractable and is due to advanced stricturing disease that is not amenable to endoscopic intervention, liver transplant should be considered as a therapeutic option.

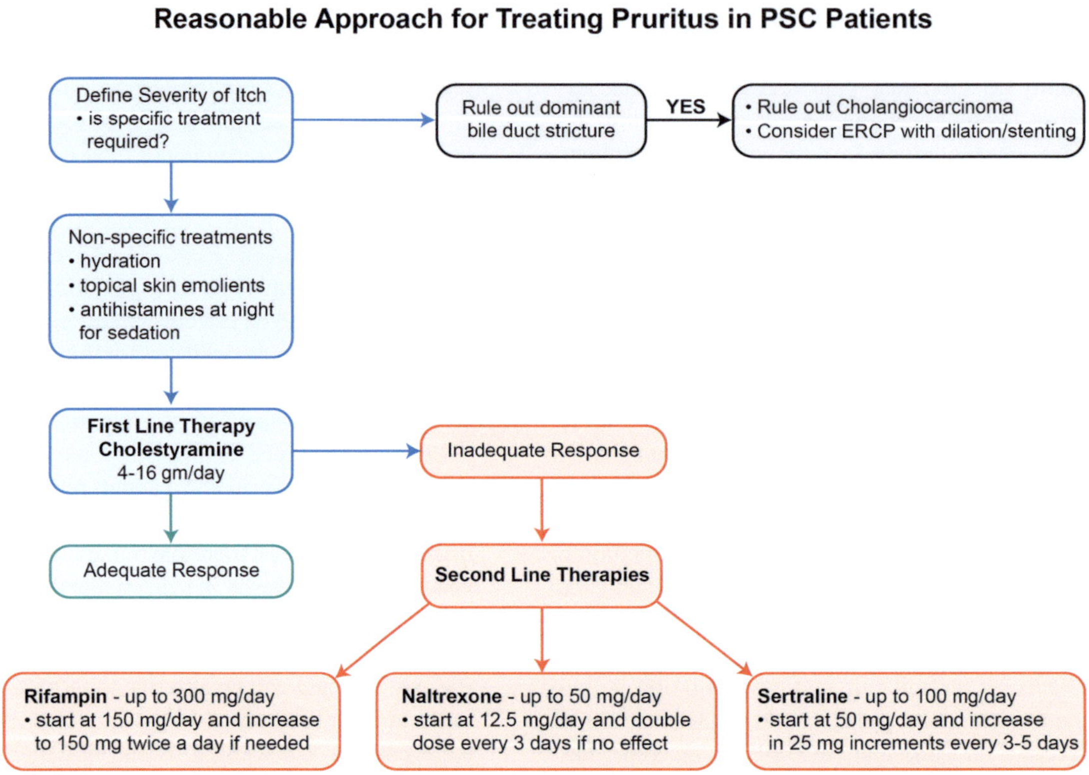

Fig. 10.2 Reasonable approach for treating pruritus in PSC patients. A reasonable approach to an itching PSC patient should include an assessment of itch severity (which can be quantitative or qualitative) to determine the impact of itch on quality of life. If the impact is minor, only nonspecific treatment may be indicated. It is important that in any PSC patient with new onset of significant pruritus, or a rapid worsening of pruritus, especially when serum cholestatic indices also deteriorate, a dominant stricture needs to be ruled out (and specifically dealt with). If pruritus is significant, first-line therapy consists of cholestyramine. If response is inadequate, then second-line therapies can be tried (instituted one at a time) and consist of either rifampin, naltrexone, or sertraline. If one of these does not work, it is reasonable to try another

Closing Remarks

Pruritus is a complex and poorly understood symptom that commonly affects patients with PSC and has a significant negative impact on their HRQOL. As we gain increasing insight into the pathways that cause and regulate itch, it is likely that more effective therapies will be developed in the near future to treat itch in PSC patients. However, for the time being, a rational stepwise approach to managing these patients can be followed that will benefit the majority of these patients.

References

1. Imam MH, Gossard AA, Sinakos E, Lindor KD. Pathogenesis and management of pruritus in cholestatic liver disease. J Gastroenterol Hepatol. 2012;27:1150–8.
2. Beuers U, Kremer AE, Bolier R, Elferink RP. Pruritus in cholestasis: facts and fiction. Hepatology. 2014;60:399–407.
3. Broome U, Olsson R, Loof L, Bodemar G, Hultcrantz R, Danielsson A, et al. Natural history and prognostic factors in 305 Swedish patients with primary sclerosing cholangitis. Gut. 1996;38:610–5.
4. Wiesner RH, Grambsch PM, Dickson ER, Ludwig J, MacCarty RL, Hunter EB, et al. Primary sclerosing cholangitis: natural history, prognostic factors and survival analysis. Hepatology. 1989;10:430–6.

5. Olsson R, Broome U, Danielsson A, Hagerstrand I, Jarnerot G, Loof L, et al. Spontaneous course of symptoms in primary sclerosing cholangitis: relationships with biochemical and histological features. Hepatogastroenterology. 1999;46:136–41.
6. Bergquist A, Said K, Broome U. Changes over a 20-year period in the clinical presentation of primary sclerosing cholangitis in Sweden. Scand J Gastroenterol. 2007; 42:88–93.
7. Smyk DS, Rigopoulou EI, Pares A, Billinis C, Burroughs AK, Muratori L, et al. Sex differences associated with primary biliary cirrhosis. Clin Dev Immunol. 2012;2012:610504.
8. Gotthardt DN, Rupp C, Bruhin M, Schellberg D, Weiss KH, Stefan R, et al. Pruritus is associated with severely impaired quality of life in patients with primary sclerosing cholangitis. Eur J Gastroenterol Hepatol. 2014;26:1374–9.
9. Benito de Valle M, Rahman M, Lindkvist B, Bjornsson E, Chapman R, Kalaitzakis E. Factors that reduce health-related quality of life in patients with primary sclerosing cholangitis. Clin Gastroenterol Hepatol Off Clin Pract J Am Gastroenterol Assoc. 2012;10:769–75.e762.
10. Dhand A, Aminoff MJ. The neurology of itch. Brain J Neurol. 2014;137:313–22.
11. Holle H, Warne K, Seth AK, Critchley HD, Ward J. Neural basis of contagious itch and why some people are more prone to it. Proc Natl Acad Sci U S A. 2012;109:19816–21.
12. Davidson S, Giesler GJ. The multiple pathways for itch and their interactions with pain. Trends Neurosci. 2010;33:550–8.
13. Schmelz M. Itch and pain. Neurosci Biobehav Rev. 2010;34:171–6.
14. Schmelz M, Schmidt R, Bickel A, Handwerker HO, Torebjork HE. Specific C-receptors for itch in human skin. J Neurosci Off J Soc Neurosci. 1997;17: 8003–8.
15. Namer B, Carr R, Johanek LM, Schmelz M, Handwerker HO, Ringkamp M. Separate peripheral pathways for pruritus in man. J Neurophysiol. 2008;100:2062–9.
16. Davidson S, Zhang X, Yoon CH, Khasabov SG, Simone DA, Giesler Jr GJ. The itch-producing agents histamine and cowhage activate separate populations of primate spinothalamic tract neurons. J Neurosci Off J Soc Neurosci. 2007;27:10007–14.
17. Jeffry J, Kim S, Chen ZF. Itch signaling in the nervous system. Physiology (Bethesda). 2011;26:286–92.
18. Kim BM, Lee SH, Shim WS, Oh U. Histamine-induced Ca(2+) influx via the PLA(2)/lipoxygenase/TRPV1 pathway in rat sensory neurons. Neurosci Lett. 2004;361:159–62.
19. Cowden JM, Zhang M, Dunford PJ, Thurmond RL. The histamine H4 receptor mediates inflammation and pruritus in Th2-dependent dermal inflammation. J Invest Dermatol. 2010;130:1023–33.
20. Reddy VB, Iuga AO, Shimada SG, LaMotte RH, Lerner EA. Cowhage-evoked itch is mediated by a novel cysteine protease: a ligand of protease-activated receptors. J Neurosci Off J Soc Neurosci. 2008;28:4331–5.
21. Tsujii K, Andoh T, Lee JB, Kuraishi Y. Activation of proteinase-activated receptors induces itch-associated response through histamine-dependent and -independent pathways in mice. J Pharmacol Sci. 2008;108: 385–8.
22. Steinhoff M, Neisius U, Ikoma A, Fartasch M, Heyer G, Skov PS, et al. Proteinase-activated receptor-2 mediates itch: a novel pathway for pruritus in human skin. J Neurosci Off J Soc Neurosci. 2003;23:6176–80.
23. Akiyama T, Carstens MI, Carstens E. Enhanced scratching evoked by PAR-2 agonist and 5-HT but not histamine in a mouse model of chronic dry skin itch. Pain. 2010;151:378–83.
24. Jordt SE, Bautista DM, Chuang HH, McKemy DD, Zygmunt PM, Hogestatt ED, et al. Mustard oils and cannabinoids excite sensory nerve fibres through the TRP channel ANKTM1. Nature. 2004;427:260–5.
25. Amadesi S, Nie J, Vergnolle N, Cottrell GS, Grady EF, Trevisani M, et al. Protease-activated receptor 2 sensitizes the capsaicin receptor transient receptor potential vanilloid receptor 1 to induce hyperalgesia. J Neurosci Off J Soc Neurosci. 2004;24:4300–12.
26. Sun YG, Chen ZF. A gastrin-releasing peptide receptor mediates the itch sensation in the spinal cord. Nature. 2007;448:700–3.
27. Koga K, Chen T, Li XY, Descalzi G, Ling J, Gu J, et al. Glutamate acts as a neurotransmitter for gastrin releasing peptide-sensitive and insensitive itch-related synaptic transmission in mammalian spinal cord. Mol Pain. 2011;7:47.
28. Akiyama T, Iodi Carstens M, Carstens E. Transmitters and pathways mediating inhibition of spinal itch-signaling neurons by scratching and other counter-stimuli. PLoS One. 2011;6:e22665.
29. Ross SE, Mardinly AR, McCord AE, Zurawski J, Cohen S, Jung C, et al. Loss of inhibitory interneurons in the dorsal spinal cord and elevated itch in Bhlhb5 mutant mice. Neuron. 2010;65:886–98.
30. Yosipovitch G, Mochizuki H. Neuroimaging of itch as a tool of assessment of chronic itch and its management. Handb Exp Pharmacol. 2015;226:57–70.
31. Gittlen SD, Schulman ES, Maddrey WC. Raised histamine concentrations in chronic cholestatic liver disease. Gut. 1990;31:96–9.
32. Wernersson S, Pejler G. Mast cell secretory granules: armed for battle. Nat Rev Immunol. 2014;14:478–94.
33. Datta DV, Sherlock S. Cholestyramine for long term relief of the pruritus complicating intrahepatic cholestasis. Gastroenterology. 1966;50:323–32.
34. Kuiper EM, van Erpecum KJ, Beuers U, Hansen BE, Thio HB, de Man RA, et al. The potent bile acid sequestrant colesevelam is not effective in cholestatic pruritus: results of a double-blind, randomized, placebo-controlled trial. Hepatology. 2010;52:1334–40.

35. Hirschfield GM, Mason A, Luketic V, Lindor K, Gordon SC, Mayo M, et al. Efficacy of obeticholic acid in patients with primary biliary cirrhosis and inadequate response to ursodeoxycholic acid. Gastroenterology. 2015;148:751–61.e758.
36. Alemi F, Kwon E, Poole DP, Lieu T, Lyo V, Cattaruzza F, et al. The TGR5 receptor mediates bile acid-induced itch and analgesia. J Clin Invest. 2013;123:1513–30.
37. Lieu T, Jayaweera G, Zhao P, Poole DP, Jensen D, Grace M, et al. The bile acid receptor TGR5 activates the TRPA1 channel to induce itch in mice. Gastroenterology. 2014;147:1417–28.
38. Hegade VS, Krawczyk M, Kremer AE, Kuczka J, Gaouar F, Kuiper EM, et al. The safety and efficacy of nasobiliary drainage in the treatment of refractory cholestatic pruritus: a multicentre European study. Aliment Pharmacol Ther. 2016;43:294–302.
39. Stapelbroek JM, van Erpecum KJ, Klomp LW, Venneman NG, Schwartz TP, van Berge Henegouwen GP, et al. Nasobiliary drainage induces long-lasting remission in benign recurrent intrahepatic cholestasis. Hepatology. 2006;43:51–3.
40. Pongcharoen P, Fleischer Jr AB. An evidence-based review of systemic treatments for itch. Eur J Pain. 2016;20:24–31.
41. Ghent CN, Carruthers SG. Treatment of pruritus in primary biliary cirrhosis with rifampin. Results of a double-blind, crossover, randomized trial. Gastroenterology. 1988;94:488–93.
42. Vesely JJ, Pien FD, Pien BC. Rifampin, a useful drug for nonmycobacterial infections. Pharmacotherapy. 1998;18:345–57.
43. Tabibian JH, Talwalkar JA, Lindor KD. Role of the microbiota and antibiotics in primary sclerosing cholangitis. Biomed Res Int. 2013;2013:389537.
44. Tabibian JH, Weeding E, Jorgensen RA, Petz JL, Keach JC, Talwalkar JA, et al. Randomised clinical trial: vancomycin or metronidazole in patients with primary sclerosing cholangitis – a pilot study. Aliment Pharmacol Ther. 2013;37:604–12.
45. Inagaki T, Moschetta A, Lee YK, Peng L, Zhao G, Downes M, et al. Regulation of antibacterial defense in the small intestine by the nuclear bile acid receptor. Proc Natl Acad Sci U S A. 2006;103:3920–5.
46. Ridlon JM, Kang DJ, Hylemon PB, Bajaj JS. Bile acids and the gut microbiome. Curr Opin Gastroenterol. 2014;30:332–8.
47. Vleggaar FP, Monkelbaan JF, van Erpecum KJ. Probiotics in primary sclerosing cholangitis: a randomized placebo-controlled crossover pilot study. Eur J Gastroenterol Hepatol. 2008;20:688–92.
48. Kremer AE, Martens JJ, Kulik W, Rueff F, Kuiper EM, van Buuren HR, et al. Lysophosphatidic acid is a potential mediator of cholestatic pruritus. Gastroenterology. 2010;139:1008–18, 1018 e1001.
49. Hashimoto T, Satoh T. Generalized pruritus in primary sclerosing cholangitis: implications of histamine release by lysophosphatidic acid. Br J Dermatol. 2015;173(5):1334–6.
50. Kremer AE, van Dijk R, Leckie P, Schaap FG, Kuiper EM, Mettang T, et al. Serum autotaxin is increased in pruritus of cholestasis, but not of other origin, and responds to therapeutic interventions. Hepatology. 2012;56:1391–400.
51. Hosonuma K, Sato K, Yamazaki Y, Yanagisawa M, Hashizume H, Horiguchi N, et al. A prospective randomized controlled study of long-term combination therapy using ursodeoxycholic acid and bezafibrate in patients with primary biliary cirrhosis and dyslipidemia. Am J Gastroenterol. 2015;110:423–31.
52. Honda A, Ikegami T, Nakamuta M, Miyazaki T, Iwamoto J, Hirayama T, et al. Anticholestatic effects of bezafibrate in patients with primary biliary cirrhosis treated with ursodeoxycholic acid. Hepatology. 2013;57:1931–41.
53. Karlsen TH, Boberg KM. Update on primary sclerosing cholangitis. J Hepatol. 2013;59:571–82.
54. Hirschfield GM, Karlsen TH, Lindor KD, Adams DH. Primary sclerosing cholangitis. Lancet. 2013;382: 1587–99.
55. Thornton JR, Losowsky MS. Plasma leucine enkephalin is increased in liver disease. Gut. 1989;30: 1392–5.
56. Nelson L, Vergnolle N, D'Mello C, Chapman K, Le T, Swain MG. Endogenous opioid-mediated antinociception in cholestatic mice is peripherally, not centrally, mediated. J Hepatol. 2006;44:1141–9.
57. Wolfhagen FH, Sternieri E, Hop WC, Vitale G, Bertolotti M, Van Buuren HR. Oral naltrexone treatment for cholestatic pruritus: a double-blind, placebo-controlled study. Gastroenterology. 1997;113:1264–9.
58. Bergasa NV, Schmitt JM, Talbot TL, Alling DW, Swain MG, Turner ML, et al. Open-label trial of oral nalmefene therapy for the pruritus of cholestasis. Hepatology. 1998;27:679–84.
59. Bergasa NV, Alling DW, Talbot TL, Swain MG, Yurdaydin C, Turner ML, et al. Effects of naloxone infusions in patients with the pruritus of cholestasis. A double-blind, randomized, controlled trial. Ann Intern Med. 1995;123:161–7.
60. Sorkin LS, Xiao WH, Wagner R, Myers RR. Tumour necrosis factor-alpha induces ectopic activity in nociceptive primary afferent fibres. Neuroscience. 1997; 81:255–62.
61. Sorkin LS, Doom CM. Epineurial application of TNF elicits an acute mechanical hyperalgesia in the awake rat. J Peripher Nerv Syst JPNS. 2000;5:96–100.
62. Spicarova D, Nerandzic V, Palecek J. Modulation of spinal cord synaptic activity by tumor necrosis factor alpha in a model of peripheral neuropathy. J Neuroinflammation. 2011;8:177.
63. Hensellek S, Brell P, Schaible HG, Brauer R, Segond von Banchet G. The cytokine TNFalpha increases the proportion of DRG neurones expressing the TRPV1 receptor via the TNFR1 receptor and ERK activation. Mol Cell Neurosci. 2007;36:381–91.
64. Sommer C, Schafers M, Marziniak M, Toyka KV. Etanercept reduces hyperalgesia in experimental

painful neuropathy. J Peripher Nerv Syst JPNS. 2001;6:67–72.
65. Lisboa LF, Asthana S, Kremer A, Swain M, Bagshaw SM, Gibney N, et al. Blood cytokine, chemokine and gene expression in cholestasis patients with intractable pruritis treated with a molecular adsorbent recirculating system: a case series. Can J Gastroenterol J Can Gastroenterol. 2012;26:799–805.
66. McCormick PA, Scott F, Epstein O, Burroughs AK, Scheuer PJ, McIntyre N. Thalidomide as therapy for primary biliary cirrhosis: a double-blind placebo controlled pilot study. J Hepatol. 1994;21:496–9.
67. Bharucha AE, Jorgensen R, Lichtman SN, LaRusso NF, Lindor KD. A pilot study of pentoxifylline for the treatment of primary sclerosing cholangitis. Am J Gastroenterol. 2000;95:2338–42.
68. Epstein MP, Kaplan MM. A pilot study of etanercept in the treatment of primary sclerosing cholangitis. Dig Dis Sci. 2004;49:1–4.
69. Hoffman W, Lakkis FG, Chalasani G. B Cells, antibodies, and more. Clin J Am Soc Nephrol CJASN. 2016;11:137–54.
70. Myers RP, Swain MG, Lee SS, Shaheen AA, Burak KW. B-cell depletion with rituximab in patients with primary biliary cirrhosis refractory to ursodeoxycholic acid. Am J Gastroenterol. 2013;108:933–41.
71. Neff GW, O'Brien CB, Reddy KR, Bergasa NV, Regev A, Molina E, et al. Preliminary observation with dronabinol in patients with intractable pruritus secondary to cholestatic liver disease. Am J Gastroenterol. 2002;97:2117–9.
72. Dvorak M, Watkinson A, McGlone F, Rukwied R. Histamine induced responses are attenuated by a cannabinoid receptor agonist in human skin. Inflamm Res Off J Eur Histamine Res Soc [et al]. 2003; 52:238–45.
73. Mayo MJ, Handem I, Saldana S, Jacobe H, Getachew Y, Rush AJ. Sertraline as a first-line treatment for cholestatic pruritus. Hepatology. 2007;45:666–74.
74. Jones EA, Molenaar HA, Oosting J. Ondansetron and pruritus in chronic liver disease: a controlled study. Hepatogastroenterology. 2007;54:1196–9.
75. McCormack HM, Horne DJ, Sheather S. Clinical applications of visual analogue scales: a critical review. Psychol Med. 1988;18:1007–19.
76. Babatin MA, Sanai FM, Swain MG. Methotrexate therapy for the symptomatic treatment of primary biliary cirrhosis patients, who are biochemical incomplete responders to ursodeoxycholic acid therapy. Aliment Pharmacol Ther. 2006;24:813–20.
77. Gotthardt D, Stiehl A. Endoscopic retrograde cholangiopancreatography in diagnosis and treatment of primary sclerosing cholangitis. Clin Liver Dis. 2010;14:349–58.

Ursodeoxycholic Acid Treatment in Primary Sclerosing Cholangitis

11

James H. Tabibian and Keith D. Lindor

Overview and Clinical Epidemiology

Primary sclerosing cholangitis (PSC) is a chronic, cholestatic disorder of the liver characterized by three major features: biliary inflammation and periductal fibrosis on liver histology, multifocal biliary strictures alternating with segmental ductal dilatation on cholangiography, and a cholestatic serum biochemical profile [1, 2]. Unlike most other cholangiopathies, i.e., disorders primarily of or affecting the biliary tract [3, 4], PSC can affect individuals of essentially all ages and racial backgrounds, remains etiopathogenically perplexing, and lacks established medical therapy despite decades of laboratory-based investigation, translational studies, and clinical trials [1, 5]. It is because of these factors that PSC has, unfortunately, been regarded as the "black box" of liver disease [6].

Although the fundamental underpinnings and optimal management approaches for PSC remain uncertain, it is clear that, as a result of these uncertainties and the generally progressive nature of PSC, there is substantial public health and patient-level burden due to this disorder. Indeed, PSC represents a major risk factor for cholangiocarcinoma (CCA) [7], carries a median liver transplantation (LT)-free survival of 15 years [8], and (despite its rarity) is a leading indication for LT in countries around the world [9]. Although LT can be curative for PSC and PSC-associated CCA, it is only performed in highly selected patients and centers, and even suitable candidates may experience recurrent disease (≈3–4 % per year) [10]. Lastly, quality of life (QOL) is also significantly impaired in patients with PSC, both pre- and post-LT, and is related to debilitating symptoms such as pruritus and fatigue as well as the unpredictable disease course and complications related to coexisting inflammatory bowel disease (IBD) [11–13].

Proposed Etiopathogenesis of and the Basis of Bile Acid Therapy in PSC

Although PSC remains an idiopathic disorder, prevailing hypotheses regarding its etiopathogenesis suggest that a disruption of gut-liver axis signaling at various levels may play a fundamental role [6]. These hypotheses are largely based on

J.H. Tabibian, MD, PhD
Division of Gastroenterology and Hepatology, University of California Davis, 4150 V St., Suite 3500, PSSB, Sacramento, CA 95817, USA
e-mail: jtabibian@ucdavis.edu

K.D. Lindor, MD (✉)
College of Health Solutions, Arizona State University, 550 North 3rd St., Phoenix, AZ 85004, USA
e-mail: keith.lindor@asu.edu

L.M. Forman (ed.), *Primary Sclerosing Cholangitis*, DOI 10.1007/978-3-319-40908-5_11

the premise that enterohepatic generation and/or circulation of microbial metabolites, derivatives, or other molecules can initiate and perpetuate aberrant or exaggerated cellular responses and subsequent biliary injury. This has been the subject of ongoing investigation over the last several decades, with the goal being to identify potentially causal molecules and pathways and develop targeted therapies accordingly.

Representing perhaps the most widely investigated molecule and certainly the most extensively studied pharmacotherapy in PSC is ursodeoxycholic acid (UDCA) [14]. First isolated over a century ago from *Thalarctos maritimus* (now known as *Ursus maritimus*), i.e., the polar bear, UDCA is a hydrophilic, 3,7-dihydroxy bile acid (BA). In most vertebrates, including *Homo sapiens*, UDCA is a secondary BA and only a minor component (<5 %) of the BA pool; the major known exception among vertebrates is the Ursidae family, particularly *Ursus americanus* (the American black bear), wherein UDCA is typically a relatively major component (>5–30 %) of the BA pool [6, 15]. BA physiology and the potential therapeutic applications of BA therapies are shown in Fig. 11.1 and discussed in greater detail in recent review articles [16, 17].

Based on studies in patients as well as various lines of experimental (e.g., model system) data, the mechanisms through which UDCA is believed to exert therapeutic effects in cholestatic disorders include dilution of hydrophobic (or otherwise "toxic") BAs, promotion of their excretion, upregulation of the biliary bicarbonate umbrella [18, 19], immunomodulation, and anti-inflammatory actions [2, 12, 15, 20–22. In addition, recent data suggest that UDCA may have anti-senescent properties [23]; while the liver has traditionally been regarded as an organ resistant to aging [24], recent studies have shown cellular senescence (in particular cholangiocyte senescence) to be increased in PSC [5], and this finding has been regarded as a marker and driver of biliary injury [23, 25].

Perhaps somewhat surprisingly, evidence supporting a therapeutic role for UDCA in PSC (or animal models thereof) has been inconsistent, with some studies even suggesting detrimental effects at high doses (discussed further below) [19, 26, 27]. As a result, because of the lack of consistently perceived benefits, in their respective practice guidelines, the American Association for the Study of Liver Diseases (AASLD) [21] and European Association for the Study of the Liver (EASL) [20] advise against and provide no specific recommendation, respectively, regarding the use of UDCA in patients with PSC.

Clinical Trials of UDCA in PSC

The earliest clinical studies of UDCA were published in the late 1980s [21, 28, 29] and, albeit uncontrolled, demonstrated promising symptomatic and objective improvements among patients with PSC [30]. These studies soon led to the first randomized controlled trial (RCT) of UDCA, which demonstrated significant improvements in multiple biochemical end points as well as in liver histology [31]. Since then, seven other RCTs have been conducted, initially with low (10–15 mg per kg body weight per day [mg/kg/d])-, then intermediate (17–23 mg/kg/day)-, and most recently high-dose (28–30 mg/kg/day) UDCA (Table 11.1) [14]. While low-dose UDCA was repeatedly shown to yield biochemical improvements, it has not been convincingly shown to improve outcomes, and thus its routine use in PSC is not recommended [21].

High-dose UDCA has been studied in PSC and shown to be associated with an increase in serious adverse outcomes. Specifically, treatment with 28–30 mg/kg/day was found to be associated with a significantly increased risk of major adverse events in a recent RCT of 150 patients with PSC, which was stopped early [19]. At the time of study termination (6 years' post-study initiation), 30 patients in the UDCA group (39 %) versus 19 patients in the placebo group (26 %) had reached one of the preestablished clinical end points, namely, development of cirrhosis, varices, CCA, LT, or death. After adjustment for baseline characteristics, the risk of a primary end point was 2.3 times greater for patients receiving UDCA compared to the placebo group ($p<0.01$) and 2.1 times greater for death, LT, or LT listing criteria ($p=0.038$). In addition, serious adverse events were more common in the UDCA group

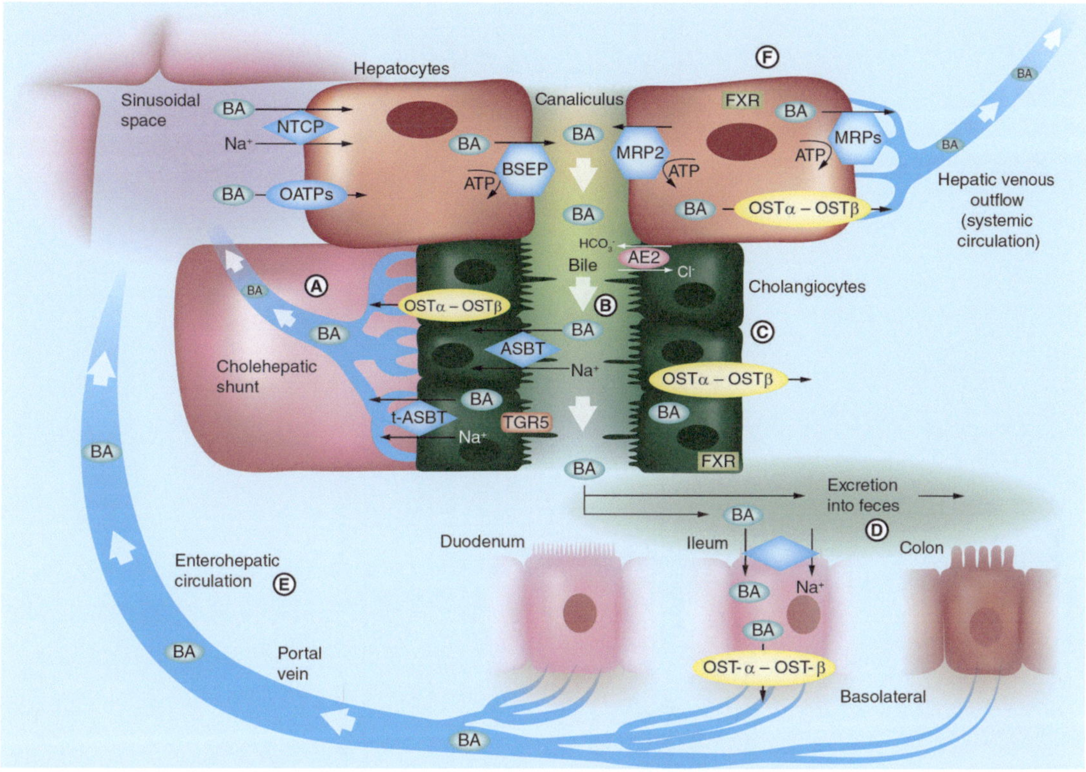

Fig. 11.1 Bile acid physiology and circulation: an avenue for therapeutic applications. Bile acids (*BAs*) are synthesized by hepatocytes and subsequently secreted into canalicular bile by means of specialized hepatocyte canalicular membrane transporters. Canalicular bile drains into the biliary tree and is modified by the epithelial cells lining it, that is, cholangiocytes. Bile then drains into the proximal small bowel, that is, duodenum, and is metabolized by enteric bacteria. Approximately 95 % of BAs are reabsorbed in the terminal ileum and enter the portal vein to be recycled back to the liver via the enterohepatic circulation. Once in the sinusoids of the liver, BAs can be taken up by hepatocytes and secreted back into bile. A fraction of (unconjugated) BAs in the biliary tree is taken up by cholangiocytes at the apical membrane (i.e., prior to reaching the small intestine) and returned to the liver sinusoids via the cholehepatic shunt. Some endogenous and synthetic BAs as well as BA analogs have considerably distinct pharmacologic properties, including but not limited to the degree to which they are cholehepatically shunted (e.g., nor-UDCA being a potent stimulator of cholehepatic shunting) or their potency for agonizing receptors such as the farnesoid X receptor (e.g., obeticholic acid being a potent FXR agonist). The unique properties of some BAs and BA analogs can be harnessed for therapeutic purposes in hepatobiliary diseases including PSC; indeed, this represents an area of ongoing biomedical research. Key: *AE2* anion exchange protein 2, *ASBT* apical sodium-dependent bile acid transporter, *BSEP* bile salt export pump, *MRP* multidrug resistance protein, *NTCP* Na+ (sodium)-taurocholate cotransporting polypeptide, *OATP* organic anion-transporting polypeptide, *OST* organic solute transporter, *t-ASBT* truncated apical sodium-dependent bile acid transporter, *TGR5* G protein-coupled bile acid receptor 1 (Adapted with permission from the Mayo Foundation for Medical Education and Research. All rights reserved)

compared to the placebo group (63 % versus 37 %, $p<0.01$). While the mechanisms of these inferior outcomes with high-dose UDCA remain uncertain, they may ostensibly be due to toxic metabolites of supratherapeutic UDCA administration and seem to be particularly affect patients with early-stage disease [27]. Based on these results, high-dose UDCA is not recommended in PSC and should not be prescribed.

To date, the most intriguing and favorable RCT-derived data supporting the role of UDCA in PSC have been with use of intermediate-dose UDCA. For example, Mitchell et al. [32] found significant improvements in serum biochemistries, hepatic fibrosis stage, and cholangiographic appearance among patients treated with intermediate-dose UDCA (Table 11.1). Subsequently, and in the largest RCT of UDCA to date, Olsson et al. [33] reported

Table 11.1 Characteristics and results of randomized trials comparing UDCA vs. placebo (or no treatment) in patients with PSC

								Outcomes					
							Study duration	Death/LT, *n* (%)		Cholangio CA		Histologic progression	
Lead author	Year	*n*	% male	% IBD	Daily dosage (mg)	Dose	(years)	UDCA	Ctrl	UDCA	Ctrl	UDCA	Ctrl
Beuers [31]	1992	14	79 %	79 %	600–800	Low	1	0 %	0 %	NA	NA	0 %	16.7 %
Lo [41]	1992	18	61 %	61 %	200	Low	2	0 %	0 %	NA	NA	NA	NA
Stiehl [42]	1994	20	NA	NA	500–1000	Low	.25	0 %	0 %	NA	NA	NA	NA
De Maria [43]	1996	40	70 %	70 %	750–1,500	Low	2	0 %	0 %	NA	NA	NA	NA
Lindor [44]	1997	102	60 %	60 %	600–800	Low	2	7.8 %	5.9 %	0 %	5.9 %	15.7 %	5.9 %
Mitchell [32]	2001	26	73 %	73 %	20/Kg	Interm.	2	0 %	7.7 %	0 %	0 %	18.2 %	50.0 %
Olsson [33]	2005	198	70 %	70 %	500–1000	Interm.	5	2.1 %	3.0 %	3.1 %	4.0 %	NA	NA
Lindor [19]	2009	149	58 %	557	750–1,500	High	6	6.6 %	4.1 %	2.6 %	2.7 %	NA	NA

Key: *Ctrl* control (placebo or no treatment), *Interm.* intermediate, *PSC* primary sclerosing cholangitis, *UDCA* ursodeoxycholic acid a 34 % relative reduction in need for LT, 31 % relative reduction in mortality, and 22 % relative reduction in diagnosis of CCA. These results did not reach statistical significance, perhaps due to the low incidence of these "hard end points" as well as inability to enroll the planned number of study participants; however, they have been regarded as showing a trend toward such by various expert investigators, many of whom continue to offer intermediate-dose UDCA to select patients with PSC (discussed in the subsequent section) [1, 6, 34]. This practice is supported by several long-term-outcome studies by our group and others from within the last several years which have shown that patients with persistently elevated ALP who achieve clinically significant improvement or normalization of ALP with UDCA therapy have decreased risk of major adverse events (e.g., CCA, need for LT, or liver-related death) [30, 35–37].

Of interest is a recent prospective European study evaluating the effects of 3 months of UDCA withdrawal on serum biochemical tests as well as QOL and symptoms among 26 patients with PSC who were receiving UDCA at a dose of 10–15 mg/kg/day [34]. At the end of UDCA withdrawal, there was a significant (76 %) increase in ALP as well as ALT, AST, bilirubin, and Mayo PSC risk score. Changes in QOL were variable across specific parameters as well as within individual patients, and the majority did not change significantly; there was, however, near doubling in pruritus rating, and this coincided with worsened fatigue in 42 % and deterioration in overall general health (a domain of the short form-36 quality of life instrument) in 60 % of patients. This study represents the largest prospective evaluation of UDCA withdrawal in PSC, and despite several limitations [6], it suggests therapeutic benefit in at least a subset of patients with PSC.

Potential Chemopreventive Properties of UDCA Against Colorectal Cancer

A small body of data suggests that UDCA may play a chemopreventive role against colorectal cancer (CRC) in individuals with PSC-IBD. For example, in a cross-sectional study of 59 patients with PSC-UC undergoing colonoscopic surveillance, UDCA use was associated with decreased prevalence of colonic dysplasia [38]. In another randomized, placebo-controlled trial of 52 patients with PSC-UC, UDCA use was associated with a relative risk of 0.26 for developing colorectal dysplasia or CRC [39]. While specific recommendations have been made regarding CRC prevention in PSC-IBD [40], routine use of UDCA for this indication has not been recommended as additional studies remain needed to confirm its putative chemopreventive properties [21].

UDCA in Clinical Practice

Use of UDCA in routine clinical practice is highly varied among gastroenterologists and even among subspecialized hepatologists within individual referral centers. This is likely a result of mixed views as to the potential benefits of UDCA therapy and the paucity of consistent, high-quality data to suggest a definite therapeutic impact. It is interesting to note that although it is well described that >20 % of patients with another cholestatic liver disease, primary biliary cirrhosis, are nonresponders to UDCA, this drug is still widely recommended as primary therapy; even in patients who are unlikely to respond (e.g., established cirrhosis) or seem to have no or minimal response to UDCA, societal guidelines do not recommend withholding it, perhaps with the hope being that some degree of benefit might still be achieved. Nevertheless, and for reasons that have not been well studied, there appears to be more reticence toward UDCA in PSC as compared to primary biliary cirrhosis, although many clinicians continue to use UDCA in patients with PSC.

Until safer and more effective pharmacotherapies become available, our current practice is to offer a trial of intermediate-dose UDCA (17–23 mg/kg/day) to patients with compensated PSC whose serum ALP remains >1.5× the upper limit of normal after 1 year since the time of diagnosis [45] or who have troublesome symptoms of cholestasis (e.g., pruritus), as shown in Fig. 11.2. If UDCA is not symptomatically well

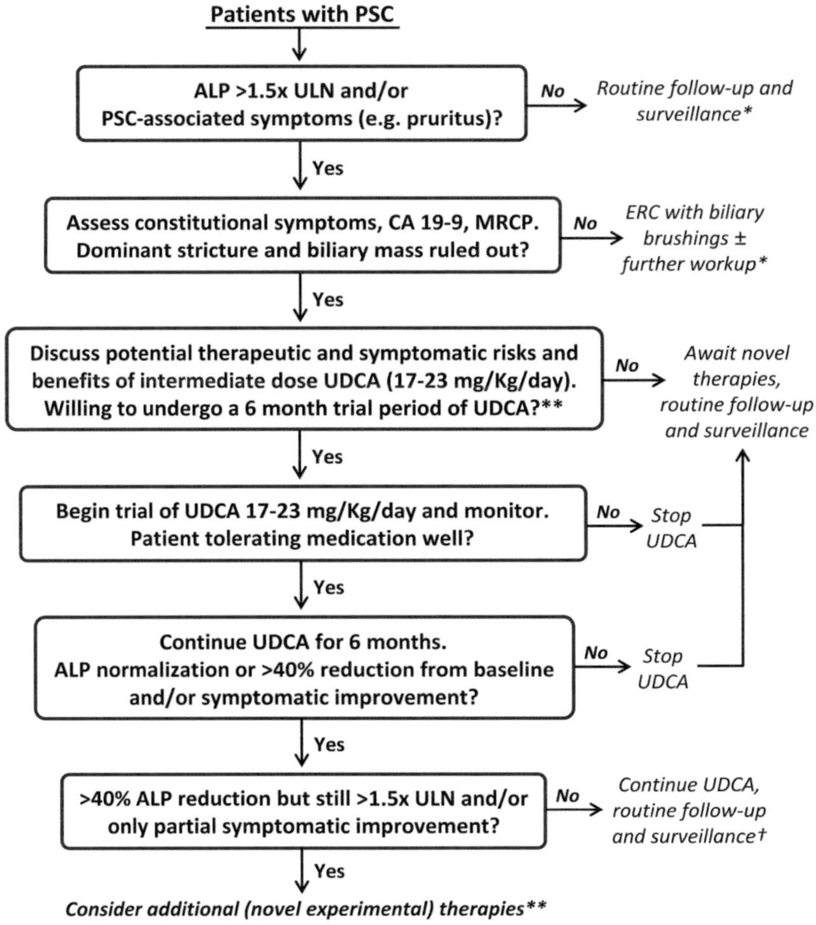

Fig. 11.2 Proposed algorithm for UDCA use in clinical practice and trials in PSC. *Surveillance and management options reviewed elsewhere [4]. **Consider referral to subspecialist in cholestatic liver disease and/or to tertiary care center. †Also consider decreasing UDCA dose to the lowest dose which maintains biochemical and/or symptomatic response on an individualized basis. Key: *ALP* serum alkaline phosphatase; *CA 19-9* carbohydrate antigen 19-9, *MRCP* magnetic resonance cholangiopancreatography, *PSC* primary sclerosing cholangitis, *UDCA* ursodeoxycholic acid, *ULN*, upper limit of normal

tolerated or if clinically significant improvement in ALP is not achieved, we discontinue UDCA treatment. These decisions are made with patients' direct involvement and input and based on careful interpretation of the available biomedical literature [6, 30–36, Ref Annals of Hep [DOI pending]]. Implementation of UDCA in this manner (1) offers patients with PSC the opportunity to potentially benefit from UDCA, (2) lends itself to prospective study in order to help expedite evidence-based treatment recommendations, and (3) can be implemented alongside novel experimental pharmacotherapies (e.g., norUDCA, the preclinical data for which indicate that it may well be more effective when used in combination with UDCA).

UDCA in PSC: Conclusions

Although many questions remain unanswered, given the morbidity and mortality of PSC, we believe that the existing evidence supports a role for judicious use of UDCA in patients with PSC, particularly in the absence of safer and more effective therapeutic options. Treatment with

UDCA can be implemented in unison with ongoing efforts to develop and rigorously test-emerging therapies through basic, translational, and clinical research endeavors.

The study of PSC pharmacotherapeutics appears to now be better positioned than ever, and with continued innovation, collaboration, and investigation, an even more broadly therapeutic treatment seems likely in the near future.

Conflicts of Interest, Disclosures James H. Tabibian – none

Keith D. Lindor – unpaid consultant for Shire and Intercept

References

1. Tabibian JH, Lindor KD. Primary sclerosing cholangitis: a review and update on therapeutic developments. Expert Rev Gastroenterol Hepatol. 2013;7(2):103–14.
2. Pollheimer MJ, Halilbasic E, Fickert P, Trauner M. Pathogenesis of primary sclerosing cholangitis. Best Pract Res Clin Gastroenterol. 2011;25(6):727–39.
3. Lazaridis KN, LaRusso NF. The cholangiopathies. Mayo Clin Proc. 2015;90(6):791–800.
4. O'Hara SP, Gradilone SA, Masyuk TV, Tabibian JH, LaRusso NF. MicroRNAs in cholangiopathies. Curr Pathobiol Rep. 2014;2(3):133–42.
5. Tabibian JH, O'Hara SP, Splinter PL, Trussoni CE, LaRusso NF. Cholangiocyte senescence by way of N-Ras activation is a characteristic of primary sclerosing cholangitis. Hepatology. 2014;59(6):2263–75.
6. Tabibian JH, Lindor KD. Ursodeoxycholic acid in primary sclerosing cholangitis: if withdrawal is bad, then administration is good (right?). Hepatology. 2014; 60(3):785–8.
7. Tabibian JH, Lindor K. Challenges of cholangiocarcinoma detection in patients with primary sclerosing cholangitis. J Anal Oncol. 2012;1:50–5.
8. Wiesner RH, Grambsch PM, Dickson ER, et al. Primary sclerosing cholangitis: natural history, prognostic factors and survival analysis. Hepatology. 1989;10(4):430–6.
9. Bjoro K, Brandsaeter B, Foss A, Schrumpf E. Liver transplantation in primary sclerosing cholangitis. Semin Liver Dis. 2006;26(1):69–79.
10. Alabraba E, Nightingale P, Gunson B, et al. A re-evaluation of the risk factors for the recurrence of primary sclerosing cholangitis in liver allografts. Liver Transpl. 2009;15(3):330–40.
11. Aberg F, Hockerstedt K, Roine RP, Sintonen H, Isoniemi H. Influence of liver-disease etiology on long-term quality of life and employment after liver transplantation. Clin Transplant. 2012;26(5):729–35.
12. Benito de Valle M, Rahman M, Lindkvist B, Bjornsson E, Chapman R, Kalaitzakis E. Factors that reduce health-related quality of life in patients with primary sclerosing cholangitis. Clin Gastroenterol Hepatol. 2012;10(7):769–775.e2.
13. Tabibian A, Tabibian JH, Beckman LJ, Raffals LL, Papadakis KA, Kane SV. Predictors of health-related quality of life and adherence in Crohn's disease and ulcerative colitis: implications for clinical management. Dig Dis Sci. 2015;60(5):1366–74.
14. Triantos CK, Koukias NM, Nikolopoulou VN, Burroughs AK. Meta-analysis: ursodeoxycholic acid for primary sclerosing cholangitis. Aliment Pharmacol Ther. 2011;34(8):901–10.
15. Hagey LR, Crombie DL, Espinosa E, Carey MC, Igimi H, Hofmann AF. Ursodeoxycholic acid in the Ursidae: biliary bile acids of bears, pandas, and related carnivores. J Lipid Res. 1993;34(11):1911–7.
16. Tabibian JH, Masyuk AI, Masyuk TV, O'Hara SP, LaRusso NF. Physiology of cholangiocytes. Compr Physiol. 2013;3(1):541–65.
17. Maillette de Buy Wenniger LJ, Oude Elferink RP, Beuers U. Molecular targets for the treatment of fibrosing cholangiopathies. Clin Pharmacol Ther. 2012;92(3):381–7.
18. Fickert P, Fuchsbichler A, Wagner M, et al. Regurgitation of bile acids from leaky bile ducts causes sclerosing cholangitis in Mdr2 (Abcb4) knockout mice. Gastroenterology. 2004;127(1):261–74.
19. Lindor KD, Kowdley KV, Luketic VA, et al. High-dose ursodeoxycholic acid for the treatment of primary sclerosing cholangitis. Hepatology. 2009;50(3):808–14.
20. European Association for the Study of the Liver. EASL clinical practice guidelines: management of cholestatic liver diseases. J Hepatol. 2009;51(2):237–67.
21. Chapman R, Fevery J, Kalloo A, et al. Diagnosis and management of primary sclerosing cholangitis. Hepatology. 2010;51(2):660–78.
22. Hofmann AF. Bile acids: trying to understand their chemistry and biology with the hope of helping patients. Hepatology. 2009;49(5):1403–18.
23. Tabibian JH, O'Hara SP, Trussoni CE, et al. Absence of the intestinal microbiota exacerbates hepatobiliary disease in a murine model of primary sclerosing cholangitis. Hepatology. 2016;63(1):185–96.
24. Verma S, Tachtatzis P, Penrhyn-Lowe S, et al. Sustained telomere length in hepatocytes and cholangiocytes with increasing age in normal liver. Hepatology. 2012;56(4):1510–20.
25. O'Hara SP, Tabibian JH, Splinter PL, LaRusso NF. The dynamic biliary epithelia: molecules, pathways, and disease. J Hepatol. 2013;58(3):575–82.
26. Fickert P, Zollner G, Fuchsbichler A, et al. Ursodeoxycholic acid aggravates bile infarcts in bile duct-ligated and Mdr2 knockout mice via disruption of cholangioles. Gastroenterology. 2002;123(4):1238–51.
27. Imam MH, Sinakos E, Gossard AA, Kowdley KV, Luketic VA, Edwyn Harrison M, McCashland T, et al. High-dose ursodeoxycholic acid increases risk of adverse outcomes in patients with early stage primary

sclerosing cholangitis. Aliment Pharmacol Ther. 2011;34(10):1185–92.
28. Chazouilleres O, Poupon R, Capron JP, et al. Ursodeoxycholic acid for primary sclerosing cholangitis. J Hepatol. 1990;11(1):120–3.
29. O'Brien CB, Senior JR, Arora-Mirchandani R, Batta AK, Salen G. Ursodeoxycholic acid for the treatment of primary sclerosing cholangitis: a 30-month pilot study. Hepatology. 1991;14(5):838–47.
30. Stanich PP, Bjornsson E, Gossard AA, Enders F, Jorgensen R, Lindor KD. Alkaline phosphatase normalization is associated with better prognosis in primary sclerosing cholangitis. Dig Liver Dis. 2011; 43(4):309–13.
31. Beuers U, Spengler U, Kruis W, et al. Ursodeoxycholic acid for treatment of primary sclerosing cholangitis: a placebo-controlled trial. Hepatology. 1992;16(3): 707–14.
32. Mitchell SA, Bansi DS, Hunt N, Von Bergmann K, Fleming KA, Chapman RW. A preliminary trial of high-dose ursodeoxycholic acid in primary sclerosing cholangitis. Gastroenterology. 2001;121(4):900–7.
33. Olsson R, Boberg KM, de Muckadell OS, et al. High-dose ursodeoxycholic acid in primary sclerosing cholangitis: a 5-year multicenter, randomized, controlled study. Gastroenterology. 2005;129(5): 1464–72.
34. Wunsch E, Trottier J, Milkiewicz M, et al. Prospective evaluation of ursodeoxycholic acid withdrawal in patients with primary sclerosing cholangitis. Hepatology. 2014;60(3):931–40.
35. Lindstrom L, Hultcrantz R, Boberg KM, Friis-Liby I, Bergquist A. Association between reduced levels of alkaline phosphatase and survival times of patients with primary sclerosing cholangitis. Clin Gastroenterol Hepatol. 2013;11(7):841–6.
36. Al Mamari S, Djordjevic J, Halliday JS, Chapman RW. Improvement of serum alkaline phosphatase to <1.5 upper limit of normal predicts better outcome and reduced risk of cholangiocarcinoma in primary sclerosing cholangitis. J Hepatol. 2013;58(2):329–34.
37. Rupp C, Rossler A, Halibasic E, et al. Reduction in alkaline phosphatase is associated with longer survival in primary sclerosing cholangitis, independent of dominant stenosis. Aliment Pharmacol Ther. 2014;40(11–12):1292–301.
38. Tung BY, et al. Ursodiol use is associated with lower prevalence of colonic neoplasia in patients with ulcerative colitis and primary sclerosing cholangitis. Ann Intern Med. 2001;134:89–95.
39. Pardi DS, et al. Ursodeoxycholic acid as a chemopreventive agent in patients with ulcerative colitis and primary sclerosing cholangitis. Gastroenterology. 2003;124:889–93.
40. Tabibian JH, Moradkhani A, Topazian MD. Colorectal cancer surveillance in primary sclerosing cholangitis and inflammatory bowel disease. Ann Hepatol. 2015;14(4):564–6.
41. Lo SK, Herrmann R, Chapman RW, et al. Ursodeoxycholic acid in primary sclerosing cholangitis: a double-blind placebo controlled trial. Hepatology. 1992;16.92A.
42. Stiehl A, Walker S, Stiehl L, et al. Effect of ursodeoxycholic acid on liver and bile duct disease in primary sclerosing cholangitis. A 3-year pilot study with a placebo-controlled study period. J Hepatol. 1994;20(1):57–64.
43. De Maria N, Colantoni A, Rosenbloom, Van Thiel DH. Ursodeoxycholic acid does not improve the clinical course of primary sclerosing cholangitis over a 2-year period. Hepatogastroenterology. 1996;43(12): 1472–9.
44. Lindor KD. Ursodiol for primary sclerosing cholangitis. Mayo Primary Sclerosing Cholangitis-Ursodeoxycholic Acid Study Group. N Engl J Med. 1997;336(10):691–5.
45. Hilscher M, Enders FB, Carey EJ, et al. Alkaline phosphatase normalization is a biomarker of improved survival in primary sclerosing cholangitis. Ann Hepatol. 2016;15(2):246–53.

Future Therapies for Primary Sclerosing Cholangitis

12

Craig Lammert and Raj Vuppalanchi

Introduction

Primary sclerosing cholangitis (PSC) is a hepatobiliary disorder characterized by bile duct destruction and hepatic fibrosis [1, 2]. It is a chronic liver disease with progression to cirrhosis and eventual liver failure [1–4]. It carries increased risk for bile duct, colorectal, and gallbladder cancer that appears to be unrelated to disease severity or stage [5–7]. There is heterogeneity in its presentation and often occurs in association with inflammatory bowel disease (IBD) [1, 2, 8, 9]. More recently, recognition of specific clinical subtypes of PSC has led to improved classification of the disease [10]. It is, therefore, imperative to recognize these clinically distinct phenotypes within the context of novel therapeutics for PSC.

A number of drugs such as colchicine, methotrexate, pencillamine, pirfenidone, azathioprine, tacrolimus, budesonide, and prednisolone have been studied in PSC patients to prevent disease progression [11]. Many of the studies that reported promising results initially were open label and performed in an uncontrolled fashion with a small number of patients. Subsequent randomized controlled trials with a larger size have unfortunately failed to reproduce the initial positive results. The most commonly studied agent is ursodeoxycholic acid (UDCA) and is believed to slow the progression of fibrosis in cholestatic liver disease based on literature from primary biliary cirrhosis clinical trials [12, 13]. The European Association for the Study of Liver (EASL) has no "specific recommendation for the general use of UDCA in PSC," whereas the American Association for the Study of Liver Diseases (AASLD) concluded that "in adult patients with PSC, we recommend against the use of UDCA,": both positions reflective of negative RCTs [14, 15]. A landmark, long-term, randomized, double-blind, placebo-controlled multi-center study using high-dose UDCA performed in the United States in 150 adults with PSC was terminated after 6 years as the frequency of adverse events (i.e., death, liver transplantation, cirrhosis, esophageal varices, and cholangiocarcinoma) was significantly higher in the active than in the placebo group, irrespective of biochemical improvement [16]. The increase in adverse events appeared to occur primarily in patients with the early stage disease compared with similar patients in the placebo group [17]. There are no current effective therapies for PSC, and unfortunately, none except dilation of biliary stricture by endoscopic retrograde cholangiography or liver transplantation have altered the course of the disease significantly [18]. Therefore, a significant unmet medical need still exists for

C. Lammert, MD • R. Vuppalanchi, MD (✉)
Division of Gastroenterology and Hepatology,
Indiana University School of Medicine,
Indianapolis, IN 46202, USA
e-mail: rvuppala@iu.edu

L.M. Forman (ed.), *Primary Sclerosing Cholangitis*, DOI 10.1007/978-3-319-40908-5_12

novel agents for the treatment of PSC and its subsequent complications.

Pathogenesis and Opportunities for Therapeutic Targets

Significant breakthroughs in the understanding the mechanisms involved in liver injury have led to several promising therapeutic agents that are currently under evaluation. Due to common downstream mechanisms of liver injury and fibrogenesis, the same therapeutic agents are undergoing evaluation for chronic liver diseases of various etiologies. A brief overview of the pathophysiology is essential to understand the rationale for investigation of the novel therapies for the treatment of PSC (Fig. 12.1).

Gut-Liver Axis in PSC and IBD

The liver plays a critical role in the immune surveillance against bacterial translocation or absorption of bacterial endotoxins into the portal circulation. Since the intestinal and biliary

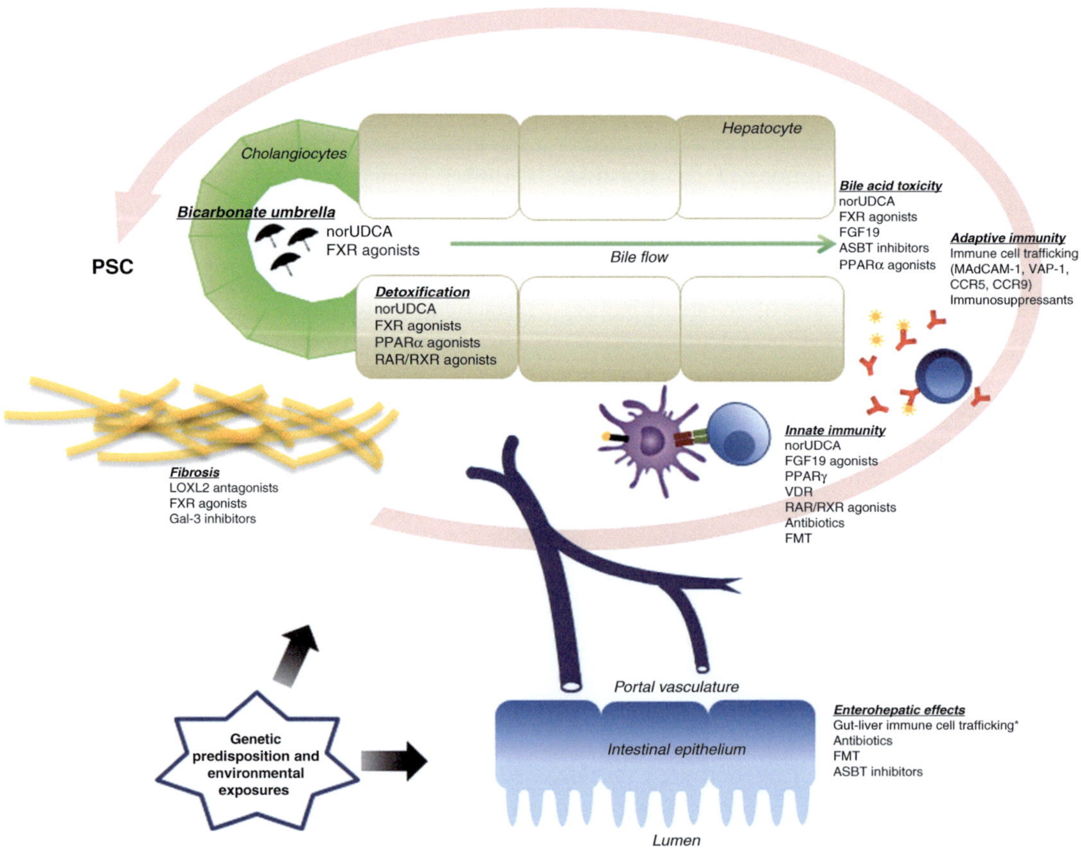

Fig. 12.1 A schematic overview of possible therapeutic targets, underlying mechanistic pathways, and pathogenesis of PSC: bile acid composition, detoxification, gut microbiota, hepatic fibrosis, adaptive and innate immune system activation, and immune cell trafficking represent areas in which a number study compounds and available drugs may exert therapeutic potential in the disease course. *FXR* farnesoid X receptor, *PPARa* peroxisome proliferator-activated receptor alpha, *VDR* vitamin D receptor, *RAR/RXR* retinoic acid receptor and retinoid X receptor, *LOXL2* lysyl oxidase-like 2, *ASBT* apical sodium-dependent bile acid transporter, *FMT* fecal microbiota transplantation, *FGF* fibroblast growth factor, *MAdCAM-1* mucosal vascular addressin cell adhesion molecule 1, *VAP* vascular adhesion protein, *CCR5* chemokine receptor type 5, *CCR9* chemokine receptor type 9

epithelia are continuous, any alterations in gut mucosal immunity ("leaky gut") or microbiome (dysbiosis) may, therefore, lead to heightened innate immune activation (liver-gut crosstalk) resulting in hepatobiliary injury (Fig. 12.1).

One of the hypotheses for the pathogenesis of PSC is the cross-reactive immunity to an antigen leading to immune-mediated gut and biliary inflammation from the enterohepatic circulation of gut-activated T lymphocytes. During intestinal inflammation, naive lymphocytes are imprinted with gut tropism by intestinal dendritic cells localized in the intestinal mucosa via integrin ligand, mucosal vascular addressin cell addressin molecule 1 (MAdCAM-1) and gut-specific chemokine, and CCL25-dependent mechanisms. Normally, these molecules are highly restricted to the gut, where they drive selective recruitment of gut-specific T and B cells and the expression the CCL25, chemokine receptor CCR9, and the integrin combination, $\alpha4\beta7$, which binds to MAdCAM-1. It is suggested that in a genetically predisposed individual, gut dysbiosis and intestinal inflammation with translocation of enteric pathogens beyond the mucosal barrier lead to activation of endogenous molecules termed damage-associated molecular patterns (DAMPS) [19–21]. Due to aberrant gut tropism seen in PSC, DAMP-associated activation of innate immunity and hepatic expression CCL25 and MAdCAM-1 result in the recruitment of mucosal effector lymphocytes bearing a "gut-trophic" phenotype. Additionally, the adhesion molecule and ectoenzyme vascular adhesion protein (VAP-1) are upregulated during chronic inflammation and support both lymphocyte adhesion through upregulation of several endothelial adhesion molecules, including MAdCAM-1, on sinusoidal endothelium [22, 23]. Also, it catabolizes amine substrates secreted by gut bacteria and contributes to reactive oxygen species generation. After entering the liver, effector cells use chemokine receptors such as CCR9 to respond to chemokines secreted by epithelial target cells resulting in cell-mediated immunological attack and bile duct destruction (Fig. 12.1). Hepatobiliary damage is likely enhanced by the action of toxic bile acids and heightened DAMP activation resulting in cellular production of inflammatory cytokines that act as ligands for chemokine receptors leading to downstream processes such as autophagy, apoptosis, and fibrosis [19, 24–26].

Therapeutic Targeting of the Gut-Liver Axis

Gut Microbiome

The importance of the commensal microbiota and its metabolites in protecting against biliary injury was recently highlighted in an animal model [27]. The critical role of gut dysbiosis is increasingly being recognized in IBD and liver disease pathogenesis through alterations in the mucosal immune system and activation of DAMPs. Gut dysbiosis represents a modifiable therapeutic target through the use of antibiotics, probiotics, or fecal microbiota transplantation. Initial positive reports with improvement in liver biochemistries after oral administration of antibiotics in combination with ursodiol have led to three prospective studies to date. In the first study, 80 patients with PSC were randomized to 3 years of UDCA (15 mg/kg per day) plus metronidazole or UDCA alone [28]. This study showed the superiority of combination therapy in the improvement in alkaline phosphatase, Mayo PSC risk score, and histology. One of the well-conducted double-blind, randomized pilot study randomized, 35 adult PSC patients to low-dose vancomycin (125 mg four times a day), high-dose vancomycin (250 mg four times a day), low-dose metronidazole (250 mg three times a day), or high-dose metronidazole (500 mg three times a day) [29]. Low-dose and high-dose vancomycin were superior to metronidazole and achieved significant decreases in serum alkaline phosphatase levels at 12 weeks [29]. In another pilot study, 16 adult patients with PSC were treated with minocycline, 100 mg orally twice daily, for a year. A modest improvement in serum alkaline phosphatase levels and Mayo risk score was observed with treatment but there was no improvement in serum bilirubin and albumin [30]. However, a recent pilot study of 16 patients PSC and UC with oral rifaximin (550 mg twice a day) has failed to show any biochemical improvement [31]. Future studies are therefore needed to understand how the antimicrobial spectra and other properties of antibiotics might determine their utility in treating PSC. Studies with oral vancomycin and fecal microbiota transplantation are currently planned (Table 12.1).

Gut Adhesion Molecules and Enterohepatic Circulation

Gut adhesion molecules are very attractive targets for pharmaceutical intervention, and given their enterohepatic expression in PSC, there is a possibility that agents that block the α4β7 – MAdCAM-1 – is expected to result in amelioration of ongoing chronic inflammation. Vedolizumab is a recombinant humanized IgG1 antibody constructed from the murine antibody Act-1, previously developed for use in patients with IBD. It inhibits adhesion and migration of leukocytes into the gastrointestinal tract by preventing the α4β7 integrin subunit from binding to MAdCAM-1. Therefore, the safety and efficacy of vedolizumab for the treatment of PSC in patients with underlying IBD is a matter of interest. Similarly, the VAP-1-blocking agent, BTT1023, is currently under investigation in phase 2 clinical trial in PSC patients with stable IBD (Table 12.1).

Bicarbonate Umbrella and Toxic Bile Acids in PSC

Bile acids are cholanic acid derivatives that act as detergents and are responsible for facilitating the absorption of dietary lipids, fat-soluble vitamins and for maintaining cholesterol homeostasis. The formation of bile acids is initiated in hepatocytes and mediated by cholesterol 7 α-hydroxylase (CYP7A1) [32]. Bile composed primarily of water, various ions, and solutes and is released into bile canaliculi on the apical side of hepatocytes. The bile acids flow through the canals of Hering before continuing through the biliary epithelium [32]. Despite continuous exposure to millimolar levels of hydrophobic bile salt monomers, the cholangiocytes are protected from damage due to a biliary HCO3- umbrella [33–37]. The formation of bicarbonate umbrella is mediated through transmembrane G-protein couple receptor (TGR5) [38]. Bile acids are stored in the gallbladder, and are then secreted into the duodenum where they are metabolized by enteric bacteria. Approximately, 95 % of these bile acids are absorbed in the terminal ileum and are then transported back to the liver via the portal vein for recycling [32]. These conjugated bile acids will be secreted back into the bile pool. This process is known as the enterohepatic shunt [32]. However, unconjugated bile acids are absorbed by the cholangiocytes and returned to the hepatocytes via the peribiliary vascular plexus in a process known as the cholehepatic shunt [32]. After synthesis, bile acids are conjugated with either glycine or taurine, which decreases the toxicity of bile and makes it more soluble [32]. In the liver, bile acids activate a nuclear receptor, farnesoid X receptor (FXR), that results in inhibition of CYP7A1 [32]. In the intestine, FXR induces an intestinal hormone, fibroblast growth factor 19 (FGF19), which activates hepatic FGF receptor 4 (FGFR4) signaling to inhibit bile acid synthesis resulting in decreased levels of 7ahydroxy-4-cholesten-3-one (C4) and endogenous bile acids (Fig. 12.1) [32].

Therapeutic Targeting of Toxic Bile

Because of the important processes that bile acids regulate through activation of receptors, bile acid derivatives and drugs that target these receptors are under development for the treatment of several diseases, including cholestatic liver disease and metabolic syndrome [39–41].

UDCA Derivative

24-norursodeoxycholic acid (*nor*UDCA) is a derivative of UDCA and is formed after removal of a methylene side group. This small alteration of the native compound establishes novel bile acid properties, enabling *nor*UDCA to overcome previous functional limitations of UDCA. *nor*UDCA is passively absorbed by cholangiocytes and subsequently undergoes extensive cho-

Table 12.1 List of novel therapeutic agents that are currently under evaluation for treatment of PSC. Brief overview of mechanism of action, route of administration, and details of the study design with primary efficacy endpoints are listed in the following table

Investigational drug (ClinicalTrials.gov identifier)	Mechanism of action	Administration	Clinical research phase	Sample size and study duration	Elevated alkaline phosphatase (AlkP) as inclusion criteria	Primary efficacy endpoint	Status	Estimated study completion date	Company
Simtuzumab (NCT01672853)	Monoclonal antibody against lysyl oxidase-like 2 (LOXL2)	Subcutaneous inj weekly	Phase 2b	$N = 225$, 96 weeks	Not required	Change from baseline in morphometric quantitative collagen on liver biopsy	Active, not recruiting	July 2016	Gilead Sciences
LUM001 (NCT02061540)	apical sodium-dependent bile acid transporter inhibitor (ASBTi)	Oral, once daily	Phase 2	$N = 20$, 14 weeks	Not required	Change from baseline in liver biochemistries, bile acids, and pruritus	Active, not recruiting	December 2015	Shire
norUDCA (NCT01755507)	Improve bicarbonate umbrella	Oral, once daily	Phase 2	$N = 160$, 12 weeks	Not required	Decrease in AlkP levels	Unknown	March 2014	Dr. Falk Pharma GmbH
Obeticholic acid (NCT02177136)	FXR agonism	Oral, once daily	Phase 2	$N = 75$, 24 weeks	AlkP at baseline ≥2xULN	Decrease in AlkP levels	Recruiting	June 2019	Intercept Pharmaceuticals
BTT1023 (NCT02239211)	Human monoclonal antibody (BTT1023) which targets the vascular adhesion protein (VAP-1)	IV infusion, every 14 days	Phase 2	$N = 41$, 120 days	AlkP at baseline >2xULN	Decrease in AlkP levels	Recruiting	March 2017	Biotie Therapies Corp
Mitomycin C (NCT01688024)	Nucleic acid synthesis inhibitors, antineoplastic agent	Delivery into biliary tree via ERCP, as needed	Phase 2	$N = 130$, 2 years	Not required	Improvement in Mayo Risk Score	Recruiting	September 2017	Investigator initiated

(continued)

Table 12.1 (continued)

Investigational drug (ClinicalTrials.gov identifier)	Mechanism of action	Administration	Clinical research phase	Sample size and study duration	Elevated alkaline phosphatase (AlkP) as inclusion criteria	Primary efficacy endpoint	Status	Estimated study completion date	Company
Vancomycin (NCT02605213)	Improve gut dysbiosis	Oral, every 6 h	Phase 4	$N=30$, 12 weeks	Not required	Decrease in AlkP levels	Recruiting	February 2016	Investigator initiated
Fecal Microbiota Transplantation (NCT02424175)	Improve gut dysbiosis	Single FMT	Phase 1, Phase 2	$N=5$, 12 weeks	AlkP at baseline >1.5xULN	>50 % improvement in liver biochemistries 3 months after intervention	Not yet recruiting	June 2017	Investigator initiated, OpenBiome
Cenicriviroc (NCT02653625)	Dual CCR2 and CCR5 receptor inhibitor	Oral, once daily	Phase 2	$N=25$, 24 weeks	AlkP at baseline >1.5xULN	Decrease in AlkP levels	Not yet recruiting	June 2017	Tobira Therapeutics
All-trans retinoic acid (ATRA) (NCT01456468)	Active metabolite of vitamin A	Oral, twice daily	Phase 1	$N=30$, 3 months	AlkP at baseline elevated	Reduction in AlkP by at least 30 %	Ongoing, but not recruiting	December 2015	Investigator initiated

lehepatic shunting [42, 43]. The physiologic result is increased cholangiocyte bicarbonate secretion and the creation of a possibly therapeutic "bicarbonate umbrella" in the biliary tree (Fig. 12.1). In fact, norUDCA resists taurine amidation, a property that increases its function in cholehepatic function compared to UDCA. *nor*UDCA has other unique features beyond UDCA, as it is more hydrophilic and thus less toxic to cholangiocytes and hepatocytes [44], but contains anti-lipotoxic, antiproliferative, antifibrotic, and anti-inflammatory effects [42, 45, 46]. Thus, *nor*UDCA has genuine potential to mitigate a number of steps in the pathogenesis of PSC and even complement mechanisms of bile acid detoxification and various overflow systems at the basolateral membrane [42, 46]. *nor*UDCA has mediated sclerosing cholangitis reversal in an experimental *Mdr2*/*Abcb4* knockout mouse model over a short study period, whereas the parent compound (UDCA) did not [45]. Human studies with norUDCA are underway, and results of phase 2 dose finding study (160 patients among 30 centers in Europe) are anticipated soon (Table 12.1). This study includes a primary outcome measure of change in serum alkaline phosphatase (AP) during the 12-week study, as well as secondary measures of the proportion of patients with at least 50% reduction in AP and rates of adverse events (NCT017555078).

Suppression of Bile Acid Biosynthesis

Bile acids, specifically those targeting the nuclear hormone receptor, FXR and the membrane associated G-protein couple receptor, TGR5 with high affinity, represent viable opportunities in the treatment of PSC [47]. Historically speaking, both targets (FXR and TGR5) have a rich history among autoimmune diseases. Specifically, TGR5 genetic polymorphisms have been associated with PSC and ulcerative colitis [48, 49], and FXR polymorphisms have been linked to inflammation and epithelial permeability in inflammatory bowel disease [50, 51]. FXR activation controls a number of downstream effects that enable cellular mechanisms to counteract biliary cholestasis via modulation of bile acid composition and inflammation. Activation of FXR not only leads to increased bile acid conjugation and excretion of bile from the hepatocyte into the canaliculi (also a bicarbonate rich choleresis) but contributes an additive role in the promotion of both phase I and phase II detoxification pathways [52–54]. UDCA and norUDCA are not ligands for FXR; however, 6-ethylchenodeoxcyholic acid (obeticholic acid (OCA) or INT-747) has strong receptor binding and activation profile [55, 56].

FXR agonist investigation in the *Mdr2*/*Abcb4* knockout mouse model has revealed significant mitigation of bile duct injury via diminished bile acid synthesis but also anti-inflammatory effects via FXR agonists (INT-767, similar FXR affinity as INT-747) [57]. Furthermore, overexpression of FXR in this model induced fibroblast growth factor 15 (or FGF19 in human) and suppressed the rate limiting enzyme-converting cholesterol to bile acids resulting in the cure of biliary injury [58]. OCA use is currently under investigation in a phase 2, blinded and randomized, placebo-controlled trial of the efficacy and safety in patients with PSC (NCT02177136). This study, estimated completion in June 2019, seeks to recruit a total of 75 subjects at 1:1:1 ratio into one of three treatment arms (Table 12.1). Two active compound groups include a daily OCA dose of 1.5 mg titrated to 3 mg and daily OCA dose of 5 mg titrated to 10 mg. The primary outcome measures include the effect of the compound on serum alkaline phosphatase as well as safety profile.

TGR5 and FGF19 also represent theoretic PSC therapeutic targets via roles in modulation of biliary composition and inflammation [59, 60]. TGR5, once activated, inhibits inflammation in part by suppression of NF-kb signaling [59] but also has a role in bile composition via cholangiocyte sensing bile sensing and bicarbonate secretion via cystic fibrosis transmembrane conductance regulator (CTFR) and anion exchange 2 (AE2) [61]. TGR5 has no current trials underway but a dual agonist of FXR, and TGR5 (INT-767) is currently undergoing preclinical evaluation. In the future, when targeted TGR5 compounds are available for treatment of cholangiopathies, off-target effects will have to be considered [62]. FGF19 expression is increased after FXR activation, resulting in a multitude of metabolic effects including suppression of bile acid synthesis and anti-inflammatory activity [63, 64]. Currently, NGM282, a recombinant protein with an amino acid sequence of 95.4 % identical to that of human FGF19, is currently under evaluation for PBC and PSC based on robust efficacy with no evidence of proliferative activity in a preclinical model (Table 12.1) [60].

Retinoic acid, an active metabolite of vitamin A, has been implicated in a number cellular processes including proliferation, differentiation, immunomodulation, and anti-inflammatory effects via activation of RXR and RAR [65, 66]. Furthermore, all-trans retinoic acid (atRA) causes an antifibrotic effect in bile duct ligation rats and carbon tetrachloride-induced liver fibrosis in vivo, yet the mechanistic pathway remains unclear [67, 68]. The administration of atRA resulted in repression of the rat CYP7A promoter, a finding that was potentiated by coadministration of UDCA. Evaluation of atRA in *Mdr2*/*Abcb4* knockout mice demonstrated reduced plasma levels of alkaline phosphatase, bile salts, duct proliferation, and inflammation in animals 12 weeks of age [69]. UDCA combined with atRA is currently being tested in an open-label trial for PSC patients with a primary outcome measure of alkaline phosphatase reduction over 3 months. Enrolled subjects continue UDCA at 15 mg/kg/day with the addition of oral atRA in two divided doses at 45 mg/m [2] (NCT01456468) (Table 12.1). Additionally, PPARα agonists have been evaluated in cholestatic liver disease since canalicular phospholipid translocator MDR3 is responsive to PPARα stimulation. Fibrates are potent PPARα agonist and increase MDR3 insertion into the canalicular membrane causing increased secretion of phosphatidylcholine resulting in the protection of cholangiocytes against bile acid toxicity. Additional mechanisms that may play a beneficial role include suppression of CYP7A1 and induction of CYP3A, each critical for bile salt synthesis and detoxification [70, 71]. Alterations in liver function and concerns related to cholestatic jaundice and cholelithiasis have unfortunately dampened the enthusiasm for the use of these agents in PSC [72].

Depletion of Bile Acid Pool

Apical sodium-dependent bile acid transport inhibitors (ASBTi) are also an exciting class of compounds that may provide another therapeutic option in PSC. Depletion of the bile acid pool through ASBTi can ultimately repress FXR-FGR signaling [73]. The action of ASBT inhibitors (LUM001, A4250 or SC-435), when tested in mouse models, was found to reduce the bile acid pool along with potentially toxic hydrophobic bile acids drastically [73, 74]. Furthermore, profibrogenic gene transcription was reduced as well as histologic fibrosis in this murine model [73]. An open-label phase II trial of LUM001, an ASBTi, in patients with PSC, is estimated to be completed in late 2015 (Table 12.1). This daily dosed compound is under evaluation with primary endpoints of safety and tolerability as well as adverse events in a 14-week study (NCT02061540).

Etiology-Independent Therapeutic Agents

Therapeutic Agents Against Fibrogenesis

Collagen cross-linking is an essential process for fibrotic matrix stabilization, a contributor to fibrosis progression, a limitation to the reversibility of liver fibrosis, and a potential therapeutic target. Lysyl oxidase-like 2 (LOXL2), a member of the LOX family with lysyl oxidase activity, is absent from adult healthy tissues and induced in disease [75]. Preclinical data using mouse models of biliary fibrosis suggested that a therapeutic anti-LOXL2 antibody significantly inhibited the progression of liver fibrosis prompting its evaluation in PSC [76]. A monoclonal antibody against lysyl oxidase-like 2 (LOXL2) in subjects with PSC is currently under evaluation (Table 12.1). Galectin-3 is a β-galactoside-binding lectin that has both intracellular effects (antiapoptotic, macrophage differentiation) and extracellular functions (chemokinetic/chemotactic factor) that are relevant to the physiopathology of PSC due to higher levels of expression of Gal-3 by in macrophages. Gal-3 is important for macrophage function in fibrotic disease including regulation of alternative activation of macrophages

[77]. Gal-3 inhibition is correlated to decreased monocyte/macrophage recruitment, cytokine production, and increased macrophage apoptosis [77]. Intravenous administration of galectin-binding drug GR-MD-02 is therefore expected to interfere with increased Gal-3-mediated inflammation and fibrogenesis seen in PSC.

Therapeutic Agents Against Inflammation and Cell Injury

The inflammation that occurs in the bile duct via translocation of enteric pathogens beyond the mucosal barrier interact with Toll-like receptors on the bile duct epithelial cells leading to increased production of inflammation cytokines, including ligands for CCR2 and CCR5 [78]. The cardinal feature of inflammation is the tissue recruitment of leukocytes, a process that is mediated predominantly by chemokines via their receptors on migrating cells. CCR2 and CCR5, two CC chemokine receptors, are important players in the trafficking of monocytes/macrophages such as monocyte chemotactic protein 1 (MCP-1) that is relevant to disease pathogenesis of PSC [79]. Overexpression of MCP-1 was observed in cholestatic liver diseases and PSC preclinical models [80, 81]. A potent, selective inhibitor of dual inhibitor of CCR2 and CCR5, currently under evaluation for the treatment of nonalcoholic steatohepatitis (NASH) and HIV may be an attractive candidate for treatment of PSC (Table 12.1) [82]. Finally, few studies have reported increased levels of serum keratin 18 fragment levels in patients with PSC suggesting the critical role of apoptosis in the pathogenesis of PSC [83, 84]. Liver-targeted caspase inhibitors could be an attractive treatment option for these patients and may be safely tolerated even in those with concomitant inflammatory bowel disease.

Safety and Tolerability of Novel Therapeutic Agents

The two key aspects of the evaluation of any investigational drug are safety – risk to the patient as assessed by laboratory testing, physical exam, adverse clinical events, and tolerability – the degree to which overt adverse effects can be tolerated by the patient.

In general, the novel therapeutic agents currently under evaluation have been previously investigated in patients with primary biliary cholangitis or non-alcoholic steatohepatitis (NASH) leading to recognition of the usual treatment-emergent adverse events (TEAEs) such as headache, abdominal pain, nausea, vomiting, diarrhea, somnolence, and elevated liver tests. In general, these TEAEs have been classified as either mild or moderate in severity. Some TEAEs, however, are drug specific and may affect the tolerability of the drug. In patients with PBC and NASH, who received treatment with OCA, a dose-dependent pruritus has been observed. Interestingly, increased liver enzymes and liver-related TEAEs including jaundice and acute cholecystitis were observed in patients with doses excess of 20 mg of OCA per day. In patients with PSC and dominant stricture resulting in inadequate bile flow, there could be an accumulation of OCA. The current study evaluating OCA for the treatment of PSC excludes patients with recent dominant stricture and also evaluates low-dose OCA between 1.5 and 10 mg per day. Alterations in lipid profile such as an increase in total cholesterol and low-density lipoprotein cholesterol were seen in NASH patients and a decrease in high-density lipoprotein cholesterol in both NASH and PBC. Although the clinical significance of these lipid changes remains unclear, the three deaths in OCA arm appear to be related to cerebro- and cardiovascular disease in the NASH (FLINT) trial. Although the main function of FGF19 is mediated through the negative control of bile acid synthesis, promotion of glycogen synthesis, lipid metabolism, and protein synthesis, there is concern about the tumorigenic potential due to high binding affinity for FGF receptor 4 whose expression correlates with progression of CCA. Another TEAE that may be of clinical relevance is diarrhea that may occur with ASBTi due to excess bile acids in the colon resulting in choleretic diarrhea. Lastly, in one study using oral minocycline for 1 year, a quarter of the study subjects withdrew due to intolerance.

Limitations of Current Approaches to the Development of Future Therapies for PSC

There is significant interindividual variability in progression, and prognosis depends on the clinical phenotype and stage of PSC at the time of initial diagnosis. For this reason, earlier attempts using any single test or a variable to predict survival in PSC patients failed due to lead time or length-time bias. Subsequent development of mathematical models of multivariable regression has allowed for an improved estimation of survival [85]. The long time required for the occurrence of sufficient hard outcomes such as death, liver failure, or cholangiocarcinoma requires the availability of a validated biomarker. Unfortunately, for a phase 2 clinical trial with novel therapeutic agents, a robust surrogate endpoint that can reliably assess response to therapy is essential to move the field forward. Alkaline phosphatase has been used as the primary endpoint in most trials but the recent termination of the multi-center study using high-dose UDCA due to increase frequency of adverse events (i.e., death, liver transplantation, cirrhosis, esophageal varices, and cholangiocarcinoma) in the active arm, despite improved alkaline phosphatase [16] has lead to major confusion. Despite this limitation, the majority of the studies require a baseline elevation in alkaline phosphatase of 1.5–2 times the upper limit of normal as the inclusion criteria to show an improvement in the clinical trial. An expert panel recently concluded that there is insufficient data to support any one biomarker and a combination of biomarkers is perhaps necessary [86]. With the exception of a few, all clinical trials are open to recruitment of patients with typical PSC and exclude other phenotypes such as small duct PSC and PSC with features of AIH (Table 12.2). Lastly, the majority of clinical trials exclude patients who are pregnant, breast feeding, hepatic decompensation, recent history of cholangitis, dominant stricture, chronic kidney disease, concomitant chronic liver disease and moderately active inflammatory

Table 12.2 Class of agents that are currently under evaluation for treatment of various phenotypes of primary sclerosing cholangitis (PSC)

	Therapeutic targeting of gut-liver axis			Therapeutic targeting of toxic bile acids					Other agents		
PSC phenotypes	Integrin α4β7 antagonist	VAP-1 blocking agent	Antibiotics and FMT	UDCA derivative	FXR agonist	ASBTi	Non-FXR nuclear receptor agonists	FGF-19 agonist	LOXL2 inhibitor	Galectin-3 inhibitor	Chemokine receptor antagonists
Typical	X	X	X	X	X	X	X	X	X	X	X
Atypical											
Small duct PSC								X			
PSC/AIH overlap											X
PSC/IBD	X	X	X	X	X			X	X	X	X

bowel disease possibly due to lack of data at this early stage of drug development.

Conclusion

PSC is a rare disease with no approved therapy. Recent breakthroughs in the understanding of the pathogenesis of PSC and other chronic liver disorders have led to several novel targets for treatment of PSC. These breakthroughs have unleashed the long-awaited arrival of novel therapeutic agents that not only delay the progression of the disease but also reverse the existing damage. It is very critical that these novel agents provide long-lasting, life-prolonging, and potentially curative treatment for patients with PSC.

References

1. Hirschfield GM, Karlsen TH, Lindor KD, et al. Primary sclerosing cholangitis. Lancet. 2013;382:1587–99.
2. LaRusso NF, Shneider BL, Black D, et al. Primary sclerosing cholangitis: summary of a workshop. Hepatology. 2006;44:746–64.
3. Porayko MK, Wiesner RH, LaRusso NF, et al. Patients with asymptomatic primary sclerosing cholangitis frequently have progressive disease. Gastroenterology. 1990;98:1594–602.
4. Olsson R, Broome U, Danielsson A, et al. Spontaneous course of symptoms in primary sclerosing cholangitis: relationships with biochemical and histological features. Hepatogastroenterology. 1999;46:136–41.
5. Broome U, Bergquist A. Primary sclerosing cholangitis, inflammatory bowel disease, and colon cancer. Semin Liver Dis. 2006;26:31–41.
6. Burak K, Angulo P, Pasha TM, et al. Incidence and risk factors for cholangiocarcinoma in primary sclerosing cholangitis. Am J Gastroenterol. 2004;99:523–6.
7. Wang R, Leong RW. Primary sclerosing cholangitis as an independent risk factor for colorectal cancer in the context of inflammatory bowel disease: a review of the literature. World J Gastroenterol. 2014;20:8783–9.
8. Boonstra K, van Erpecum KJ, van Nieuwkerk KM, et al. Primary sclerosing cholangitis is associated with a distinct phenotype of inflammatory bowel disease. Inflamm Bowel Dis. 2012;18:2270–6.
9. Olsson R, Danielsson A, Jarnerot G, et al. Prevalence of primary sclerosing cholangitis in patients with ulcerative colitis. Gastroenterology. 1991;100:1319–23.
10. Eaton JE, Talwalkar JA, Lazaridis KN, et al. Pathogenesis of primary sclerosing cholangitis and advances in diagnosis and management. Gastroenterology. 2013;145:521–36.
11. Karlsen TH, Vesterhus M, Boberg KM. Review article: controversies in the management of primary biliary cirrhosis and primary sclerosing cholangitis. Aliment Pharmacol Ther. 2014;39:282–301.
12. Lammers WJ, Hirschfield GM, Corpechot C, et al. Development and validation of a scoring system to predict outcomes of patients With primary biliary cirrhosis receiving ursodeoxycholic acid therapy. Gastroenterology. 2015;149:1804–12.e4.
13. Lee J, Belanger A, Doucette JT, et al. Transplantation trends in primary biliary cirrhosis. Clin Gastroenterol Hepatol. 2007;5:1313–5.
14. EASL. Clinical practice guidelines: management of cholestatic liver diseases. J Hepatol. 2009;51:237–67.
15. Chapman R, Fevery J, Kalloo A, et al. Diagnosis and management of primary sclerosing cholangitis. Hepatology. 2010;51:660–78.
16. Lindor KD, Kowdley KV, Luketic VA, et al. High-dose ursodeoxycholic acid for the treatment of primary sclerosing cholangitis. Hepatology. 2009;50:808–14.
17. Imam MH, Sinakos E, Gossard AA, et al. High-dose ursodeoxycholic acid increases risk of adverse outcomes in patients with early stage primary sclerosing cholangitis. Aliment Pharmacol Ther. 2011;34:1185–92.
18. Narumi S, Roberts JP, Emond JC, et al. Liver transplantation for sclerosing cholangitis. Hepatology. 1995;22:451–7.
19. Ganz M, Szabo G. Immune and inflammatory pathways in NASH. Hepatol Int. 2013;7:771–81.
20. Frazier TH, DiBaise JK, McClain CJ. Gut microbiota, intestinal permeability, obesity-induced inflammation, and liver injury. JPEN J Parenter Enteral Nutr. 2011;35:14S–20.
21. Chait A, Kim F. Saturated fatty acids and inflammation: who pays the toll? Arterioscler Thromb Vasc Biol. 2010;30:692–3.
22. Liaskou E, Karikoski M, Reynolds GM, et al. Regulation of mucosal addressin cell adhesion molecule 1 expression in human and mice by vascular adhesion protein 1 amine oxidase activity. Hepatology. 2011;53:661–72.
23. Weston CJ, Shepherd EL, Claridge LC, et al. Vascular adhesion protein-1 promotes liver inflammation and drives hepatic fibrosis. J Clin Invest. 2015;125:501–20.
24. Alisi A, Carsetti R, Nobili V. Pathogen- or damage-associated molecular patterns during nonalcoholic fatty liver disease development. Hepatology. 2011;54:1500–2.
25. Gauley J, Pisetsky DS. The translocation of HMGB1 during cell activation and cell death. Autoimmunity. 2009;42:299–301.
26. Nakanuma Y, Sasaki M, Harada K. Autophagy and senescence in fibrosing cholangiopathies. J Hepatol. 2015;62:934–45.
27. Tabibian JH, O'Hara SP, Trussoni CE, et al. Absence of the intestinal microbiota exacerbates hepatobiliary disease in a murine model of primary sclerosing cholangitis. Hepatology. 2016;63:185–96.

28. Farkkila M, Karvonen AL, Nurmi H, et al. Metronidazole and ursodeoxycholic acid for primary sclerosing cholangitis: a randomized placebo-controlled trial. Hepatology. 2004;40:1379–86.
29. Tabibian JH, Weeding E, Jorgensen RA, et al. Randomised clinical trial: vancomycin or metronidazole in patients with primary sclerosing cholangitis – a pilot study. Aliment Pharmacol Ther. 2013;37:604–12.
30. Silveira MG, Torok NJ, Gossard AA, et al. Minocycline in the treatment of patients with primary sclerosing cholangitis: results of a pilot study. Am J Gastroenterol. 2009;104:83–8.
31. Tabibian JH, Gossard A, El-Youssef M, et al. Prospective clinical trial of rifaximin therapy for patients with primary sclerosing cholangitis. Am J Ther. 2014. [Epub ahead of print].
32. Reshetnyak VI. Physiological and molecular biochemical mechanisms of bile formation. World J Gastroenterol. 2013;19:7341–60.
33. Jones H, Alpini G, Francis H. Bile acid signaling and biliary functions. Acta Pharm Sin B. 2015;5:123–8.
34. Erlinger S. A HCO(3)(-)umbrella protects human cholangiocytes against bile salt-induced injury. Clin Res Hepatol Gastroenterol. 2012;36:7–9.
35. Beuers U, Maroni L, Elferink RO. The biliary HCO(3)(-) umbrella: experimental evidence revisited. Curr Opin Gastroenterol. 2012;28:253–7.
36. Hohenester S, Maillette de Buy Wenniger L, Jefferson DM, et al. Biliary bicarbonate secretion constitutes a protective mechanism against bile acid-induced injury in man. Dig Dis. 2011;29:62–5.
37. Erlinger S. Chronic fibrosing cholangiopathies: a consequence of a defective HCO(3)(-) "umbrella"? Clin Res Hepatol Gastroenterol. 2011;35:85–8.
38. Keitel V, Reich M, Haussinger D. TGR5: pathogenetic role and/or therapeutic target in fibrosing cholangitis? Clin Rev Allergy Immunol. 2015;48:218–25.
39. Li T, Apte U. Bile acid metabolism and signaling in cholestasis, inflammation, and cancer. Adv Pharmacol. 2015;74:263–302.
40. Li T, Chiang JY. Bile acids as metabolic regulators. Curr Opin Gastroenterol. 2015;31:159–65.
41. Halilbasic E, Claudel T, Trauner M. Bile acid transporters and regulatory nuclear receptors in the liver and beyond. J Hepatol. 2013;58:155–68.
42. Trauner M, Halilbasic E, Claudel T, et al. Potential of nor-ursodeoxycholic acid in cholestatic and metabolic disorders. Dig Dis. 2015;33:433–9.
43. Halilbasic E, Fuchs C, Hofer H, et al. Therapy of primary sclerosing cholangitis – today and tomorrow. Dig Dis. 2015;33 Suppl 2:149–63.
44. Hofmann AF, Zakko SF, Lira M, et al. Novel biotransformation and physiological properties of norursodeoxycholic acid in humans. Hepatology. 2005; 42:1391–8.
45. Fickert P, Wagner M, Marschall HU, et al. 24-norUrsodeoxycholic acid is superior to ursodeoxycholic acid in the treatment of sclerosing cholangitis in Mdr2 (Abcb4) knockout mice. Gastroenterology. 2006;130:465–81.
46. Moustafa T, Fickert P, Magnes C, et al. Alterations in lipid metabolism mediate inflammation, fibrosis, and proliferation in a mouse model of chronic cholestatic liver injury. Gastroenterology. 2012;142: 140–51.e12.
47. Beuers U, Kullak-Ublick GA, Pusl T, et al. Medical treatment of primary sclerosing cholangitis: a role for novel bile acids and other (post-)transcriptional modulators? Clin Rev Allergy Immunol. 2009;36: 52–61.
48. Hov JR, Keitel V, Schrumpf E, et al. TGR5 sequence variation in primary sclerosing cholangitis. Dig Dis. 2011;29:78–84.
49. Hov JR, Keitel V, Laerdahl JK, et al. Mutational characterization of the bile acid receptor TGR5 in primary sclerosing cholangitis. PLoS One. 2010;5:e12403.
50. Nijmeijer RM, Gadaleta RM, van Mil SW, et al. Farnesoid X receptor (FXR) activation and FXR genetic variation in inflammatory bowel disease. PLoS One. 2011;6:e23745.
51. Stanimirov B, Stankov K, Mikov M. Bile acid signaling through farnesoid X and TGR5 receptors in hepatobiliary and intestinal diseases. Hepatobiliary Pancreat Dis Int. 2015;14:18–33.
52. Thomas C, Pellicciari R, Pruzanski M, et al. Targeting bile-acid signalling for metabolic diseases. Nat Rev Drug Discov. 2008;7:678–93.
53. Gnerre C, Blattler S, Kaufmann MR, et al. Regulation of CYP3A4 by the bile acid receptor FXR: evidence for functional binding sites in the CYP3A4 gene. Pharmacogenetics. 2004;14:635–45.
54. Barbier O, Torra IP, Sirvent A, et al. FXR induces the UGT2B4 enzyme in hepatocytes: a potential mechanism of negative feedback control of FXR activity. Gastroenterology. 2003;124:1926–40.
55. Pellicciari R, Fiorucci S, Camaioni E, et al. 6alpha-ethyl-chenodeoxycholic acid (6-ECDCA), a potent and selective FXR agonist endowed with anticholestatic activity. J Med Chem. 2002;45:3569–72.
56. Ali AH, Carey EJ, Lindor KD. Recent advances in the development of farnesoid X receptor agonists. Ann Transl Med. 2015;3:5.
57. Baghdasaryan A, Claudel T, Gumhold J, et al. Dual farnesoid X receptor/TGR5 agonist INT-767 reduces liver injury in the Mdr2-/- (Abcb4-/-) mouse cholangiopathy model by promoting biliary HCO(-)(3) output. Hepatology. 2011;54:1303–12.
58. Modica S, Petruzzelli M, Bellafante E, et al. Selective activation of nuclear bile acid receptor FXR in the intestine protects mice against cholestasis. Gastroenterology. 2012;142:355–65.e1-4.
59. Pols TW, Noriega LG, Nomura M, et al. The bile acid membrane receptor TGR5 as an emerging target in metabolism and inflammation. J Hepatol. 2011;54: 1263–72.
60. Luo J, Ko B, Elliott M, et al. A nontumorigenic variant of FGF19 treats cholestatic liver diseases. Sci Transl Med. 2014;6:247ra100.
61. Keitel V, Cupisti K, Ullmer C, et al. The membrane-bound bile acid receptor TGR5 is localized in the epi-

thelium of human gallbladders. Hepatology. 2009;50: 861–70.
62. Beuers U, Trauner M, Jansen P, et al. New paradigms in the treatment of hepatic cholestasis: from UDCA to FXR, PXR and beyond. J Hepatol. 2015;62:S25–37.
63. Bhatnagar S, Damron HA, Hillgartner FB. Fibroblast growth factor-19, a novel factor that inhibits hepatic fatty acid synthesis. J Biol Chem. 2009;284:10023–33.
64. Kir S, Beddow SA, Samuel VT, et al. FGF19 as a postprandial, insulin-independent activator of hepatic protein and glycogen synthesis. Science. 2011;331:1621–4.
65. Cai SY, He H, Nguyen T, et al. Retinoic acid represses CYP7A1 expression in human hepatocytes and HepG2 cells by FXR/RXR-dependent and independent mechanisms. J Lipid Res. 2010;51:2265–74.
66. He H, Mennone A, Boyer JL, et al. Combination of retinoic acid and ursodeoxycholic acid attenuates liver injury in bile duct-ligated rats and human hepatic cells. Hepatology. 2011;53:548–57.
67. Wang H, Dan Z, Jiang H. Effect of all-trans retinoic acid on liver fibrosis induced by common bile duct ligation in rats. J Huazhong Univ Sci Technolog Med Sci. 2008;28:553–7.
68. Hisamori S, Tabata C, Kadokawa Y, et al. All-trans-retinoic acid ameliorates carbon tetrachloride-induced liver fibrosis in mice through modulating cytokine production. Liver Int. 2008;28:1217–25.
69. Cai SY, Mennone A, Soroka CJ, et al. All-trans-retinoic acid improves cholestasis in alpha-naphthylisothiocyanate-treated rats and Mdr2-/- mice. J Pharmacol Exp Ther. 2014;349:94–8.
70. Ghonem NS, Assis DN, Boyer JL. Fibrates and cholestasis. Hepatology. 2015;62:635–43.
71. Honda A, Ikegami T, Nakamuta M, et al. Anticholestatic effects of bezafibrate in patients with primary biliary cirrhosis treated with ursodeoxycholic acid. Hepatology. 2013;57:1931–41.
72. Parra JL, Reddy KR. Hepatotoxicity of hypolipidemic drugs. Clin Liver Dis. 2003;7:415–33.
73. Miethke AG, Zhang W, Simmons J, et al. Pharmacological inhibition of apical sodium-dependent bile acid transporter changes bile composition and blocks progression of sclerosing cholangitis in multidrug resistance 2 knockout mice. Hepatology. 2016;63:512–23.
74. Baghdasaryan A, Fuchs CD, Osterreicher CH, et al. Inhibition of intestinal bile acid absorption improves cholestatic liver and bile duct injury in a mouse model of sclerosing cholangitis. J Hepatol. 2016;64(3):674–81.
75. Barry-Hamilton V, Spangler R, Marshall D, et al. Allosteric inhibition of lysyl oxidase-like-2 impedes the development of a pathologic microenvironment. Nat Med. 2010;16:1009–17.
76. Ikenaga N, Yoshida S, Liu SB, et al. Selective inhibition of lysyl oxidase like 2 (LOXL2) using a therapeutic monoclonal antibody suppresses the progression of biliary fibrosis in novel PSC-like mouse model. Hepatology. 2013;58:581A–2.
77. Hsieh WC, Mackinnon AC, Lu WY, et al. Galectin-3 regulates hepatic progenitor cell expansion during liver injury. Gut. 2015;64:312–21.
78. Harada K, Nakanuma Y. Innate immunity in the pathogenesis of cholangiopathy: a recent update. Inflamm Allergy Drug Targets. 2012;11:478–83.
79. Marra F, Romanelli RG, Giannini C, et al. Monocyte chemotactic protein-1 as a chemoattractant for human hepatic stellate cells. Hepatology. 1999;29:140–8.
80. Tsuneyama K, Harada K, Yasoshima M, et al. Monocyte chemotactic protein-1, -2, and -3 are distinctively expressed in portal tracts and granulomata in primary biliary cirrhosis: implications for pathogenesis. J Pathol. 2001;193:102–9.
81. Tabibian JH, O'Hara SP, Splinter PL, et al. Cholangiocyte senescence by way of N-ras activation is a characteristic of primary sclerosing cholangitis. Hepatology. 2014;59:2263–75.
82. Thompson M, Saag M, Dejesus E, et al. A 48-week randomized Phase 2b study evaluating cenicriviroc vs. efavirenz in treatment-naive HIV-infected adults with CCR5-tropic virus. AIDS. 2016;30(6):869–78.
83. Tinmouth J, Lee M, Wanless IR, et al. Apoptosis of biliary epithelial cells in primary biliary cirrhosis and primary sclerosing cholangitis. Liver. 2002;22: 228–34.
84. Masuoka HC, Vuppalanchi R, Deppe R, et al. Individuals with primary sclerosing cholangitis have elevated levels of biomarkers for apoptosis but not necrosis. Dig Dis Sci. 2015;60:3642–6.
85. Talwalkar JA, Lindor KD. Natural history and prognostic models in primary sclerosing cholangitis. Best Pract Res Clin Gastroenterol. 2001;15:563–75.
86. Ponsioen CY, Chapman RW, Chazouilleres O, et al. Surrogate endpoints for clinical trials in primary sclerosing cholangitis; review and results from an International PSC Study Group consensus process. Hepatology. 2016;63(4):1357–67.

Noninvasive Imaging of Primary Sclerosing Cholangitis: A Radiologic Perspective

13

Paul D. Russ

Abbreviations

^{18}F-FDG	Fluorodeoxyglucose
CBD	Common bile duct
CCA	Cholangiocarcinoma
CHD	Common hepatic duct
CT	Computed tomography
ERC	Endoscopic retrograde cholangiography
GBC	Gallbladder carcinoma
HCC	Hepatocellular carcinoma
IHD	Intrahepatic bile duct
kPa	Kilopascal
LSM	Liver stiffness measurement
LT	Liver transplantation
METAVIR	Meta-analysis of histological data in viral hepatitis
MRI	Magnetic resonance imaging
MRC	Magnetic resonance cholangiography
MRE	Magnetic resonance elastography
PET	Positron emission tomography
PET/CT	Positron emission tomography/computed tomography
PHTN	Portal hypertension
PSC	Primary sclerosing cholangitis
PTC	Percutaneous transhepatic cholangiography
SUV	Standardized uptake value
T1W	T1-weighted
T2W	T2-weighted
US	Transabdominal ultrasound
UTE	1-D transient elastography
VCTE™	Vibration-controlled transient elastography
VRT	Volume rendering technique

P.D. Russ, MD, FACR
Professor Emeritus, Department of Radiology, University of Colorado Hospital, University of Colorado Denver, Anschutz Medical Campus, 12605 E. 16th Ave, Aurora CO 80045, USA
e-mail: paul.russ@ucdenver.edu

Introduction

Primary sclerosing cholangitis (PSC) is an uncommon, but nonetheless significant chronic cholestatic liver disease. It occurs in a relatively young patient population, frequently progresses to end-stage liver disease, and is highly associated with cholangiocarcinoma (CCA). Because of low disease prevalence, but frequent complications, PSC patients often receive care at institutions with advanced multidisciplinary hepatobiliary and liver transplantation services. Radiologic tests are routinely performed in the diagnosis, management, and treatment of PSC. Noninvasive modalities used include transabdominal ultrasound (US), computed tomography (CT), magnetic resonance imaging (MRI), magnetic resonance cholangiography (MRC), and positron emission tomography/computed tomography (PET/CT).

L.M. Forman (ed.), *Primary Sclerosing Cholangitis*, DOI 10.1007/978-3-319-40908-5_13

Imaging of the biliary tree contributes to the diagnosis of PSC. The diagnosis of PSC is made not only from clinical history, laboratory results, and liver biopsy but also based on radiologic findings [26]. This chapter reviews the role of noninvasive imaging in PSC.

Radiologic-Pathologic Correlation

The utility of noninvasive diagnostic radiology is primarily based on the detection and demonstration of characteristic macroscopic morphologic changes of disease. By the time of presentation and diagnosis, PSC has caused macroscopic damage and morphologic alterations of the biliary tree that are relatively unique to PSC compared to other cholangiopathies. This reflects the histopathology of PSC.

PSC is a fibroinflammatory, fibroobliterative disease that nonuniformly involves the larger intrahepatic bile ducts and/or the extrahepatic bile duct. PSC causes morphologic distortion of these larger bile ducts that were initially described using percutaneous transhepatic cholangiography (PTC) and endoscopic retrograde cholangiography (ERC). The basic macroscopic finding of PSC is the presence of multiple biliary strictures separated by normal caliber or only mildly dilated bile duct segments. The nonuniformity of PSC causes asymmetries in duct morphology and disease distribution. Features of PSC as originally demonstrated by PTC and ERC include bile duct strictures, beading, mural irregularity, diverticula, pruning, focal dilatation, and duct wall thickening [4].

Of note, the normal biliary tree is difficult to demonstrate with noninvasive imaging because of its relatively small caliber. In PSC, obstructing strictures result in the upstream accumulation of bile. The increased volume of bile within at least mildly distended intra- and/or extrahepatic bile ducts results in much greater conspicuity of ducts and associated pathologic changes. Although the biophysical principles and technology of noninvasive modalities differ substantially, US, CT, MRI, and MRC all depend on contrast differences inherent in normal and pathologic tissues to generate images. Because the contrast difference between fluid bile (water) and the liver (soft tissue) is pronounced, the cholestatic pathophysiology of PSC is fundamental to its depiction.

Transabdominal Ultrasound (US)

US likely impacts the diagnosis of PSC more than it is realized. In one study, the mean age at diagnosis was 40 years [46]. The majority of PSC patients present with symptoms. The most prevalent symptom is right upper quadrant or abdominal pain. Other symptoms and signs include pruritus, jaundice, fever, and weight loss [43]. Biochemical tests are usually cholestatic, often with a disproportionately elevated alkaline phosphatase, consistent with bile duct obstruction [20]. In this clinical scenario, US is often the first test ordered, and can be the first to demonstrate the biliary tree abnormalities of PSC.

The pathophysiology of PSC contributes to its depiction at US. Inflammatory infiltration of the bile duct wall and periductal fibrosis [7, 22] results in thickening, irregularity, and increased echogenicity. Fibrosis is strongly echogenic at sonography. Superimposed obstruction can cause at least mild upstream dilatation. Fluid is anechoic at sonography. As a result, US contrast resolution is increased by the pathologic changes of PSC, and US can depict the findings of PSC (Fig. 13.1) [5, 21]. However, it should be emphasized that a negative US examination does not exclude the presence of PSC.

PSC can lead to cirrhosis and US can assess cirrhosis. Changes in hepatic shape, surface morphology, and increased parenchymal echogenicity from fibrosis can be used to suspect or establish a diagnosis of cirrhosis. Surface morphology is particularly amenable to US evaluation in the setting of perihepatic ascites, which acts as an acoustic window. Other findings of portal hypertension (PHTN) can be appreciated to include umbilical vein collaterals and splenomegaly. Spectral and color Doppler US are very useful in evaluating flow directionality and velocity, waveform morphology, and patency of hepatic vessels. Many findings at Doppler US are characteristic of cirrhosis and PHTN.

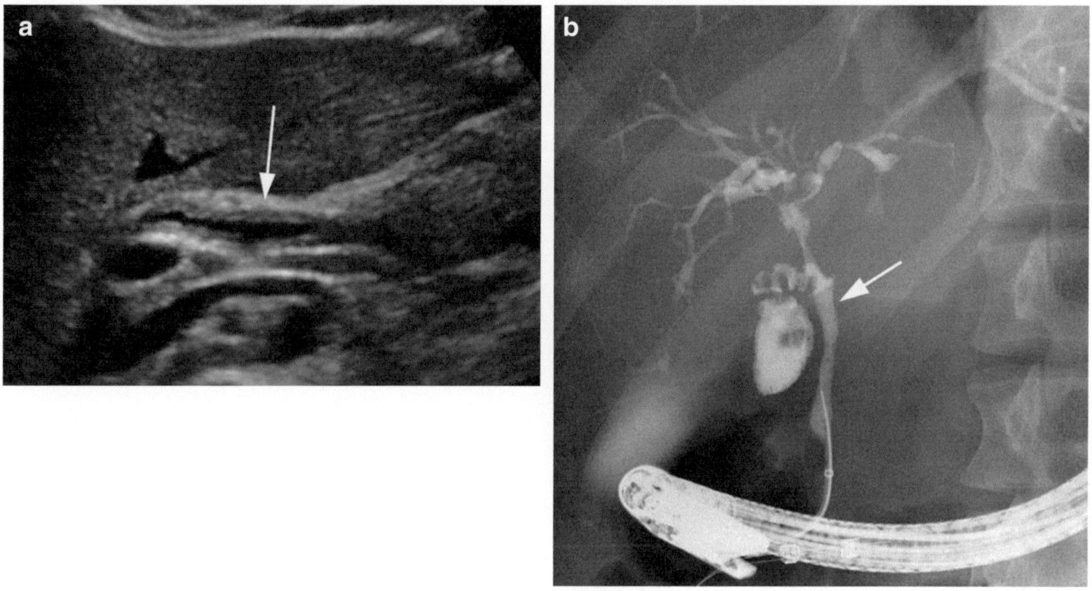

Fig. 13.1 US of a 24-year-old female with PSC. (**a**) US shows anechoic bile in mildly dilated extrahepatic bile duct, mucosal irregularity, and diffuse bile duct wall thickening (*arrow*). (**b**) Her ERC demonstrates typical luminal findings of PSC (*arrow*). Note IHD involvement

One of the most significant complications of PSC is CCA, developing in 8–14 % of PSC patients [43]. CCA can be suspected or detected by US. Intrahepatic CCAs are depicted as solid mass lesions that can be either hyperechoic or less frequently hypoechoic [32]. Intrinsic sonographic features usually do not distinguish mass-forming CCA from other intrahepatic benign or malignant neoplasms. Although the level of biliary obstruction can be correctly identified in 96 % of CCAs [31], direct demonstration of distal common bile duct (CBD) CCAs by US is limited by bowel-related gas that usually obscures the suprapancreatic and intrapancreatic CBD segments.

Perihilar CCAs (Klatskin tumors) can be demonstrated sonographically. The modified Bismuth-Corlette classification system [3] emphasizes the relationship of perihilar CCAs to the common hepatic duct (CHD). The CHD is consistently demonstrable by US. As a result, intrahepatic bile duct (IHD) obstruction to the level of the CHD is often apparent in cases of perihilar CCA [31]. Isolation of the right hepatic duct and/or left hepatic duct, nonvisualization of the CHD, abnormal CHD thickening, and abnormal soft tissue or a mass at the level of the CHD are highly suggestive of perihilar CCA, as is an associated collapsed, nondistended gallbladder in a fasting patient.

PSC patients are also at an increased risk for gallbladder carcinoma (GBC). GBC is thought to be associated with carcinogenesis induced by chronic PSC-related gallbladder inflammation and a neoplastic field effect involving the gallbladder and bile ducts [23, 30]. The prevalence of gallbladder mass lesions in PSC patients is estimated to be 3–14 % compared to 0.35 % in the general population [30]. In PSC, 56 % of mass lesions have dysplasia or are GBC. Lewis et al. pathologically evaluated 72 whole gallbladder specimens from 66 cholecystectomies performed at liver transplantation (LT) and 6 cholecystectomies performed prior to LT in PSC patients [23]. GBC was found in 14 % of the gallbladders. In addition, gallbladder intestinal metaplasia, low-grade dysplasia, and high-grade dysplasia were identified as significant associated risk factors. A metaplasia-flat dysplasia-carcinoma sequence was proposed for GBC in PSC patients.

US is the best modality to evaluate the gallbladder. Because of the risk of GBC in PSC, both the American Association for the Study of Liver

Diseases (AASLD) and the European Association for the Study of the Liver (EASL) recommend annual abdominal ultrasound for the detection of gallbladder lesions [30]. It is recommended that cholecystectomy be performed for all polyps ≥0.8 cm and probably for all polyps < 0.8 cm, unless the patient is a very poor cholecystectomy candidate, in which case the lesion should be sonographically reevaluated every 3–6 months.

Computed Tomography (CT)

CT is a readily available noninvasive imaging modality with significant impact in PSC. Current multi-detector scanners generate images with high spatial resolution and high temporal resolution. High spatial resolution results from thin slices (~1 mm) and fast acquisition speed. Thin slices increase image sharpness and anatomic detail. Thin slices allow for the postprocessing of data sets using multiplanar reformatting (MPR), maximum intensity projection (MIP), and volume rendering techniques (VRT). These postprocessing algorithms produce nonaxial images displayed in coronal, sagittal, and nonorthogonal projections. VRT images can be rotated and tumbled in contiguous conventional and nonconventional projections for optimal anatomic display. For surgical planning, advanced software and an independent 3-D workstation can be used for lobar and segmental volumetrics and to display the anatomy of the hepatic veins, portal vein, and hepatic artery. High temporal resolution allows for bolus tracking of exogenously administered contrast with segmented time frames of image acquisition used to generate arterial, portal venous, and delayed phases of enhancement. Unfortunately, CT cholangiography with positive-contrast excretion into the bile ducts can no longer be performed. The contrast material used, Cholografin®, is no longer available in the United States.

Analogous to US, CT is often performed in patients with abdominal pain and jaundice. It is not uncommon for CT to be the first test to detect PSC. The CT findings of PSC, especially early in its course, can be subtle. Mildly dilated IHDs have a disconnected "dot-dash" pattern corresponding to end-on and longitudinally oriented distended duct segments separated by intervening soft tissue density strictures [42]. Even small, peripheral IHDs can be conspicuous within the background liver, being filled with low-density bile, which intrinsically increases the otherwise moderate contrast resolution of CT. The fibroinflammatory and fibroobliterative changes of PSC manifest as duct wall thickening, irregularity, and narrowing, with the degree of duct wall enhancement being variable and inconsistent [38]. Mural changes are most apparent at the level of the CHD. By CT, the CHD is large enough to be consistently demonstrated in patients without or with PSC. Low-density fat in the hepatic hilum delineates its outer wall, and low-density bile within the CHD lumen defines its inner wall. The CHD is discernible as a ring-like structure on axial images and is normally of uniform thickness ≤1.5 mm. In PSC, the CHD becomes irregular with wall thickening potentially ≥2.0 mm (Fig. 13.2) [38].

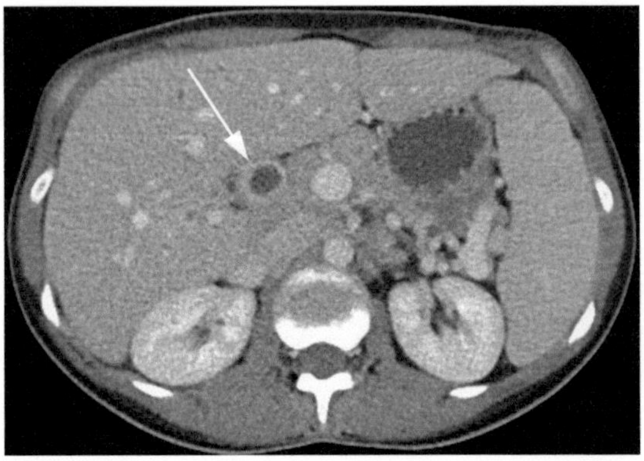

Fig. 13.2 CT of a 37-year-old female with PSC. CT shows common hepatic duct dilatation with intraluminal bile, wall thickening, and bile duct wall enhancement (*arrow*)

CCA can be suspected or detected by CT. Intrahepatic CCA can present as a mass lesion. Intrahepatic CCAs do have neovascularity. In larger intrahepatic CCAs, macroscopic neovascularity tends to be sparse, stringy, and peripheral. Mass-forming intrahepatic CCAs tend to be dominated by an abundant, central fibrous stroma with scant tumor cellularity. At

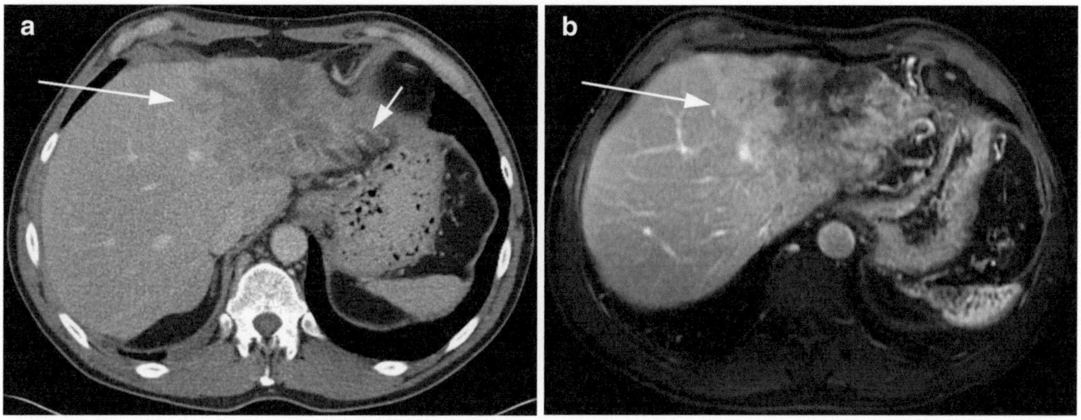

Fig. 13.3 Cholangiocarcinoma in a 52-year-old male with PSC. (**a**) Portal venous phase CT depicts a large, poorly marginated, heterogeneous intrahepatic mass-forming cholangiocarcinoma (*long arrow*) in the left hepatic lobe associated with obstructed peripheral bile ducts (*short arrow*). (**b**) Intrahepatic mass-forming cholangiocarcinoma in same patient demonstrated by portal venous phase MRI (*arrow*)

arterial phase CT, these CCAs tend to have no discernible to mild peripheral enhancement with central iso- to hypodensity. During the portal venous and delayed phases, there can be centripetal enhancement with contrast retention in the extracellular matrix of the central fibrous tissue, which can be subtle [14]. These lesions tend to be rounded, somewhat poorly marginated in non-cirrhotic livers, but pseudoencapsulated in cirrhosis; they can be associated with overlying capsular retraction, adjacent dilated IHDs, and satellite nodules (Fig. 13.3a) [10, 37, 39]. With intrahepatic mass-forming CCAs, vascular encasement is common, but macroscopic thrombus is unusual [10]. The features of intrahepatic CCA can overlap with those of hepatocellular carcinoma (HCC), particularly poorly differentiated HCCs or larger HCCs with central necrosis.

Small intrahepatic CCAs can appear as arterial phase hypervascular nodules [8, 9]. These CCAs tend to accumulate contrast, and enhance during the portal venous and delayed phases of multiphasic imaging. This is compared to typical small HCCs which wash out and become hypodense during the portal venous and delayed phases. However, arterial phase hypervascular CCAs with subsequent washout do occur.

PSC patients with cirrhosis are at an increased risk of HCC, which is estimated to be up to 2 % per year [30]. This is probably related to the association of HCC and cirrhosis. Given the overlap of imaging features, HCC should be considered in PSC patients with cirrhosis.

Of perihilar CCAs, 70 % are of the periductal infiltrating morphologic subtype [14]. These can be difficult to demonstrate by CT and can appear only as a stricture. Although some features such as duct wall thickening >5 mm, stricture length ≥18–22 mm, shouldering, portal venous or delayed phase enhancement, and soft tissue stranding within portal fat planes suggest perihilar periductal infiltrating CCA, these findings are insufficient to reliably differentiate dominant benign strictures from malignant strictures in PSC [14, 38]. Of note, malignant lymphadenopathy is common in cases of perihilar infiltrating CCA [14].

Of perihilar CCAs, 12–22 % are of the mass-forming morphologic subtype [14]. Perihilar masses measuring 1–9 cm can occur with features analogous to intrahepatic mass-forming CCAs. Small lesions can be seen as hypervascular arterial phase nodules. Larger lesions tend to have less pronounced arterial phase rim enhancement and can have portal venous or delayed phase washin and contrast retention within the central fibrous stroma. Portal vein invasion with visible thrombus can be seen.

Distal CCAs are anatomically defined as involving the CBD between the cystic duct origin and the ampulla of Vater [29]. Approximately 89 % are periductal infiltrating, and 11 % are intraductal growing [19]. CBD dilatation is present in 96 % of cases. Imaging findings are usually limited to CBD dilatation with abrupt downstream narrowing, irregular wall thickening, and enhancement. Because these lesions tend not to be mass forming, only 11 % have associated main pancreatic duct dilatation. Main pancreatic duct dilatation occurs when the tumor extends into the downstream ampulla of Vater or into the surrounding pancreatic parenchyma [19].

Magnetic Resonance Imaging (MRI)

Dynamic multiphasic abdominal MRI with an exogenous intravascular-extracellular contrast agent provides anatomic and enhancement characterization of PSC and its complications that are analogous to CT. An advantage of MRI is better contrast resolution compared to CT. A disadvantage of MRI is decreased spatial and temporal resolution compared to CT. Decreased spatial resolution and increased noise from physiological motion is also worse with MRI because of its relatively slower data acquisition time compared to CT. However, because of the differences in image content, CT and MRI are unpredictably complementary, and both are often used in cases of PSC.

Noncontrast MRI is used to generate two fundamentally different types of images. T2-weighted (T2W) images are based on differences in the micromagnetic environment of water-associated protons in fluid versus solid tissue. T2W MRI displays fluid as markedly hyperintense compared to an intermediate to hypointense soft tissue background. T1-weighted (T1W) images are derived from differences in the macromolecular environment of water-associated protons in fluid versus soft tissue. Using T1W MRI, fluid appears hypointense compared to mild to moderately hyperintense soft tissue. Because T1W images can be acquired faster, spatial resolution is better than with T2W scanning.

The inherently high contrast resolution of MRI can be augmented by intravenously administered exogenous contrast material. With the exception of hepatobiliary-specific agents, the pharmacokinetics of gadolinium-based MRI contrast is equivalent to iodinated CT contrast material. Intravenously administered gadolinium-based MRI contrast, which is not hepatobiliary specific, is used to generate a multiphasic dynamic series of T1W images that are analogous to multiphasic dynamic CT. Gadolinium-based agents increase the contrast resolution and signal-to-noise ratio, improving spatial resolution and lesion conspicuity. Because of its intravascular-extracellular distribution, gadolinium contrast demonstrates the same enhancement features of focal and diffuse pathology and of normal background anatomic structures as does iodinated CT contrast. As a result, a dynamic multiphasic T1W MRI series can be generated with arterial, portal venous, and delayed phases, with hypervascular lesions appearing hyperintense and hypovascular lesions being hypointense. With routine MRI scanning protocols, gadolinium contrast does not produce clinically significant changes in T2W images; postcontrast T2W scans are not obtained.

Using conventional contrast-enhanced MRI, the depicted features of PSC and its complications are the same as with CT (Fig. 13.3b). With multiphasic T1W MRI, the bile duct changes of PSC are shown as wall irregularity, thickening, and enhancement. Biliary obstruction is shown as duct dilatation accentuated by retained intraluminal bile that remains hypointense to the liver. Intrahepatic or perihilar mass-forming CCA can show arterial phase rim enhancement with centripetal washin during the portal venous and delayed phases. On T2W images, biliary obstruction is shown as duct dilatation accentuated by retained intraluminal bile that is hyperintense to the liver. Mass-forming CCA tends to be mild to moderately hyperintense compared to background hepatic parenchyma on T2W scans.

Magnetic Resonance Cholangiography (MRC)

The initial detection and diagnosis of PSC by US, CT, and MRI are usually limited to previously undiagnosed patients presenting with unexplained

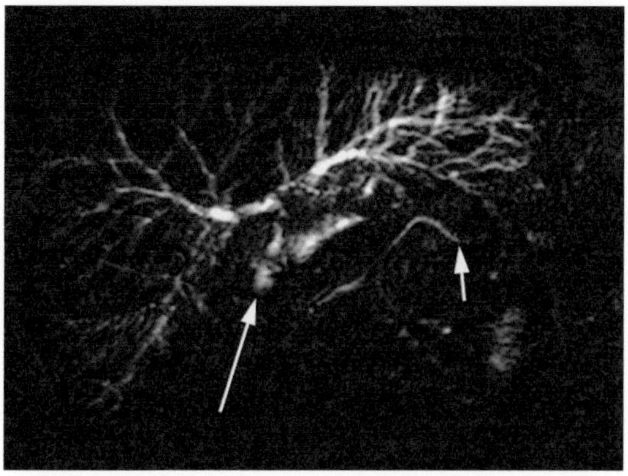

Fig. 13.4 Recurrent PSC in an allograft of a 59-year-old male, 7 years after LT with Roux-en-Y anastomosis for PSC. MRC shows recurrent PSC in the allograft. Note fluid in the Roux loop (*long arrow*). Incidentally, main pancreatic duct segment demonstrated (*short arrow*)

abdominal pain and jaundice. When PSC and/or its complications are clinically suspected or established, MRC becomes an important noninvasive imaging modality. MRC is a heavily T2W MRI technique that generates high signal intensity from fluid bile. The intrinsic T2W hyperintensity of bile outlines the luminal morphology of normal and abnormal bile ducts against such an extremely hypointense background that solid tissue becomes indiscernible. Several sets of MRC images are acquired using different parameters to optimally demonstrate the biliary tree. Data sets can be directly obtained or indirectly produced by postprocessing in any anatomic plane for display. Directly acquired thick-slab coronal images with multiple obliquities around the sagittal axis and high resolution 3-D images reconstructed with postprocessing into a coronal rotational VRT data set result in images that are equivalent to invasive positive-contrast cholangiography (ERC and PTC). The multiprojectional and rotational features of MRC are optimal for the display of significant bile duct findings that could otherwise be obscured by the overlap of structures.

The MRC findings of PSC are the same as those described for ERC and PTC (Fig. 13.4) [25, 45]. Dave et al. reported a meta-analysis of the diagnostic performance of MRC compared to ERC and PTC [13]. Studies were selected only if they included a control group of patients with other hepatobiliary diseases. Of the manuscripts that fulfilled criteria for analysis, the overall prevalence of PSC among the study patients was 185/456 (41 %). MRC interpretations were compared to ERC or PTC as the reference standards. MRC had results comparable to conventional cholangiography with a sensitivity in detecting PSC of 86 % and a specificity of 94 %. In addition, three clinical scenarios were simulated to evaluate the impact of pretest probability on the results. When the pretest probability of PSC was 25 % (low clinical suspicion), the posttest probability of PSC given a negative MRC was 5 % (considered sufficient to exclude PSC). When the pretest probability was 75 % (high clinical suspicion), the posttest probability of PSC given a positive MRC was 98 % (considered sufficient to diagnose PSC). In what was considered the worst-case scenario, a pretest probability of 50 %, the posttest probability of PSC given a positive MRC was 94 %, and the posttest probability of PSC given a negative MRC was 13 %. MRC can be quickly performed in conjunction with dynamic multiphasic MRI providing additive information in cases of PSC and its complications [27, 34, 37].

In a retrospective study of 64 PSC patients, Ruiz et al. suggested that MRC features combined with multiphasic liver MRI findings can be used to predict PSC disease progression [34]. All patients had at least two MRCs separated by at least a 1-year interval with multiple scans performed in some patients. A semiquantitative method was used to systematically score both MRI and MRC findings to assess PSC disease severity. Scores from the first and last MRI and MRC were compared, with an interval increase in score considered disease worsening, no score change considered disease stability, and a decrease in score to be considered improvement. At mean follow-up of 4 years (range, 1–9), 58 % showed radiologic worsening, 42 % remained stable, and no patient showed improvement. Using data derived from the subgroup with interval worsening, two MRI progression risk score equations were developed, one for studies performed without contrast and another for studies performed with contrast. It was noted that nearly 90 % of patients with radiologic worsening had an elevated progression risk score, compared to a low progression risk score in nearly 85 % of patients with stable disease. In addition, over the study interval, 5/64 (8 %) patients were diagnosed with PSC-associated malignancies, CCA ($n=2$), GBC ($n=2$), and HCC ($n=1$). Ruiz et al. concluded that risk score analysis could predict PSC disease progression and suggested that annual MRI and MRC were useful for PSC surveillance [34].

The MRC findings of PSC-related CCA are the same as those described for ERC and PTC, viz., a dominant stricture with malignant features. Compared to benign strictures, malignant strictures tend to be longer (≥18–22 mm) with asymmetric narrowing, irregular margins, and shouldering [14]. These findings, however, are relatively nonspecific. Irregular margins and asymmetric narrowing are found in 30 % of benign strictures. Gradual tapering and abrupt narrowing are seen equally in benign and malignant strictures. The most common cholangiographic finding in PSC-related CCA is progressive stricture formation with increased upstream bile duct dilatation [37]. Low-risk, noninvasive serial MRC is particularly suitable for detecting progressive stricture formation [34]. Although useful for detecting suspicious findings and providing a roadmap for subsequent ERC, MRC cannot replace ERC for brush cytology or therapeutic interventions such as stenting. It is important to note, however, that noninvasive imaging should be performed before interventional procedures to avoid postprocedural changes, pneumobilia, and stent-associated artifact that can and do degrade radiologic results.

MR Elastography (MRE)

Morbidity and mortality from biliary cirrhosis, PHTN, and liver failure affect a large proportion of PSC patients [43, 46]. As reported by Wiesner et al., among a group of 174 PSC patients, liver biopsy showed septal fibrosis (Stage 3) or cirrhosis (Stage 4) in 43 % of asymptomatic patients and in 69 % of symptomatic patients [46]. During a mean follow-up of 5.2 years, 22 % of initially asymptomatic PSC patients developed liver failure. During a mean follow-up of 6.2 years, 49 % of symptomatic patients developed liver failure or died, with 93 % of deaths attributable to liver disease; 9 % of symptomatic patients were referred for or underwent LT. Therefore, monitoring the development and progression of hepatic fibrosis/cirrhosis in PSC has a significant impact on patient management.

Elastography is now used to quantitatively measure liver stiffness, a surrogate biomarker for hepatic fibrosis/cirrhosis in lieu of subjective cross-sectional imaging assessment and/or liver biopsy [41]. Elastography can be performed using either US or MRE. A commonly used US implementation is 1-D transient elastography (UTE). FibroScan® uses UTE with proprietary technology termed vibration-controlled transient elastography (VCTE™) [28]. A US probe is used to intermittently deliver compression waves to a region of interest in the right hepatic lobe with a volume 100 times larger than liver biopsy. Within the hepatic parenchyma, compression waves generate shear waves based on the viscoelastic properties of the liver tissue. Shear wave speed increases with liver stiffness, which increases with hepatic fibrosis. The ultrasound transducer tracks and measures shear wave velocity in meters per second, which is then converted into a liver stiffness measurement (LSM) expressed in kilopascals (kPa). In a cohort of 73 PSC patients who underwent liver biopsy, Corpechot et al. verified that a METAVIR-derived histologic fibrosis score correlated with VCTE LSMs [11]. Values predictive of fibrosis stages ≥F1, ≥F2, ≥F3, and F4 were 7.4 kPa, 8.6 kPa, 9.6 kPa, and 14.4 kPa, respectively.

Commercially available FDA-approved proprietary MRE technology is currently manufactured by Resoundant, Inc. It can be implemented as an upgrade on currently available MRI scanners manufactured by GE Healthcare, Philips Healthcare, and Siemens Healthcare [41]. An external flexible membrane attached to the right upper quadrant is used to generate continuous compression waves that are converted to shear waves within the liver [12, 41, 44]. Intrahepatic shear waves are tracked and displayed as axial maps of the liver at four separate slice locations; color-coded MR elastograms are used to generate results reported as shear stiffness in kilopascals (kPa) [41]. It should be noted that UTE and MRE use different algorithms to quantify liver stiffness. The liver stiffness measurement by UTE in kPa is not equivalent to the shear stiffness measurement by MRE in kPa; the UTE value is numerically three-times larger than the MRE value [17].

Huwart et al. verified that the histologic METAVIR fibrosis scoring system correlated with MRE measurements of shear elasticity in a cohort of 96 consecutive patients who underwent liver biopsy for suspected chronic liver disease [17]. Values predictive of fibrosis stages ≥F1, ≥F2, ≥F3, and F4 were 2.4 kPa, 2.5 kPa, 3.1 kPa, and 4.3 kPa, respectively. MRE needs to be verified in a cohort of PSC patients.

Some studies suggest that MRE has performance characteristics that exceed those of UTE and other sonographic methodologies [12, 18, 41]. Machine time for MRE data acquisition is 1–2 min; MRE can be performed along with routine dynamic MRI and MRC. The technical success rate of MRE is significantly higher than UTE (94 % vs. 84 %, $P=0.016$) [18]. MRE can be accurately performed in patients with ascites and obesity. UTE cannot be used when there is perihepatic ascites because shear waves do not propagate through liquids. A 4.5 % UTE failure rate (no LSM value obtainable) correlates with a body mass index >28 kg/m^2 [16]. When correlated with histology, using area under receiver operating characteristic curve analysis to compare predictive performance, MRE was significantly better than UTE for METAVIR fibrosis stages F ≥1, F ≥2, F ≥3, and F=4 among a heterogeneous group of chronic liver disease patients [18]. It is suggested that the increased accuracy of MRE is related to the large tissue volume and the noncontiguity of the four 10-mm-thick cross sections through the liver, which reduces sampling error introduced by inhomogeneously distributed fibrosis [40].

Positron Emission Tomography/ Computed Tomography (PET/CT)

PET/CT is a noninvasive imaging modality that coregisters the results of a whole-body PET scan with CT. PET is a nuclear medicine study that is most commonly performed using the radionuclide fluorodeoxyglucose, ^{18}F-FDG, to map the cellular metabolism of glucose. Inflammation and malignant growth increases the uptake and retention of intracellular ^{18}F-FDG. The radioactive decay of ^{18}F-FDG is used to generate a scan of differential metabolic activity. Relative differences in radioactivity are semiquantitatively measured as a function of standardized uptake value (SUV), and hypermetabolic foci are displayed as areas of increased saturation on a color map. With PET/CT, the PET color map is superimposed or fused onto images from a conventional CT performed sequentially before or after the PET acquisition to colocalize the areas of increased metabolism to anatomic structures.

In PSC patients, PET/CT can be used in primary tumor (CCA) detection, but is more often incorporated into the staging of patients who are being considered for tumor resection or LT. Annunziata et al. recently published a meta-analysis of ^{18}F-FDG PET alone or PET/CT in the evaluation of the primary tumor in cases of suspected or documented intrahepatic, perihilar, and distal CCA in a spectrum of patients [2]. Both PET alone and PET/CT were shown to be accurate in the diagnosis of primary CCA. For PET/CT, overall sensitivity and specificity in the detection of primary CCA was 82 % and 75 %, respectively. For the detection of hilar CCA, using either PET or PET/CT, sensitivity and specificity were 84 % and 95 %, respectively. However, the authors noted that additional studies were needed to verify the findings in perihilar CCA, given the small number of cases in the meta-analysis.

Alkhawaldeh et al. reported the ^{18}F-FDG PET/CT results of a PSC cohort, 47/65 (72 %) with CCA [1]. Using semiquantitative SUV analysis, sensitivity and specificity for primary tumor detection were 94 % and 83 %, respectively. There were six false-positive studies, four from inflammatory strictures of PSC and two related to stent placement.

Li et al. reported on the utility of ^{18}F-FDG PET/CT in the preoperative staging of 17 patients, with perihilar CCA (background liver disease if present not specified), who underwent exploratory laparotomy with the intent of radical resection [24]. Histologic confirmation of primary tumor, regional lymphadenopathy, and distant metastases was available in all cases. The sensitivity of whole-body PET/CT in detecting the primary perihilar CCA was 58.8 %.

As noted by Ruys et al., data regarding the role of ^{18}F-FDG PET/CT in detecting malignant locoregional lymphadenopathy and distant metastases is sparse [36]. In the study by Li et al., the sensitivity and specificity in detecting lymph node metastases were 41.7 % and 80 %, respectively, with PET-avid malignant nodes ranging in size from 4 to 30 mm [24]. For distant metastases involving the liver and peritoneum, sensitivity and specificity were 55.6 % and 87.5 %, respectively.

Presurgical Staging of Cholangiocarcinoma

There are two potentially curative surgical options for de novo and PSC-related CCA, radical resection and LT [33]. Noninvasive imaging is especially important in perihilar CCA because tumor involvement of the bile ducts, hepatic artery, and portal vein at the hepatic hilum determines resectability, and radial tumor diameter ≤3 cm is required for LT. Imaging is also used to evaluate for locoregional lymphadenopathy and distant metastases.

As noted by Ruys et al., published data describing the diagnostic performance of CT, MRI, US, and PET/CT for the preoperative staging of perihilar CCA is limited [36]. CT was found to be the most frequently used radiologic test. Meta-analysis was not feasible for MRI, US, or PET/CT because of the small number of patients in the data sets. Abstracted results for longitudinal ductal involvement, portal vein involvement, hepatic artery involvement, lymph node metastases, and distant metastases are presented in Table 13.1 [36].

In the staging of perihilar CCA, CT is usually performed because of its high spatial resolution, anatomic detail, and temporal resolution. Primary tumor radial diameter, longitudinal ductal extension, portal vein involvement, and hepatic artery involvement can be evaluated. Given their high contrast resolution, MRI and MRC can provide complementary information to CT results with regard to tumor size, hilar/perihilar extension, and bile duct involvement, but MRI usually has poorer spatial and temporal resolution of the hepatic artery and the portal vein, which can be worsened by MRI flow-related artifact.

The accuracy of CT is limited in the evaluation of locoregional nodes in perihilar CCA. The meta-analysis by Ruys et al. yielded a summary estimate of 61 % sensitivity and 88 % specificity for detecting metastatic lymphadenopathy [36]. In routine CT interpretation, a short-axis diameter >10 mm is used to define metastatic nodal enlargement. However, in a pathologic study of resected nodes in perihilar CCA, Ruys et al. noted 65 % sensitivity and 61 % specificity for nodal positivity using a cutoff value of 10.5 mm [35]. In one study, PET/CT had 41.7 % sensitivity

Table 13.1 Diagnostic performance values for CT, MRI, US, and PET/CT in the preoperative staging of perihilar cholangiocarcinoma [36]

	Accuracy (%)	Sensitivity (%), specificity (%)			
	Bile duct	Portal vein	Hepatic artery	Lymph node	Distant
CT[a]	86	89, 92	84, 93	61, 88	67, 94[c]
MRI[b]	71–80	79, 0[c]	–	–	–
US[b]	59–82	75–83, 93–100	0–43, 100	–	–
PET/CT[b]	–	–	–	42, 80[c]	56, 88[c]

– no data, *Bile duct* longitudinal bile duct extension, *portal vein* portal vein involvement, *hepatic artery* hepatic artery involvement, *lymph node* lymph node metastases, *distant* distant metastases

[a]Summary estimates except for distant metastases

[b]Non-pooled ranges

[c]Single study

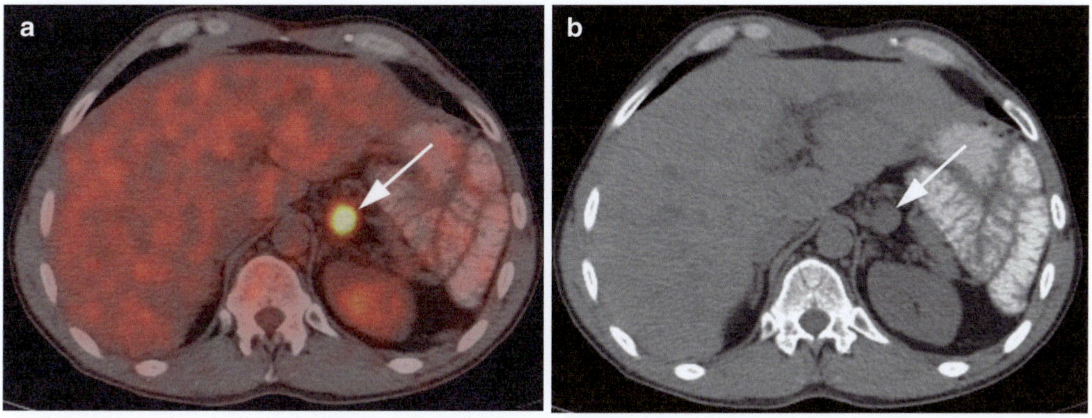

Fig. 13.5 ^{18}F-FDG PET/CT in a 45-year-old male with PSC. (**a**) Markedly PET-avid nonmalignant, reactive gastrohepatic lymph node (*arrow*) depicted by fused PET/CT. (**b**) Concurrent CT scan without intravenous contrast shows the enlarged node (*arrow*). This node decreased in size during 7 years of follow-up imaging

and 80% specificity in detecting malignant lymphadenopathy [24]. Limited results are usually attributed to the high prevalence of PSC inflammatory lymphadenopathy (Fig. 13.5) [35]. Therefore, lymph node sampling by staging laparoscopy or laparotomy is performed prior to definitive surgery [14, 33].

Extranodal metastases to the liver, peritoneum, lung, adrenal glands, and bones occur in perihilar CCA [14]. Because multiphasic liver CT can be incorporated into a complete CT examination of the chest, abdomen, and pelvis, CT is useful to screen for distant metastases. In one study, CT had a 67% sensitivity and 94% specificity for detecting distant metastases [15]. In one study, PET/CT had a 56% sensitivity and 88% specificity in demonstrating distant metastases [24]. However, in both of these studies, the evaluation of distant metastatic disease was limited to the liver and peritoneum. Although staging laparoscopy or laparotomy is important to diagnose peritoneal carcinomatosis, laparoscopy and laparotomy are limited to evaluating metastatic disease within the abdomen. Complete CT of the chest, abdomen, and pelvis or whole-body PET/CT (usual coverage from calvarial vertex through the upper thighs) could show extra-abdominal disease in the noninvasive preoperative staging of patients with perihilar CCA. In addition, there is evidence that ^{18}F-FDG PET/CT is accurate in detecting bone metastases and is superior to conventional whole-body bone scintigraphy, especially in the axial skeleton [6].

Conclusion

US, CT, MRI, MRC, and PET/CT are noninvasive radiologic tests used in the care of patients with PSC and its complications. All of these modalities can depict the findings of PSC. Any could be the first exam to detect PSC in subclinical cases. In established cases of PSC, US is used to annually screen PSC patients because of their high risk for gallbladder adenocarcinoma.

MRC is accurate in the diagnosis of PSC. MRC findings parallel those of ERC, with potentially better display of intrahepatic bile duct changes. Because MRC is noninvasive and does not involve the use of ionizing radiation, its utility for surveillance of disease progression and PSC-related complications is being recognized. However, the demonstration of a dominant stricture by MRC still requires follow-up ERC for therapeutic management and for evaluation of malignancy.

CT remains the noninvasive radiologic workhorse in patients with an established diagnosis of PSC. It is used to evaluate cholangitis (e.g., cholangitic abscess formation), deteriorating liver function, fibrosis/cirrhosis, PHTN, and malignancy (CCA, HCC, or GBC). Important in tumor staging, CT helps to characterize the primary malignancy with regard to size, radial and longitudinal spread, invasion of the hepatic artery and portal vein, associated bile duct dilatation, and involvement of contiguous structures such as the hepatoduodenal ligament and duodenum [14, 15, 36]. Although limited in assessing malignant lymphadenopathy and peritoneal carcinomatosis, multiphasic dynamic liver CT performed in conjunction with CT of the chest, abdomen, and pelvis can be used to screen for distant metastases.

PET/CT can provide additional information in PSC, especially in cases complicated by malignancy. Although the data is limited, PET/CT can contribute to the detection of the primary tumor, malignant lymph nodes, and distant metastases. False-positive results associated with the fibroinflammation and reactive lymphadenopathy of PSC are noted as a potential limitation (Fig. 13.5).

Among the more investigative technologies, MRE is the most likely to be incorporated next into the routine evaluation of PSC patients. Quickly performed along with MRI and MRC, MRE can accurately quantitate fibrosis in both hepatic lobes. Because MRE is noninvasive, unlike liver biopsy, potentially more accurate than liver biopsy and sonographic elastography, and does not use ionizing radiation, MRE could become the study of choice to evaluate hepatic fibrosis, progression of hepatic fibrosis, and response to evolving antifibrotic therapies.

In summary, US, CT, MRI, MRC, and PET/CT are routinely used in the care of PSC patients. Each modality is unique. None demonstrate all of the findings of PSC and its complications. Depending on the clinical situation, the judicious use of more than one of these complementary studies is likely to provide the most complete information for the best care of PSC patients.

References

1. Alkhawaldeh K, Faltten S, Biersack HJ, Ezziddin S. The value of F-18 FDG PET in patients with primary sclerosing cholangitis and cholangiocarcinoma using visual and semiquantitative analysis. Clin Nucl Med. 2011;36:879–83.
2. Annunziata S, Caldarella C, Pizzuto DA, Galiandro F, Sadeghi R, Giovanella L, et al. Diagnostic accuracy of fluorine-18-fluorodeoxyglucose positron emission tomography in the evaluation of the primary tumor in patients with cholangiocarcinoma: a meta-analysis. Biomed Res Int. 2014;2014:247693. doi:10.1155/2014/247693. Epub 2014 May 13.
3. Bismuth H, Nakache R, Diamond T. Management strategies in resection for hilar cholangiocarcinoma. Ann Surg. 1992;215:31–8.
4. Campbell WL, Ferris JV, Holbert BL, Thaete FL, Baron RL. Biliary tract carcinoma complicating primary sclerosing cholangitis: evaluation with CT, cholangiography, US and MR imaging. Radiology. 1998;207:41–50.
5. Carroll BA, Oppenheimer DA. Sclerosing cholangitis: sonographic demonstration of bile duct wall thickening. AJR Am J Roentgenol. 1982;139:1016–8.
6. Chang CY, Gill CM, Simeone FJ, Taneja AK, Huang AJ, Torriani M, et al. Comparison of the diagnostic accuracy of 99 m-Tc-MDP bone scintigraphy and 18 F-FDG PET/CT for the detection of skeletal metastases. Acta Radiol. 2016;57(1):58–65. doi:10.1177/0284185114564438.
7. Chapman RWG, Arborgh BAM, Rhodes JM, Summerfield JA, Dick R, Scheuer PJ, et al. Primary sclerosing cholangitis: a review of its clinical features, cholangiography, and hepatic histology. Gut. 1980;21:870–7.
8. Choi JY, Lee JM, Sirlin CB. CT and MR imaging diagnosis and staging of hepatocellular carcinoma: part I. Development, growth, and spread: key pathologic and imaging aspects. Radiology. 2014;272:635–54.
9. Choi JY, Lee JM, Sirlin CB. CT and MR imaging diagnosis and staging of hepatocellular carcinoma: part II. Extracellular agents, hepatobiliary agents, and ancillary imaging features. Radiology. 2014;273:30–50.
10. Chung YE, Kim MJ, Park YN, Choi JY, Pyo JY, Kim YC, et al. Varying appearances of cholangiocarcinoma: radiologic-pathologic correlation. Radiographics. 2009;29:683–700.
11. Corpechot C, Gaouar F, Naggar AE, Kemgang A, Wendum D, Poupon R, et al. Baseline values and changes in liver stiffness measured by transient elastography are associated with severity of fibrosis and outcomes of patients with primary sclerosing cholangitis. Gastroenterology. 2014;146:970–9.
12. Cui J, Heba E, Hernandez C, Haufe W, Hooker J, Andre MP, et al. MRE is superior to ARFI for the diagnosis of fibrosis in patients with biopsy-proven NAFLD: a prospective study. Hepatology. 2016;63(2):453–61. doi:10.1002/hep.28337.
13. Dave M, Elmunzer BJ, Dwamena BA, Higgins PDR. Primary sclerosing cholangitis: meta-analysis of diagnostic performance of MR cholangiopancreatography. Radiology. 2010;256:387–96.
14. Engelbrecht MR, Katz SS, van Gulik TM, Lameris JS, van Delden OM. Imaging of perihilar cholangiocarcinoma. AJR Am J Roentgenol. 2015;204:782–91.

15. Engels JT, Balfe DM, Lee JKT. Biliary carcinoma: CT evaluation of extrahepatic spread. Radiology. 1989; 172:35–40.
16. Foucher J, Castera L, Bernard PH, Adhoute X, Laharie D, Bertet J, et al. Prevalence and factors associated with failure of liver stiffness measurement using FibroScan in a prospective study of 2114 examinations. Eur J Gastroenterol Hepatol. 2006;18:411–2.
17. Huwart L, Sempoux C, Salameh N, Jamart J, Annet L, Sinkus R, et al. Liver fibrosis: noninvasive assessment with MR elastography versus aspartate aminotransferase-to-platelet ratio index. Radiology. 2007;245:458–66.
18. Huwart L, Sempoux C, Vicaut E, Salameh N, Annet L, Danse E, et al. Magnetic resonance elastography for the noninvasive staging of liver fibrosis. Gastroenterology. 2008;135:32–40.
19. Kim JH, Kim MJ, Chung JJ, Lee WJ, Yoo HS, Lee JT. Differential diagnosis of periampullary carcinomas at MR imaging. Radiographics. 2002;22:1335–52.
20. Krones E, Graziadei I, Trauner M, Fickert P. Evolving concepts in primary sclerosing cholangitis. Liver Int. 2012;32:352–69.
21. Laing FC, Jeffrey Jr RB, Wing VW, Nyberg DA. Biliary dilatation: defining the level and cause by real-time US. Radiology. 1986;160:39–42.
22. Lee YM, Kaplan MM. Primary sclerosing cholangitis. N Engl J Med. 1995;332:924–33.
23. Lewis JT, Talwalkar JA, Rosen CB, Smyrk TC, Abraham SC. Prevalence and risk factors for gallbladder neoplasia in patients with primary sclerosing cholangitis: evidence for a metaplasia-dysplasia-carcinoma sequence. Am J Surg Pathol. 2007;31:907–13.
24. Li J, Kuehl H, Grabellus F, Muller SP, Radunz S, Antoch G, et al. Preoperative assessment of hilar cholangiocarcinoma by dual-modality PET/CT. J Surg Oncol. 2008;98:438–43.
25. MacCarty RL, LaRusso NF, Wiesner RH, Ludwig J. Primary sclerosing cholangitis: findings on cholangiography and pancreatography. Radiology. 1983;149: 39–44.
26. Nakanuma Y, Zen Y, Portmann BC. Diseases of the bile ducts. In: Burt AD, Portmann BC, Ferrell LD, editors. MacSween's pathology of the liver. Edinburgh: Churchill Livingstone/Elsevier; 2012. p. 491–562.
27. Park HS, Lee JM, Choi JY, Lee MW, Kim HJ, Han JK, et al. Preoperative evaluation of bile duct cancer: MRI combined with MR cholangiopancreatography versus MDCT with direct cholangiography. AJR Am J Roentgenol. 2008;190:396–405.
28. Patel K, Wilder J. Fibroscan. Clin Liver Dis. 2014;4: 97–100.
29. Razumilava N, Gores GJ. Cholangiocarcinoma. Lancet. 2014;383:2168–79.
30. Razumilava N, Gores GJ, Lindor KD. Cancer surveillance in patients with primary sclerosing cholangitis. Hepatology. 2011;54:1842–52.
31. Robledo R, Muro A, Prieto ML. Extrahepatic bile duct carcinoma: US characteristics and accuracy in demonstration of tumors. Radiology. 1996;198: 869–73.
32. Ros PR, Buck JL, Goodman ZD, Ros AM, Olmsted WW. Intrahepatic cholangiocarcinoma: radiologic-pathologic correlation. Radiology. 1988;167:689–93.
33. Rosen CB, Heimbach JK, Gores GJ. Liver transplantation for cholangiocarcinoma. Transpl Int. 2010;23: 692–7.
34. Ruiz A, Lemoinne S, Carrat F, Corpechot C, Chazouilleres O, Arrive L. Radiologic course of primary sclerosing cholangitis: assessment by three-dimensional magnetic resonance cholangiography and predictive features of progression. Hepatology. 2014;59:242–50.
35. Ruys AT, Kate FJ, Busch OR, Engelbrecht MR, Gouma DJ, van Gulik TM. Metastatic lymph nodes in hilar cholangiocarcinoma: does size matter? HPB (Oxford). 2011;13:881–6.
36. Ruys AT, van Beem BE, Engelbrecht MRW, Bipat S, Stoker J, van Gulik TM. Radiological staging in patients with hilar cholangiocarcinoma: a systematic review and meta-analysis. Br J Radiol. 2012;85: 1255–62.
37. Sainani NI, Catalano OA, Holalkere NS, Zhu AX, Hahn PF, Sahani DV. Cholangiocarcinoma: current and novel imaging techniques. Radiographics. 2008;28:1263–87.
38. Schulte SJ, Baron RL, Teefey SA, Rohrmann Jr CA, Freeny PC, Shuman WP. CT of the extrahepatic bile ducts: wall thickness and contrast enhancement in normal and abnormal ducts. AJR Am J Roentgenol. 1990;154:79–85.
39. Soyer P, Bluemke DA, Reichle R, Calhoun PS, Bliss DF, Scherrer A, et al. Imaging of intrahepatic cholangiocarcinoma: 1. peripheral cholangiocarcinoma. AJR Am J Roentgenol. 1995;165:1427–31.
40. Talwalkar JA. Elastography for detecting hepatic fibrosis: options and considerations. Gastroenterology. 2008;135:299–302.
41. Tang A, Cloutier G, Szeverenyi NM, Sirlin CB. Ultrasound elastography and MR elastography for assessing liver fibrosis: part I, principles and techniques. AJR Am J Roentgenol. 2015;205:22–32.
42. Teefey SA, Baron RL, Rohrmann CA, Shuman WP, Freeny PC. Sclerosing cholangitis: CT findings. Radiology. 1988;169:635–9.
43. Tischendorf JJW, Geier A, Trautwein C. Current diagnosis and management of primary sclerosing cholangitis. Liver Transpl. 2008;14:735–46.
44. Venkatesh SK, Yin M, Ehman RL. Magnetic resonance elastography of liver: technique, analysis and clinical applications. J Magn Reson Imaging. 2013;37: 544–55.
45. Vitellas KM, Keogan MT, Freed KS, Enns RA, Spritzer CE, Baillie JM, et al. Radiologic manifestations of sclerosing cholangitis with emphasis on MR cholangiopancreatography. Radiographics. 2000;20:959–75.
46. Wiesner RH, Grambsch PM, Dickson ER, Ludwig J, MacCarty RL, Hunter EB, et al. Primary sclerosing cholangitis: natural history, prognostic factors and survival analysis. Hepatology. 1989;10:430–6.

Endoscopic Evaluation and Management of Primary Sclerosing Cholangitis

14

Hazem T. Hammad and Raj J. Shah

Introduction

Primary sclerosing cholangitis (PSC) is a chronic inflammatory cholestatic liver disease that is characterized by fibrosis and progressive destruction of the intra- and extrahepatic bile ducts with an increased risk for cholangiocarcinoma (CCA) and eventual development of cirrhosis in the majority of patients [1]. In this chapter we review the central role of endoscopy in the initial diagnosis of PSC, endoscopic evaluation and endotherapy for dominant strictures, endoscopic evaluation for development of CCA, and endoscopic evaluation and management of recurrent PSC after liver transplantation.

Endoscopic Evaluation of PSC

PSC diagnosis is usually pursued after the incidental finding of persistent abnormal cholestatic liver function tests (most commonly, alkaline phosphatase) or presentation with suspicious symptoms (later in the course of the disease) such as abdominal pain, pruritus, fatigue, and weight loss [2].

Endoscopic retrograde cholangiography (ERC) was previously the de facto diagnostic tool in patients with suspected PSC; however, many studies have shown that magnetic resonance cholangiography (MRC) performs equally well with sensitivity and specificity of ≥80 % and ≥87 %, respectively, for the diagnosis of PSC. Given the noninvasive nature and lack of radiation exposure, MRC is currently considered the diagnostic modality of choice in patient with suspected PSC [3, 4].

Nonetheless, ERC may still have a role as a diagnostic tool in PSC, particularly in patients with early changes of PSC that could be missed by MRC, or when MRC visualization of the bile ducts is limited or equivocal [4] (Fig. 14.1).

The typical findings on cholangiography include multifocal, short, annular strictures alternating with normal or slightly dilated segments resulting in a "beaded" appearance (Fig. 14.2).

Confluent long strictures can also sometimes be seen and are worrisome for the development of CCA. Typically, both intra- and extrahepatic bile ducts are involved, although a subset of patients (<25 %) may have intrahepatic disease only. The gallbladder, cystic duct, and pancreatic duct may also be associated with PSC [5]. The classic cholangiographic findings mentioned above are not entirely specific and can sometimes be seen in secondary causes of sclerosing cholangitis such

H.T. Hammad, MD
R.J. Shah, MD, FASGE, AGAF (✉)
Section of Interventional Endoscopy,
Division of Gastroenterology and Hepatology,
University of Colorado Anschutz Medical Campus,
1635 Aurora Ct. Mail Stop F735, Rm. AIP 2.031,
Aurora, CO 80045, USA
e-mail: Raj.shah@ucdenver.edu

L.M. Forman (ed.), *Primary Sclerosing Cholangitis*, DOI 10.1007/978-3-319-40908-5_14

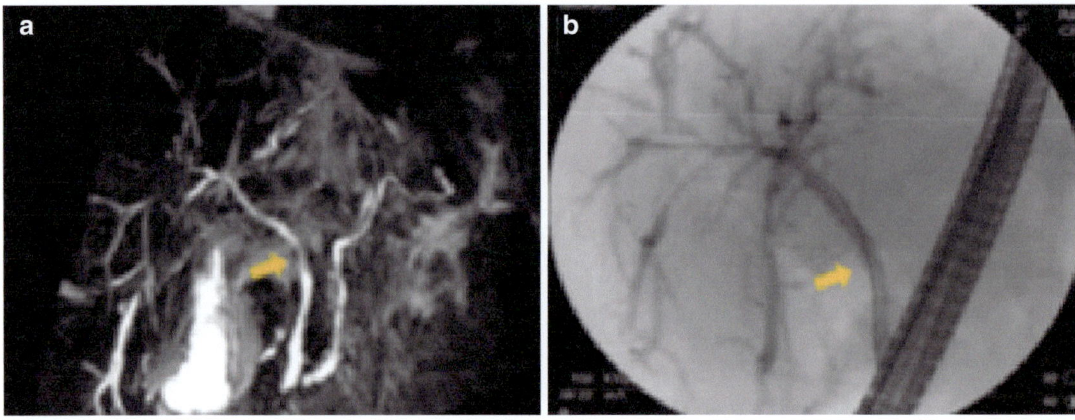

Fig. 14.1 (**a**) MRC images suspicious for a dominant stenosis in the mid bile duct (*arrow*). (**b**) Follow-up ERCP showed no evidence of stenosis in the bile duct (*arrow*)

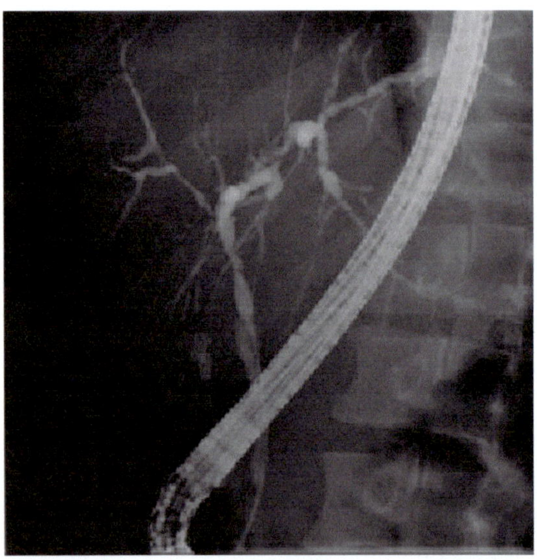

Fig. 14.2 Typical cholangiographic features of multifocal, short, annular strictures alternating with normal or slightly dilated segments resulting in a "beaded" appearance

as autoimmune pancreatitis, portal biliopathy, eosinophilic cholangitis, mast cell cholangitis, hepatic inflammatory pseudotumor, recurrent pyogenic cholangitis, primary immune deficiency, and AIDS-related cholangiopathy [6].

Endoscopic ultrasound (EUS) has also been studied as a minimally invasive tool for the diagnosis of extrahepatic PSC. Lutz et al. evaluated four sonographic parameters that are suspicious for PSC: wall thickening (≥1.5 mm), irregular wall structure (≥1 mm thickening in a duct length of maximum 5 mm), significant changes of the caliber of the common bile duct (≥2 mm change in a duct length of maximum 5 mm), and perihilar lymphadenopathy (≥10 mm). When two of these parameters were met, the sensitivity and specificity of predicting PSC were 76 % and 100 %, with positive and negative predictive values of 100 % and 79 %, respectively [7]. EUS-guided liver biopsy has been gaining more popularity as a safe and efficacious method to get adequate liver tissue samples and may be utilized more in the future when radiologic and endoscopic evaluation for PSC is inconclusive [8, 9].

Endoscopic Therapy for PSC

Endoscopic biliary therapy for PSC is primarily performed as a palliative measure and to exclude neoplasia. The presence of worsening symptoms (pruritus and RUQ abdominal pain), jaundice, cholangitis, rising cholestatic liver enzymes, or CA 19-9 in patients with PSC are typical indications for endoscopic retrograde cholangiopancreatography (ERCP) with the main goal of targeting a dominant biliary stricture for tissue sampling and endotherapy. If mass lesion or abscess is clinically suspected, abdominal ultrasound or MRI can be more helpful initial diagnostic tests.

A reasonable goal with endoscopic treatment is improving symptoms and excluding malignancy. A surrogate marker for improved biliary drainage is serum alkaline phosphatase. Improvement of serum alkaline phosphatase to <1.5 upper limit of normal was found to predict a better outcome and reduce the risk of CCA in PSC [10, 11]. Predictors for successful clinical and laboratory improvement after therapeutic ERCP include a high bilirubin level and the presence of a dominant stricture, especially in the common bile duct location [12].

Although randomized, controlled data to evaluate the effectiveness of endoscopic therapy in PSC is not available, multiple uncontrolled case series have suggested favorable outcomes. Gotthardt et al. followed 171 PSC patients for up to 20 years. Patients with dominant stenoses underwent serial endoscopic dilations. The 5- and 10-year survival free of liver transplantation was 81 % and 52 %, respectively [13]. Another study that evaluated the impact of endoscopic therapy in PSC patients reported a significantly higher 5-year survival rate in patients undergoing endoscopic therapy than what was predicted by the Mayo risk score (83 % vs. 65 %). Multiple studies have supported this finding with 4- or 5-year survival rates that are 12–18 % higher than what was predicted by the Mayo risk score [14–16].

Endoscopic Sphincterotomy

Although the biliary sphincter could be involved by the inflammatory/fibrotic process in PSC and may contribute to biliary obstruction, sphincterotomy alone is seldom used as a sole treatment modality in PSC but rather to facilitate further interventions such as tissue sampling, stone extraction, balloon dilation, or stent placement [17].

Balloon Dilation vs. Stenting of Dominant Stenoses

Balloon dilation without stenting has been shown to be an effective modality to treat dominant strictures in PSC. In a prospective single-center study from Germany, 96 patients with dominant stenoses were treated with endoscopic balloon dilations, only five of which needed a short-term (1–2 week) stent due to complete biliary obstruction and cholangitis. Over the 20-year study duration, an average of 5.2 balloon dilations per patient were performed (range 1–17). Endoscopic balloon dilations allowed the preservation of a functioning common bile duct and of at least one hepatic duct up to 2 cm above the bifurcation in all patients. Progression of liver disease led to the need for liver transplantation in 23 % of patients [13].

Some experts, including our institution, advocate for endoscopic stenting to treat benign dominant stenoses in a similar fashion as benign postoperative biliary strictures [18] (Fig. 14.3).

One of the early reports of stent therapy in PSC revealed technical success in 21 out of 25 patients (84 %) with dominant stenosis. Stents were exchanged or removed either electively at 2–3 month intervals or because of symptoms attributed to clogging. Endoscopic stenting was followed by clinical and biochemical improvement in 16 of 21 patients (76 %) over a median follow-up of 29 months. However, it was noted that about half of the follow-up ERCPs were performed on a nonelective basis because of jaundice or cholangitis attributable to early clogging of stents [19]. As a result, most centers advocate earlier removal (e.g., 2–4 weeks) of indwelling biliary stents, though our practice has been to perform stent exchanges at 6–8-week intervals until the dominant stenosis has resolved. Etiology for stent failure in PSC may include the rapid occlusion of stents by inflammatory debris shed from the biliary tree. Moreover, in patients with dominant stenoses near the bifurcation, placement of one stent into a hepatic duct could potentially worsen the drainage of the unstented hepatic duct; thus, if a dominant stenosis extends into both the right and left hepatic ducts, we would advocate for bilateral stenting.

To compare balloon dilation and stenting, a retrospective single-center study of 71 patients found no significant difference in cholestatic parameters between patients who underwent endoscopic dilation alone versus those who received stenting in addition to dilation. However,

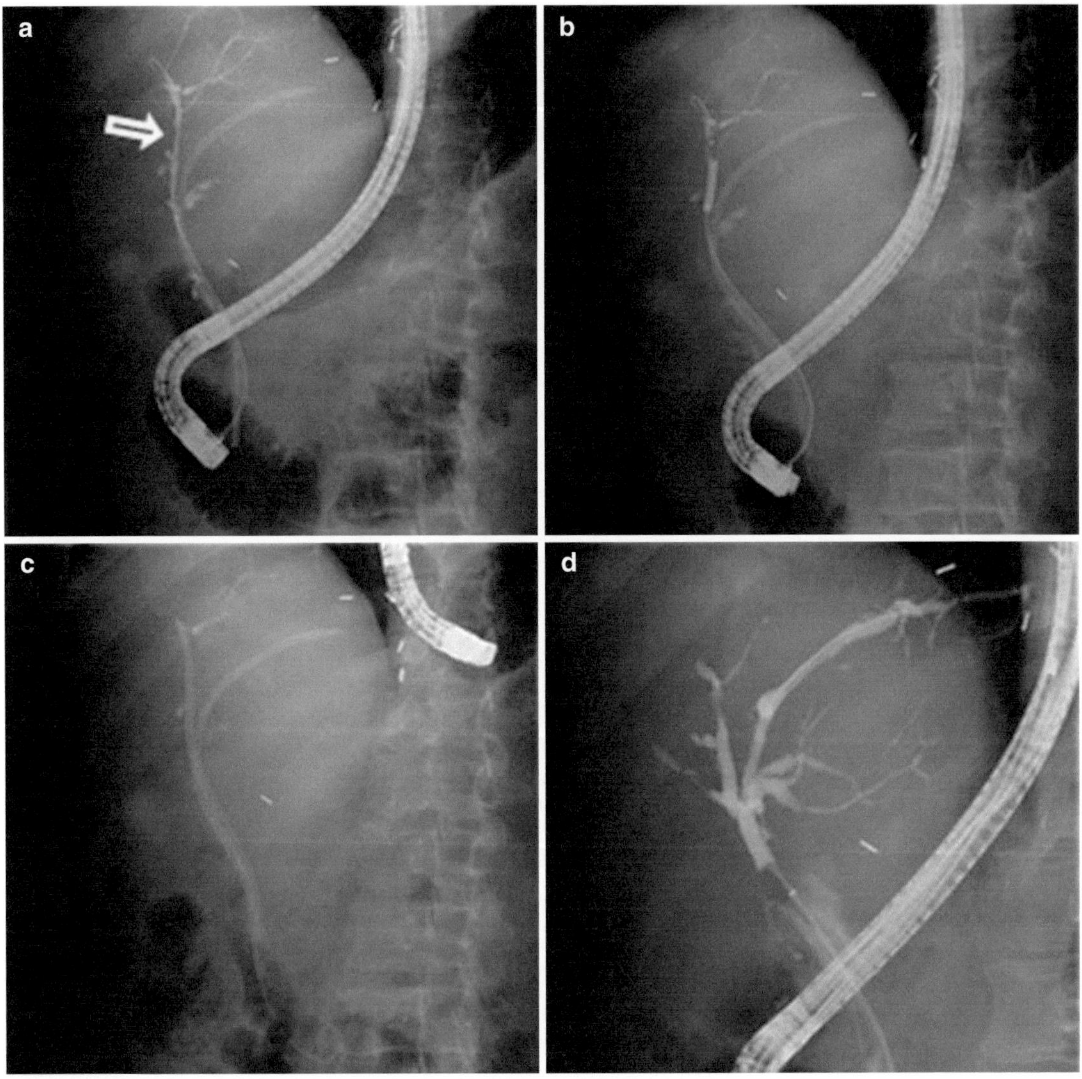

Fig. 14.3 Moderate localized biliary stricture in the right hepatic ducts (**a**) treated with balloon dilation (**b**) and stent placement (**c**) with resulting improvement of the stricture after 8 weeks (**d**)

a significantly higher rate of adverse events (AEs) such as cholangitis was noted in the stent group [20]. The authors concluded that there was no additional benefit from stenting after balloon dilation and that stenting was associated with more AEs. However, in this cohort of patients, stents were only placed in patients for whom biliary drainage was not adequate with endoscopic balloon dilation alone. Therefore, the patients in the stent group may have had more severe disease compared to the balloon-dilation-only group. It is also noteworthy that a subgroup analysis showed significantly higher AEs related to percutaneous biliary drains (such as cholangitis, bleeding, and bile duct perforation) compared to endoscopic stenting [20].

To overcome the problem of premature clogging of stents and resulting adverse events (AEs), some studies focused on reducing the duration of stent placement. In one study, sixteen patients with symptomatic PSC and dominant stenoses were treated with short-term stent placement (median duration, 9 days) and found that 81 % of patients remained asymptomatic over a 19-month follow-up without recurrence of cholestasis [21]. In another study, 32 patients with dominant strictures were treated with short-term stenting (mean duration 11 days, range 1–23 days). Serum bilirubin normalized in 12 of 14 patients (86 %) who initially presented with jaundice, and 80 % of the patients remained intervention-free after 1 year [22].

Temporary plastic stents are the only type of stents used currently for the treatment of dominant strictures in PSC [23]. We would avoid the use of fully covered self expanding metal stent (SEMS) in this patient population due to often small diameter of ducts and risk of stent-associated changes that may be seen with indwelling fully covered SEMS.

Endoscopic Evaluation for Malignancy in PSC

The incidence of CCA in patients with PSC is higher than in the general population. Population-based studies show that the annual risk is about 2 % with cumulative 10-year and 30-year incidences of 6–11 % and 20 %, respectively [24–26].

CCA in PSC is usually detected at an advanced stage and has a very poor prognosis with a dismal overall median survival of just 5 months [27]. In appropriate candidates, if CCA is detected in an early stage, expedited consideration for curative liver transplantation may be pursued.

Patient- or disease-related risk factors that seem to increase the risk of CCA in PSC include older age at time of PSC diagnosis, longer duration of inflammatory bowel disease, history of colorectal cancer or dysplasia, history of variceal bleeding, tobacco smoking, and alcohol consumption [24, 26, 28–33].

If suspected, confirming (or excluding) CCA in PSC patients can be clinically challenging to the endoscopist. The presence of segmental fibrotic strictures throughout the biliary tree makes access to the areas of concern and adequate tissue sampling very challenging.

If CCA is suspected due to abnormal imaging studies, increasing LFTs or CA 19-9 the biliary tree should be evaluated for the presence of dominant strictures, as they appear to be a major risk factor for CCA [34]. A "dominant stricture" is defined as a stenosis with a diameter of 1.5 mm in the common bile duct or of 1 mm in the right or left main hepatic ducts (within 2 cm of the bifurcation) [35].

The prevalence of dominant bile duct strictures in PSC is 36–57 %, and up to one quarter of dominant strictures is malignant [35, 36]. Hence, these are the primary targets for tissue sampling at time of ERCP. One study that clearly showed the importance of dominant strictures in PSC followed 128 patients for a mean duration of 9.8 years. The survival was reduced in patients with dominant strictures (13 %) compared to those without (23 %). The difference in survival was mostly due to the development of CCA in patients with dominant strictures [36]. In the early stages of PSC, CCA may still develop without the presence of a dominant stricture. Further, according to population-based studies, around one-third of the hepatobiliary malignancies are diagnosed within the first year after the diagnosis of PSC [24, 26].

Diagnostic Workup

Non-endoscopic methods to diagnose CCA in PSC such as serum tumor markers and imaging studies lack both sensitivity and specificity for the detection of CCA.

The most commonly used tumor marker in clinical practice is CA 19-9. In a prospective observational study from Germany that included a cohort of 106 patients who were followed for a median of 5 years, CA 19-9 was elevated (>100 ng/ml) in 24 % of patients; however, CCA developed in only 3 %. It is also not uncommon to see a drop in CA 19-9 level after treatment of biliary obstruction and caution should be exercised in its interpretation in the setting of acutely worsening cholestasis (e.g., cholangitis or jaundice) as it may inappropriately alarm both patient and provider [37]. Moreover, it is noteworthy that CA 19-9 testing will have no value in patients with negative Lewis antigen (7 % of the general population) as they cannot express CA 19-9 [38].

Imaging studies seem to perform poorly as well. A study that followed 230 patients over 6 years reported sensitivity to ultrasound, computed tomography, and magnetic resonance imaging for CCA of 57 %, 75 %, and 63 %, respectively [39].

Endoscopic Evaluation of Dominant Biliary Strictures in PSC

Brush Cytology

This includes the use of conventional cytology brush during ERCP to obtain cells from a concerning stricture for cytology analysis (Fig. 14.4).

This method is considered relatively easy and has a very high specificity (95–100 %), but unfortunately has a disappointing low sensitivity that ranges from 29 to 73 % [40, 41].

These findings were confirmed by a meta-analysis of 54 studies that revealed a pooled specificity of 97 % but a pooled sensitivity of only 43 % [42]. It is likely that the low sensitivity is due to severe periductular fibrosis and stricturing in PSC limiting access and adequate sampling of concerning areas.

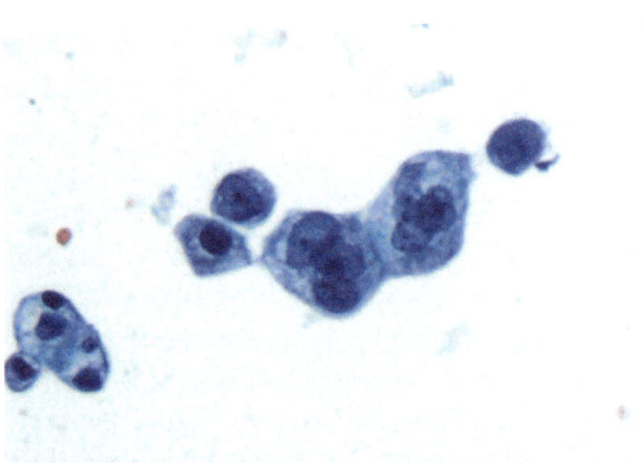

Fig. 14.4 Cluster of malignant cells from a common bile duct brushing (*arrow*) in PSC. In comparison to the adjacent benign cells (*arrow head*), the malignant cells are larger, with dark nuclei and high nucleus to cytoplasmic ratios than the benign cells. Papanicolaou stain, 200× (Image courtesy of Paul Dimaggio, MD, University of Colorado Department of Pathology)

Endoscopic Ultrasound

EUS-guided fine needle aspiration (EUS-FNA) can be a valuable diagnostic tool for suspected malignant biliary stricture when brush cytology and biopsy are inconclusive with a sensitivity and specificity up to 89 % and 100 %, respectively [43, 44]. EUS-FNA can also be utilized for evaluation and sampling of suspicious lymph nodes. Given the rare possibility of tumor seeding with FNA [45], most institutions feel that EUS-FNA of suspicious biliary strictures is a contraindication to liver transplantation.

Fluorescence In Situ Hybridization (FISH)

In this technique, fluorescently labeled DNA probes are used to assess cells obtained using biliary brushings for chromosomal abnormalities. At our center, we provide two brushing specimens of the stricture and submit to cytology who will then divide the specimens for routine cytology and FISH evaluation. The probe set used assesses the pericentromeric regions on chromosomes 3, 7, and 17, and a locus-specific probe on chromosome 9p21 [46, 47]. The results of FISH testing can be classified as normal, polysomy (if five or more cells show gains of two or more of the four probes), tetrasomy (if 10 or more cells showed four copies of all probes), and trisomy (if 10 or more cells showed three copies of chromosome 7 or 3 and two or fewer copies of the other three probes) [46] (Fig. 14.5).

FISH polysomy is highly associated with CCA; however, trisomy and tetrasomy are not considered independent predictors for CCA, and patients with these changes seem to have a similar outcome to patients with normal FISH testing [46–49].

In a Mayo clinic study of 235 PSC patients, FISH polysomy had a sensitivity of 46 % and specificity of 88 % for the diagnosis of CCA [46]. These findings were confirmed by a meta-analysis of eight studies involving 828 patients [50]. An interesting subsequent study from the same center showed that in patients with an index

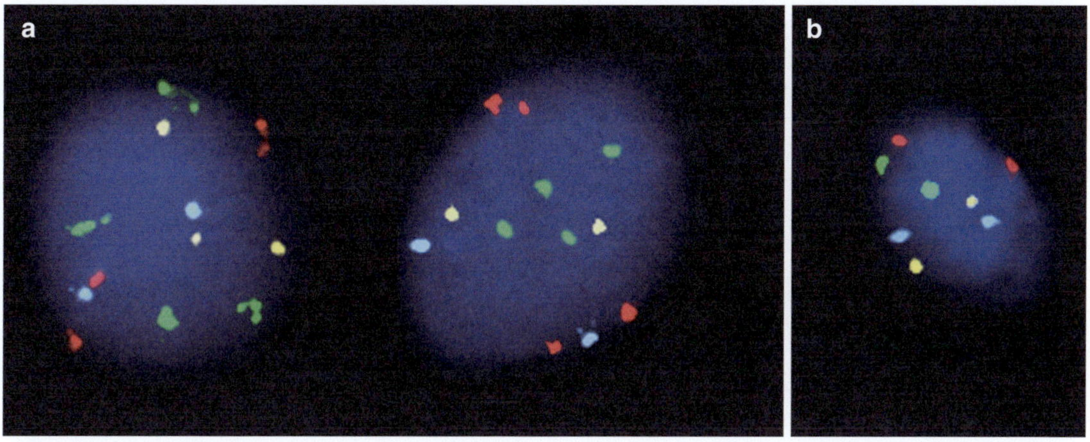

Fig. 14.5 A chromosome enumeration assay for interphase cells was performed using a mixture of DNA sequence probes specific for the centromeres of chromosome 3 (*red*), 7 (*green*), and 17 (*aqua*) and for the 9p21 (p16) locus on chromosome 9 (*gold*) along with a DAPI counterstain on ThinPrep slides of bile duct brushings. (Panel **a**) Two polyploid interphase cells from the same patient demonstrating four copies of chromosome 3, four copies 7 centromere, and two copies of 9p16 and 17 centromere sequences. (Panel **b**) A normal interphase cell with two copies of each signal for 3, 7, and 17 centromere and 9p21 (p16) sequences (Image courtesy of Billie Carstens, Colorado Genetics Laboratory)

polysomy FISH study who had subsequent non-polysomy results, only 18 % ended up developing CCA. For those patients with subsequent positive polysomy FISH (so-called serial polysomy), 69 % subsequently developed CCA [47]. This study emphasizes the limitation of a single polysomy FISH result and the importance of repeating the FISH testing for risk stratification. Further, in liver transplant centers that propose treating PSC patients with suspected CCA utilizing the Mayo protocol, the proposal is based on suspicious cholangiographic appearance of a stricture, elevated CA 19-9 (greater than 100), and/or FISH polysomy to support the upgraded listing [51].

Another study that attempted to improve the utility of FISH testing in PSC showed that finding of positive FISH testing in multiple areas of the biliary tree, so-called multifocal polysomy (MFP), was the strongest predictor of CCA (when compared to unifocal polysomy and suspicious cytology). The 1- and 3-year cumulative incidence rates of CCA among MFP patients were 65 % and 83 %, respectively. This study suggested that brushing multiple areas of the biliary tree (even without the presence of dominant stricture) and placing the specimens in separate jars help risk stratify these patients and may improve the ability to detect CCA. Interestingly, this study did not find an elevated CA 19-9 (>129 U/ml) to be an independent predictor of CCA [48].

Intraductal Endoscopy

Cholangioscopy provides direct visualization into the biliary tree. However, it has a limited role in PSC due to narrowed ducts and inability to traverse strictures without pre-inspection dilation, which could alter mucosal characteristics [52]. Further, inflammatory changes in the setting of PSC or stent changes could make it difficult to distinguish from malignant changes and nodular mass-like villiform changes are not uncommon in benign PSC [52, 53]. However, select studies have suggested that cholangioscopy might increase the ability to differentiate between malignant and benign strictures in PSC [54]. In a prospective observational study from Germany that included 53 PSC patients, cholangioscopy (2D-Microendoscope ERCP, Almikro Ltd., Bad Krozingen, Germany) had a higher sensitivity (92 % vs. 66 %; $P=0.25$) and specificity (93 % vs. 51 %; $P<0.001$) for detecting CCA, when compared to endoscopic brush cytology alone [55]. However this degree of neoplasia detection utilizing cholangioscopy has not yet been duplicated. Liu et al. reported a sensitivity of 75 % and specificity of 55 % for cholangioscopy (SpyGlass system, Boston Scientific, Natick, MA, USA) in 18 PSC patients with suspected CCA [54]. Another recent small report described the use of video cholangioscopy and NBI (Olympus Tokyo, Inc) during cholangioscopy. Despite a 48 % increase in the rate of detecting suspicious lesions that led to more biopsy specimens being obtained, NBI-directed biopsies did not improve the dysplasia detection rate compared with white-light imaging and overall did not confirm a true value for the use of cholangioscopy in this patient population [56]. Further, we reported our data on the use of cholangioscopy in 41 patients with PSC. Cholangioscopy identified one extrahepatic CCA but missed two intrahepatic CCAs. In this report, cholangioscopy was very helpful to detect biliary stones in 56 % of patients (30 % of which were missed on cholangiography) which could contribute to recurrent cholangitis [52].

Transpapillary intraductal ultrasound was used to analyze dominant strictures in 40 PSC patients and showed a sensitivity of 87.5 % and specificity of 90.6 % for detection of CCA. Larger studies are needed to confirm the utilization of this technique in PSC patients and fragility of the probes have limited its use [57].

Probe-Based Confocal Laser Endomicroscopy (pCLE)

Due to the limitations of conventional tissue sampling and direct visual inspection of mucosal changes by cholangioscopy, investigation in the subepithelial changes that may help exclude malignancy has been sought. The technique of pCLE provides a real-time in vivo microscopic images of the bile duct epithelium using a small (2.8 F) diameter probe but requires direct contact to the mucosa and a minimally tangential approach for optimal imaging. Due to the probe size, pre-inspection dilation is generally not required. The probe can be placed either through a cholangioscope or through the lumen of a standard cannula that permits tip deflection (Swing Tip, Olympus America, Inc). The Miami classification was developed for indeterminate non-PSC biliary stricture. It includes five malignant imaging characteristics: thick white bands (>20 μms), thick dark bands (>40 μms), epithelial structures, dark clumps, and fluorescein leakage [58, 59] (Fig. 14.6).

Our group evaluated a total of 20 strictures specifically in patients with PSC. The use of pCLE was feasible in 95 % of examinations. The sensitivity was 100 %; however, specificity was only 61.1 %. This was likely due to inflammatory ductal changes in the setting of PSC. Interestingly, in two patients with positive pCLE but only

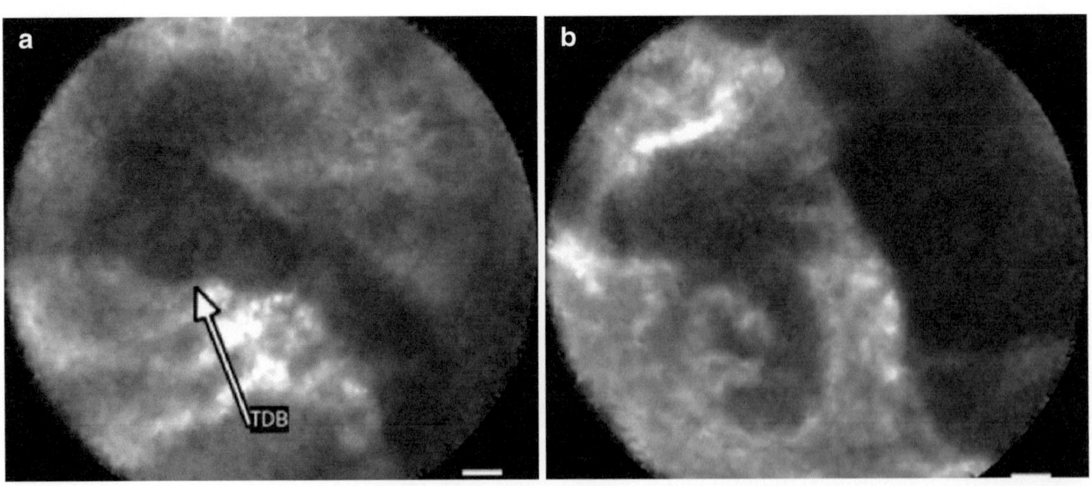

Fig. 14.6 pCLE images in malignant dominant stricture. (**a**) Showing thick dark band and (**b**) showing dark clumps

"atypical" cytopathology who underwent liver transplantation, dysplasia was noted in the segment of the explanted duct that corresponded to the location of abnormality during pCLE examination [60]. A multicenter study of 102 of indeterminate pancreaticobiliary strictures (PSC patients were excluded) showed that combining two or more of the Miami criteria significantly increased the sensitivity and predictive values. The sensitivity, specificity, positive predictive value, and negative predictive value were found to be 97 %, 33 %, 80 %, and 80 %, respectively. So, if a dominant stenosis shows benign pCLE features, then it is more reassuring to reduce the frequency of surveillance sampling required [59]. Another study supporting the above findings included 10 pCLE experts who reviewed pCLE findings from 46 patients with PSC strictures. Combining pCLE and tissue sampling yielded sensitivity and negative predictive value of 100 % [61].

A multicenter registry study utilizing pCLE specifically in PSC patients with dominant stenoses is ongoing.

The Paris classification attempts to take into account inflammatory or reactive changes that may be seen in biliary strictures. It included criteria for benign inflammatory conditions (vascular congestion, dark granular patterns with scales, increased inter-glandular space, and thickened reticular structure) that may help improve the specificity of pCLE findings and may be more relevant in patients with PSC [62].

Antibiotic Prophylaxis

Given the often diffuse, segmental intrahepatic structuring associated with PSC, injecting contrast during ERCP into obstructed ducts may increase the risk for post-ERCP cholangitis. Cholangitis in PSC can be life-threatening and lead to liver decompensation due to an inability to decompress intrahepatic segmental biliary obstruction [63]. Thus, pre-procedure IV antibiotics or oral antibiotics started 48 h prior to ERCP followed by a 3- to 5-day course post-ERCP are considered the standard of care and despite randomized, controlled data [64, 65]. At our institution, we routinely administer an IV dose of a quinolone or ampicillin/sulbactam prior to ERCP and give a 5- to 7-day course of quinolone or amoxicillin-clavulanate after the procedure. Further, in patients who have had post-ERCP cholangitis, we will provide oral antibiotics for 48 h prior to a repeat ERCP and anecdotally have found it to help reduce the risk of cholangitis in these more susceptible individuals.

Adverse Events of ERCP in PSC

The largest reported series of PSC patients with long-term follow-up reported an AE rate of 7.3 % among 317 ERCPs performed on 117 PSC patients over a mean duration of 8 years. The most common AEs were post-ERCP pancreatitis, cholangitis, sepsis, biliary tract perforation, post-sphincterotomy bleeding, and liver abscess. The complications were mild without a need for surgical intervention. There were no procedure-related deaths [15].

Role of Endoscopy in Recurrent PSC After Liver Transplantation

A German study that followed 335 PSC patients for 98.8 months after liver transplantation showed that recurrent PSC was diagnosed in 20.3 % of the patients after 4.6 years. Risk factors for recurrent PSC were older donor age, IBD, and INR at time of transplantation [66]. Diagnosis of recurrent PSC can be challenging, particularly in differentiating it from many other conditions that could cause biliary strictures (ischemia, hepatic artery thrombosis, chronic ductopenic rejection, ABO incompatibility, bacterial/fungal cholangitis, etc.). Biliary strictures after liver transplant can be classified into anastomotic and non-anastomotic strictures. Non-anastomotic biliary strictures occur more often after liver transplantation for PSC than for other indications [67]. Given involvement of extrahepatic bile ducts in PSC, Roux-en-Y choledocho- or hepaticojejunostomy (as opposed to duct-to-duct anastomosis) or more recently choledochoduodenostomy is considered the method of choice for biliary reconstruction [68]. The Roux-en-Y anatomy makes endoscopic access for diagnostic and therapeutic purposes challenging; however, the recent advances in biliary endoscopy using balloon-assisted deep enteroscopy (single and double balloon) after Roux-en-Y reconstruction was shown to be feasible and highly efficacious [69]. These techniques are not widely available and are mostly performed in specialized tertiary centers. Given the aforementioned factors, MRC is considered the first choice for evaluation of biliary strictures after liver transplantation. Anastomotic strictures can be treated successfully with balloon dilation and stenting [70]. Non-anastomotic strictures can also be treated with balloon dilation and stenting but appear to be more difficult to treat [71]. Most of the published data, however, are for complications involving liver transplantation with duct-to-duct anastomosis. Percutaneous transhepatic biliary drainage (PTBD) can also be used for the management of biliary strictures after liver transplantation, particularly if endoscopic approach is not successful [72]. Preliminary data from our institution (DDW 2016, Poster Tu1572) showed that at a median 2-year follow-up, deep enteroscopy ERC compared to percutaneous transhepatic biliary drain is associated with fewer procedures, fewer post-procedure hospitalization days, and a shorter time to resolve anastomotic strictures in patients with long limb surgical biliary bypass including Roux-en-Y reconstruction after liver transplantation.

There are no published data to show the overall efficacy of endoscopic treatment on the progression of recurrent PSC aside from symptomatic management of biliary strictures and their complications. Retransplantation for progressive, recurrent disease is often an unfortunate consequence.

Conclusions and Future Directions

The best approach to treat dominant strictures in PSC is still unknown. Endoscopic balloon dilation (along with short-term stenting for severe strictures and patients presenting with cholangitis) seems to be the best approach. We perform serial upsizing of stents to treat dominant stenoses until their resolution. Studies are underway to clearly define and compare the role of each modality in treatment of PSC (Short-term Stenting Versus Balloon Dilatation for Dominant Strictures in Primary Sclerosing Cholangitis, NCT01398917).

Despite the availability of multiple diagnostic tests for CCA, confirming or excluding CCA in PSC is still a major challenge to clinicians. There have been some exciting developments in finding biomarkers for CCA that could play a role in the future. Among those are promising early studies for markers that can be studied in the bile aspirated at the time of ERCP such as oxidized phospholipids, volatile organic compounds, and DNA methylation [73–75]. For now, we advocate the use of brush cytology, biopsy/histology, and FISH analyses and consider pCLE for all dominant stenoses [76].

Recurrent PSC following liver transplantation is problematic, but advances in deep enteroscopy techniques provide minimally invasive options for symptomatic patients.

Conflict of Interest Dr. Shah is on the medical advisory board and has received unrestricted educational grants from Boston Scientific, unrestricted educational grants and prototype endoscope loans from Olympus, Inc. and unrestricted educational grants and honoraria from Mauna Kea Technologies, Inc.

References

1. Tischendorf JJ, Hecker H, Kruger M, Manns MP, Meier PN. Characterization, outcome, and prognosis in 273 patients with primary sclerosing cholangitis: a single center study. Am J Gastroenterol. 2007;102(1):107–14.
2. Broome U, Olsson R, Loof L, Bodemar G, Hultcrantz R, Danielsson A, et al. Natural history and prognostic factors in 305 Swedish patients with primary sclerosing cholangitis. Gut. 1996;38(4):610–5.
3. Berstad AE, Aabakken L, Smith HJ, Aasen S, Boberg KM, Schrumpf E. Diagnostic accuracy of magnetic resonance and endoscopic retrograde cholangiography in primary sclerosing cholangitis. Clin Gastroenterol Hepatol. 2006;4(4):514–20.
4. Angulo P, Pearce DH, Johnson CD, Henry JJ, LaRusso NF, Petersen BT, et al. Magnetic resonance cholangiography in patients with biliary disease: its role in

primary sclerosing cholangitis. J Hepatol. 2000;33(4):520–7.

5. MacCarty RL, LaRusso NF, Wiesner RH, Ludwig J. Primary sclerosing cholangitis: findings on cholangiography and pancreatography. Radiology. 1983;149(1):39–44.
6. Abdalian R, Heathcote EJ. Sclerosing cholangitis: a focus on secondary causes. Hepatology. 2006;44(5):1063–74.
7. Lutz HH, Wasmuth HE, Streetz K, Tacke F, Koch A, Luedde T, et al. Endoscopic ultrasound as an early diagnostic tool for primary sclerosing cholangitis: a prospective pilot study. Endoscopy. 2012;44(10):934–9.
8. Gor N, Salem SB, Jakate S, Patel R, Shah N, Patil A. Histological adequacy of EUS-guided liver biopsy when using a 19-gauge non-Tru-Cut FNA needle. Gastrointest Endosc. 2014;79(1):170–2.
9. Diehl DL, Johal AS, Khara HS, Stavropoulos SN, Al-Haddad M, Ramesh J, et al. Endoscopic ultrasound-guided liver biopsy: a multicenter experience. Endosc Int Open. 2015;3(3):E210–5.
10. Al Mamari S, Djordjevic J, Halliday JS, Chapman RW. Improvement of serum alkaline phosphatase to <1.5 upper limit of normal predicts better outcome and reduced risk of cholangiocarcinoma in primary sclerosing cholangitis. J Hepatol. 2013;58(2):329–34.
11. Lindstrom L, Hultcrantz R, Boberg KM, Friis-Liby I, Bergquist A. Association between reduced levels of alkaline phosphatase and survival times of patients with primary sclerosing cholangitis. Clin Gastroenterol Hepatol. 2013;11(7):841–6.
12. Enns R, Eloubeidi MA, Mergener K, Jowell PS, Branch MS, Baillie J. Predictors of successful clinical and laboratory outcomes in patients with primary sclerosing cholangitis undergoing endoscopic retrograde cholangiopancreatography. Can J Gastroenterol. 2003;17(4):243–8.
13. Gotthardt DN, Rudolph G, Kloters-Plachky P, Kulaksiz H, Stiehl A. Endoscopic dilation of dominant stenoses in primary sclerosing cholangitis: outcome after long-term treatment. Gastrointest Endosc. 2010;71(3):527–34.
14. Baluyut AR, Sherman S, Lehman GA, Hoen H, Chalasani N. Impact of endoscopic therapy on the survival of patients with primary sclerosing cholangitis. Gastrointest Endosc. 2001;53(3):308–12.
15. Gluck M, Cantone NR, Brandabur JJ, Patterson DJ, Bredfeldt JE, Kozarek RA. A twenty-year experience with endoscopic therapy for symptomatic primary sclerosing cholangitis. J Clin Gastroenterol. 2008;42(9):1032–9.
16. Stiehl A, Rudolph G, Kloters-Plachky P, Sauer P, Walker S. Development of dominant bile duct stenoses in patients with primary sclerosing cholangitis treated with ursodeoxycholic acid: outcome after endoscopic treatment. J Hepatol. 2002;36(2):151–6.
17. Johnson GK, Geenen JE, Venu RP, Schmalz MJ, Hogan WJ. Endoscopic treatment of biliary tract strictures in sclerosing cholangitis: a larger series and recommendations for treatment. Gastrointest Endosc. 1991;37(1):38–43.
18. Costamagna G, Tringali A, Mutignani M, Perri V, Spada C, Pandolfi M, et al. Endotherapy of postoperative biliary strictures with multiple stents: results after more than 10 years of follow-up. Gastrointest Endosc. 2010;72(3):551–7.
19. van Milligen de Wit AW, van Bracht J, Rauws EA, Jones EA, Tytgat GN, Huibregtse K. Endoscopic stent therapy for dominant extrahepatic bile duct strictures in primary sclerosing cholangitis. Gastrointest Endosc. 1996;44(3):293–9.
20. Kaya M, Petersen BT, Angulo P, Baron TH, Andrews JC, Gostout CJ, et al. Balloon dilation compared to stenting of dominant strictures in primary sclerosing cholangitis. Am J Gastroenterol. 2001;96(4):1059–66.
21. van Milligen de Wit AW, Rauws EA, van Bracht J, Mulder CJ, Jones EA, Tytgat GN, et al. Lack of complications following short-term stent therapy for extrahepatic bile duct strictures in primary sclerosing cholangitis. Gastrointest Endosc. 1997;46(4):344–7.
22. Ponsioen CY, Lam K, van Milligen de Wit AW, Huibregtse K, Tytgat GN. Four years experience with short term stenting in primary sclerosing cholangitis. Am J Gastroenterol. 1999;94(9):2403–7.
23. Abu-Wasel B, Keough V, Renfrew PD, Molinari M. Biliary stent therapy for dominant strictures in patients affected by primary sclerosing cholangitis. Pathobiology. 2013;80(4):182–93.
24. Boonstra K, Weersma RK, van Erpecum KJ, Rauws EA, Spanier BW, Poen AC, et al. Population-based epidemiology, malignancy risk, and outcome of primary sclerosing cholangitis. Hepatology. 2013;58(6):2045–55.
25. Kornfeld D, Ekbom A, Ihre T. Survival and risk of cholangiocarcinoma in patients with primary sclerosing cholangitis. A population-based study. Scand J Gastroenterol. 1997;32(10):1042–5.
26. Bergquist A, Ekbom A, Olsson R, Kornfeldt D, Loof L, Danielsson A, et al. Hepatic and extrahepatic malignancies in primary sclerosing cholangitis. J Hepatol. 2002;36(3):321–7.
27. Rosen CB, Nagorney DM, Wiesner RH, Coffey Jr RJ, LaRusso NF. Cholangiocarcinoma complicating primary sclerosing cholangitis. Ann Surg. 1991;213(1):21–5.
28. de Valle MB, Bjornsson E, Lindkvist B. Mortality and cancer risk related to primary sclerosing cholangitis in a Swedish population-based cohort. Liver Int. 2012;32(3):441–8.
29. Boberg KM, Bergquist A, Mitchell S, Pares A, Rosina F, Broome U, et al. Cholangiocarcinoma in primary sclerosing cholangitis: risk factors and clinical presentation. Scand J Gastroenterol. 2002;37(10):1205–11.
30. Burak K, Angulo P, Pasha TM, Egan K, Petz J, Lindor KD. Incidence and risk factors for cholangiocarcinoma in primary sclerosing cholangitis. Am J Gastroenterol. 2004;99(3):523–6.
31. Chalasani N, Baluyut A, Ismail A, Zaman A, Sood G, Ghalib R, et al. Cholangiocarcinoma in patients with primary sclerosing cholangitis: a multicenter case-control study. Hepatology. 2000;31(1):7–11.

32. Bergquist A, Glaumann H, Persson B, Broome U. Risk factors and clinical presentation of hepatobiliary carcinoma in patients with primary sclerosing cholangitis: a case-control study. Hepatology. 1998;27(2):311–6.
33. Broome U, Lofberg R, Veress B, Eriksson LS. Primary sclerosing cholangitis and ulcerative colitis: evidence for increased neoplastic potential. Hepatology. 1995;22(5):1404–8.
34. Rudolph G, Gotthardt D, Kloeters-Plachky P, Rost D, Kulaksiz H, Stiehl A. In PSC with dominant bile duct stenosis, IBD is associated with an increase of carcinomas and reduced survival. J Hepatol. 2010; 53(2):313–7.
35. Bjornsson E, Lindqvist-Ottosson J, Asztely M, Olsson R. Dominant strictures in patients with primary sclerosing cholangitis. Am J Gastroenterol. 2004;99(3): 502–8.
36. Chapman MH, Webster GJ, Bannoo S, Johnson GJ, Wittmann J, Pereira SP. Cholangiocarcinoma and dominant strictures in patients with primary sclerosing cholangitis: a 25-year single-centre experience. Eur J Gastroenterol Hepatol. 2012;24(9):1051–8.
37. Petersen-Benz C, Stiehl A. Impact of dominant stenoses on the serum level of the tumor marker CA19-9 in patients with primary sclerosing cholangitis. Z Gastroenterol. 2005;43(6):587–90.
38. Nehls O, Gregor M, Klump B. Serum and bile markers for cholangiocarcinoma. Semin Liver Dis. 2004;24(2):139–54.
39. Charatcharoenwitthaya P, Enders FB, Halling KC, Lindor KD. Utility of serum tumor markers, imaging, and biliary cytology for detecting cholangiocarcinoma in primary sclerosing cholangitis. Hepatology. 2008;48(4):1106–17.
40. Levy MJ, Baron TH, Clayton AC, Enders FB, Gostout CJ, Halling KC, et al. Prospective evaluation of advanced molecular markers and imaging techniques in patients with indeterminate bile duct strictures. Am J Gastroenterol. 2008;103(5):1263–73.
41. Aljiffry M, Renfrew PD, Walsh MJ, Laryea M, Molinari M. Analytical review of diagnosis and treatment strategies for dominant bile duct strictures in patients with primary sclerosing cholangitis. HPB (Oxford). 2011;13(2):79–90.
42. Trikudanathan G, Navaneethan U, Njei B, Vargo JJ, Parsi MA. Diagnostic yield of bile duct brushings for cholangiocarcinoma in primary sclerosing cholangitis: a systematic review and meta-analysis. Gastrointest Endosc. 2014;79(5):783–9.
43. Fritscher-Ravens A, Broering DC, Knoefel WT, Rogiers X, Swain P, Thonke F, et al. EUS-guided fine-needle aspiration of suspected hilar cholangiocarcinoma in potentially operable patients with negative brush cytology. Am J Gastroenterol. 2004;99(1):45–51.
44. Ohshima Y, Yasuda I, Kawakami H, Kuwatani M, Mukai T, Iwashita T, et al. EUS-FNA for suspected malignant biliary strictures after negative endoscopic transpapillary brush cytology and forceps biopsy. J Gastroenterol. 2011;46(7):921–8.
45. Paquin SC, Gariepy G, Lepanto L, Bourdages R, Raymond G, Sahai AV. A first report of tumor seeding because of EUS-guided FNA of a pancreatic adenocarcinoma. Gastrointest Endosc. 2005;61(4):610–1.
46. Bangarulingam SY, Bjornsson E, Enders F, Barr Fritcher EG, Gores G, Halling KC, et al. Long-term outcomes of positive fluorescence in situ hybridization tests in primary sclerosing cholangitis. Hepatology. 2010;51(1):174–80.
47. Barr Fritcher EG, Kipp BR, Voss JS, Clayton AC, Lindor KD, Halling KC, et al. Primary sclerosing cholangitis patients with serial polysomy fluorescence in situ hybridization results are at increased risk of cholangiocarcinoma. Am J Gastroenterol. 2011; 106(11):2023–8.
48. Eaton JE, Barr Fritcher EG, Gores GJ, Atkinson EJ, Tabibian JH, Topazian MD, et al. Biliary multifocal chromosomal polysomy and cholangiocarcinoma in primary sclerosing cholangitis. Am J Gastroenterol. 2015;110(2):299–309.
49. Barr Fritcher EG, Voss JS, Jenkins SM, Lingineni RK, Clayton AC, Roberts LR, et al. Primary sclerosing cholangitis with equivocal cytology: fluorescence in situ hybridization and serum CA 19-9 predict risk of malignancy. Cancer Cytopathol. 2013;121(12): 708–17.
50. Navaneethan U, Njei B, Venkatesh PG, Vargo JJ, Parsi MA. Fluorescence in situ hybridization for diagnosis of cholangiocarcinoma in primary sclerosing cholangitis: a systematic review and meta-analysis. Gastrointest Endosc. 2014;79(6):943–50.e3.
51. Rizvi S, Gores GJ. Pathogenesis, diagnosis, and management of cholangiocarcinoma. Gastroenterology. 2013;145(6):1215–29.
52. Awadallah NS, Chen YK, Piraka C, Antillon MR, Shah RJ. Is there a role for cholangioscopy in patients with primary sclerosing cholangitis? Am J Gastroenterol. 2006;101(2):284–91.
53. Chen YK, Pleskow DK. SpyGlass single-operator peroral cholangiopancreatoscopy system for the diagnosis and therapy of bile-duct disorders: a clinical feasibility study (with video). Gastrointest Endosc. 2007;65(6):832–41.
54. Liu R, Cox Rn K, Siddiqui A, Feurer M, Baron T, Adler DG. Peroral cholangioscopy facilitates targeted tissue acquisition in patients with suspected cholangiocarcinoma. Minerva Gastroenterol Dietol. 2014;60(2):127–33.
55. Tischendorf JJ, Kruger M, Trautwein C, Duckstein N, Schneider A, Manns MP, et al. Cholangioscopic characterization of dominant bile duct stenoses in patients with primary sclerosing cholangitis. Endoscopy. 2006;38(7):665–9.
56. Azeem N, Gostout CJ, Knipschield M, Baron TH. Cholangioscopy with narrow-band imaging in patients with primary sclerosing cholangitis undergoing ERCP. Gastrointest Endosc. 2014;79(5):773–9.e2.
57. Tischendorf JJ, Meier PN, Schneider A, Manns MP, Kruger M. Transpapillary intraductal ultrasound in

the evaluation of dominant bile duct stenoses in patients with primary sclerosing cholangitis. Scand J Gastroenterol. 2007;42(8):1011–7.
58. Meining A, Chen YK, Pleskow D, Stevens P, Shah RJ, Chuttani R, et al. Direct visualization of indeterminate pancreaticobiliary strictures with probe-based confocal laser endomicroscopy: a multicenter experience. Gastrointest Endosc. 2011;74(5):961–8.
59. Meining A, Shah RJ, Slivka A, Pleskow D, Chuttani R, Stevens PD, et al. Classification of probe-based confocal laser endomicroscopy findings in pancreaticobiliary strictures. Endoscopy. 2012;44(3):251–7.
60. Heif M, Yen RD, Shah RJ. ERCP with probe-based confocal laser endomicroscopy for the evaluation of dominant biliary stenoses in primary sclerosing cholangitis patients. Dig Dis Sci. 2013;58(7):2068–74.
61. Shah RJ, Chennat JS, Cesaro P, Slivka A, Sejpal DV, Jamidar PA, et al. Distinguishing benign from malignant dominant biliary strictures in patients with primary sclerosing cholangitis utilizing probe-based confocal LASER endomicroscopy (pCLE): a multicenter, expert consensus review. Gastrointest Endosc. 2013;77(5):AB164.
62. Caillol F, Filoche B, Gaidhane M, Kahaleh M. Refined probe-based confocal laser endomicroscopy classification for biliary strictures: the Paris Classification. Dig Dis Sci. 2013;58(6):1784–9.
63. Bangarulingam SY, Gossard AA, Petersen BT, Ott BJ, Lindor KD. Complications of endoscopic retrograde cholangiopancreatography in primary sclerosing cholangitis. Am J Gastroenterol. 2009;104(4):855–60.
64. Lindor KD, Kowdley KV, Harrison ME, American College of G. ACG clinical guideline: primary sclerosing cholangitis. Am J Gastroenterol. 2015;110(5):646–59; quiz 60.
65. Committee ASoP, Khashab MA, Chithadi KV, Acosta RD, Bruining DH, Chandrasekhara V, et al. Antibiotic prophylaxis for GI endoscopy. Gastrointest Endosc. 2015;81(1):81–9.
66. Hildebrand T, Pannicke N, Dechene A, Gotthardt DN, Kirchner G, Reiter FP, et al. Biliary strictures and recurrence after liver transplantation for primary sclerosing cholangitis: a retrospective multicenter analysis. Liver Transpl. 2016;22(1):42–52.
67. Sheng R, Zajko AB, Campbell WL, Abu-Elmagd K. Biliary strictures in hepatic transplants: prevalence and types in patients with primary sclerosing cholangitis vs those with other liver diseases. AJR Am J Roentgenol. 1993;161(2):297–300.
68. Welsh FK, Wigmore SJ. Roux-en-Y Choledochojejunostomy is the method of choice for biliary reconstruction in liver transplantation for primary sclerosing cholangitis. Transplantation. 2004;77(4):602–4.
69. Shah RJ, Smolkin M, Yen R, Ross A, Kozarek RA, Howell DA, et al. A multicenter, U.S. experience of single-balloon, double-balloon, and rotational overtube-assisted enteroscopy ERCP in patients with surgically altered pancreaticobiliary anatomy (with video). Gastrointest Endosc. 2013;77(4):593–600.
70. Kim TH, Lee SK, Han JH, Park do H, Lee SS, Seo DW, et al. The role of endoscopic retrograde cholangiography for biliary stricture after adult living donor liver transplantation: technical aspect and outcome. Scand J Gastroenterol. 2011;46(2):188–96.
71. Rizk RS, McVicar JP, Emond MJ, Rohrmann Jr CA, Kowdley KV, Perkins J, et al. Endoscopic management of biliary strictures in liver transplant recipients: effect on patient and graft survival. Gastrointest Endosc. 1998;47(2):128–35.
72. Kim ES, Lee BJ, Won JY, Choi JY, Lee DK. Percutaneous transhepatic biliary drainage may serve as a successful rescue procedure in failed cases of endoscopic therapy for a post-living donor liver transplantation biliary stricture. Gastrointest Endosc. 2009;69(1):38–46.
73. Navaneethan U, Gutierrez NG, Venkatesh PG, Jegadeesan R, Zhang R, Jang S, et al. Lipidomic profiling of bile in distinguishing benign from malignant biliary strictures: a single-blinded pilot study. Am J Gastroenterol. 2014;109(6):895–902.
74. Navaneethan U, Parsi MA, Lourdusamy V, Bhatt A, Gutierrez NG, Grove D, et al. Volatile organic compounds in bile for early diagnosis of cholangiocarcinoma in patients with primary sclerosing cholangitis: a pilot study. Gastrointest Endosc. 2015;81(4):943–9.e1.
75. Andresen K, Boberg KM, Vedeld HM, Honne H, Jebsen P, Hektoen M, et al. Four DNA methylation biomarkers in biliary brush samples accurately identify the presence of cholangiocarcinoma. Hepatology. 2015;61(5):1651–9.
76. Shah RJ. Cholangiocarcionoma and primary sclerosing cholangitis: the answer lies within. Gastrointest Endosc. 2014;79(5):780–2.

Percutaneous Biliary Intervention in Patients with Primary Sclerosing Cholangitis

15

Thor Johnson and Janette D. Durham

Indications for Percutaneous Intervention

Diagnosis of PSC

Percutaneous transhepatic cholangiography (PTC) for the purpose of diagnosis is reserved for patients in whom MRC followed by second-line ERC is inadequate to assess cholangiographic anatomy or to demonstrate a suspected dominant stricture. Recent improvements in both technologies make this necessity increasingly uncommon. Both techniques have sensitivities for PSC diagnosis in the 80 % range [1]. ERC failure occurs for multiple reasons including unfavorable postoperative anatomy, inability to access the bile duct due to anatomic variation, and severe, diffuse intra- and extrahepatic biliary disease. Assessment for posttransplant PSC recurrence in patients with a biliary enteric anastomosis is one example where ERC may fail and PTC is pursued.

T. Johnson, MD (✉) • J.D. Durham, MD
Division of Interventional Radiology,
University of Colorado School of Medicine,
Aurora, CO, USA
e-mail: Thor.johnson@ucdenver.edu;
Janette.durham@ucdenver.edu

Treatment of Cholangitis Refractory to Medical or Endoscopic Therapy

Controlling infection, stone disease, and abscess helps manage the clinical course of PSC patients. Dominant strictures occur in 45–70 % of PSC patients referred for endoscopy [2–5]. Strictures provide an unclear contribution to the development of cholestasis, the fluctuation of symptoms, and the development of liver fibrosis [5]; however, dilation of dominate strictures in noncirrhotic patients leads to biochemical and symptomatic improvement in most reports. Drainage of one or multiple liver segments along with antimicrobial therapy is appropriate to treat cholangitis. When endoscopy fails to control severe symptoms of cholestasis or refractory cholangitis, percutaneous transhepatic drainage (PTD) and stricture dilation are appropriate. Transhepatic access may be utilized for choledochoscopy with or without electrohydraulic lithotripsy to fragment intraductal stones. Small abscesses may respond to biliary drainage combined with medical therapy; otherwise, percutaneous drainage is pursued.

Diagnosis and Palliation of Biliary Obstruction in Patients with CCA

Dominant strictures are associated with reduced mean survival, 13.7 years compared to 23 years without dominant strictures, primarily due to

L.M. Forman (ed.), *Primary Sclerosing Cholangitis*, DOI 10.1007/978-3-319-40908-5_15

underlying CCA [4]. The 10-year cumulative incidence of cancer is 6–11 % and the 30-year incidence is 20 % [6]. Evaluation of strictures with fluoroscopically guided cytological sampling and forceps biopsy is therefore important for early detection of cancer. When endoscopic and/or percutaneous approaches are unsuccessful, a combined approach with visualized endoscopic biopsy via a transhepatic access may be useful and more sensitive for diagnosis.

PTD is performed in PSC patients with CCA to relieve biliary obstruction and control symptoms either as a pretransplant strategy or as a palliative therapy. In patients who develop CCA, prior intervention with external drains may increase the incidence of peritoneal seeding, although this has not been demonstrated [7]. As a result, percutaneous biopsy and/or percutaneous drainage are considered contraindications to liver transplantation in some centers. PTD is frequently performed as a preoperative intervention prior to resection in non-PSC patients who develop CCA, with some attention paid to limiting the duration of drainage prior to surgery. Drain placement not only improves symptoms and helps control infection, but in-place drains for some surgeons may facilitate biliary anastomosis creation.

Procedural Description

Percutaneous Transhepatic Cholangiography

The non-dilated bile ducts in PSC patients make percutaneous access challenging and limit the utility of ultrasound for guidance. Procedures are often prolonged and painful with multiple needle punctures necessary to access small ducts. General anesthesia for the initial procedure is helpful for both patient comfort and to ensure patient breathing cooperation when a small duct is eventually opacified and subsequently needs to be catheterized.

Preoperative antibiotics should be administered an hour before the procedure, unless the patient presents with cholangitis, in which case antibiotics should be started 24 h prior. If cholangitis is not part of the presentation, a single dose of antibiotics is sufficient. Antibiotics should be chosen to cover gram-negative and enteric bacteria, and if possible an antibiotic with biliary excretion is preferred. Coagulation parameters should be corrected as close to normal as possible, with platelet count greater than 50,000 per uL. All heparin (unfractionated and low molecular weight) should be discontinued prior to the procedure and withheld for 12–48 h depending on the complexity of the procedure and whether drainage is performed.

Axial imaging with CT or MRI is evaluated to determine the optimum segment to enter for upstream access to a stricture or to optimize drainage. Ultrasound imaging is inadequate for evaluation, as careful assessment of ducts of each liver segment is required. Cholangiography is performed in multiple obliquities to allow complete assessment of ducts with 300 mg or less iodinated contrast so as not to obscure stones. With the patient supine, there is the tendency to underfill the anterior right and left biliary ducts. If the procedure is performed on a side-tilting gantry, the patient can be positioned to facilitate anterior filling; otherwise, complete cholangiography may require inflation of a balloon in the extrahepatic duct, placed through a peripheral sheath that is then injected upstream. In patients presenting with cholangitis, this degree of intervention should be postponed for several days after a drain is placed, in order to permit initial duct decompression and to avoid sepsis from contrast/infected bile intravasation.

Percutaneous Transhepatic Drainage and Stricture Dilation

When cholangiographic findings confirm a stricture or stone, PTD is entertained. If possible, access is directed to a peripheral duct to optimize drainage of a large portion of the liver and prevent complications associated with central puncture. A two-stick procedure may be required, targeting first a more central, larger, first-order intrahepatic duct for cholangiography and then,

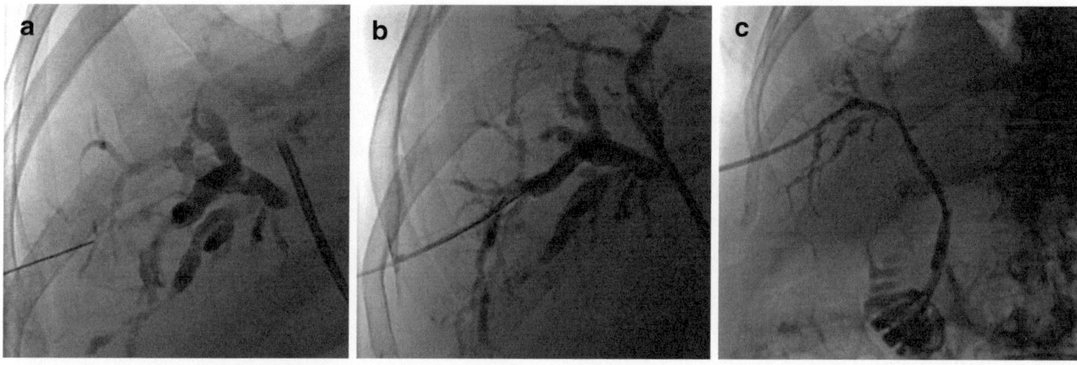

Fig. 15.1 (**a–c**) The typical steps of percutaneous transhepatic drainage. Needle passes are performed with injection of contrast until the biliary system is identified, often from access of a relatively central duct. A peripheral duct is then selected for puncture that will optimize drainage of multiple liver segments (**a**). An .018-in. torqueable guide wire is passed through the needle into the biliary system. This permits placement of a catheter that is used to advance a wire into the bowel (**b**). After serial dilation of the transhepatic tract and sometimes the ducts themselves, a percutaneous biliary drainage catheter is placed through the liver and into the small bowel (**c**)

once opacified, a second more peripheral duct for drainage.

The goal for the first drainage session is placement, at minimum, of a secure external drain, when internal-external drainage requires extensive intervention to negotiate diseased ducts. If a catheter cannot be passed into the bowel at initial tube placement, the patient returns at 2 days for conversion to internal-external drainage (Fig. 15.1a–c). Strictures are often easier to traverse after external drainage and biliary decompression. Drainage typically requires placement of 5–8 Fr. catheters. A transhepatic tract dictates drain placement for a minimum of several weeks in the face of biliary obstruction, to avoid cholangitis and/or sepsis, as well as bile leak.

After the tract matures, typically 2 weeks, dominant strictures are evaluated with both brush cytology including fluorescence in situ hybridization (FISH) and forceps biopsy under fluoroscopic guidance. When these results are negative but suspicion for cancer remains, transhepatic cholangioscopic evaluation is planned. Transhepatic fine-needle aspiration biopsy is no longer performed due to concern for peritoneal seeding and exclusion from future transplantation.

Balloon dilation of both dominant strictures and long intrahepatic strictures is then performed at 6-week intervals followed by biliary catheter exchange until symptoms improve. Unlike endoscopy where intervention is usually limited to hilar and extrahepatic duct strictures, peripheral strictures may be treated without additional morbidity, as many strictures in the opposite lobe reachable by contralateral access or adjacent lobe by ipsilateral access are dilated. Stricture dilation with long inflation times, utilizing high pressure (20 atm) balloons of 4–6 mm diameter intrahepatically or 10 mm at the hilum or extrahepatically, is followed by placement of an 8 Fr. internal-external drainage catheter. In patients with PSC, larger drains often obstruct downstream ducts, and serial drain enlargement, as is often employed when treating other benign strictures, is not appropriate. Three-month evaluation for drain removal is planned; clinical response in addition to stricture appearance dictates removal. Because most extrahepatic strictures are successfully managed with endoscopy, percutaneously placed metallic stents are not part of the treatment paradigm in PSC patients.

Post-procedurally, patients are admitted for pain control and treatment of cholangitis. Patients will have drain-related pain for 2–3 weeks that often requires oral narcotics. Management requires patient education and training, particularly in the first 6 weeks when pain may be severe and drain complications frequently arise.

Results

Percutaneous Transhepatic Cholangiography for PSC Diagnosis

Cholangiographic findings in PSC are not specific. The differential includes a long list of secondary causes of biliary inflammation and obstruction that result in similar bile duct abnormalities. Interpretation of cholangiography is therefore made in conjunction with the clinical presentation (most often in young and middle-aged serologically negative males with inflammatory bowel disease) of cholestasis (elevation of alkaline phosphatase and gamma-glutamyl transferase) without identification of secondary cause. Small duct PSC, a PSC variant, can have a similar clinical presentation but normal cholangiography.

MacCarty et al. described the cholangiographic findings in 86 patients with PSC in whom secondary causes of cholangitis were excluded and compared them to the cholangiographic findings in 82 patients with bile duct carcinoma and 16 patients with primary biliary cirrhosis (PBC) [8]. PSC was characterized by multifocal, short, annular strictures of both the intra- and extrahepatic bile ducts alternating with normal or slightly dilated segments to produce a "beaded" appearance. Confluent long strictures were found with advanced disease (Fig. 15.2). A specific finding, occurring in 27 % of patients, was diverticulum of the extrahepatic duct with or without associated band-like strictures. The lack of extrahepatic disease in PBC patients can differentiate PBC from PSC. Typical patient populations are also different as PBC is most likely to present in young to middle-aged female patients with positive serology (anti-mitochondrial antibody). Bile duct cancer in patients without PSC tended to be focal or multifocal at presentation.

Interpretation of cholangiograms requires a methodical segmental duct assessment. Isolated segmental or lobar ducts can be readily missed without careful assessment. Dominant strictures, defined by Stiehl et al., include an extrahepatic stricture of ≤ 1.5 mm in the common bile duct or ≤ 1.0 mm in the hepatic duct within 2 cm of the bifurcation [9].

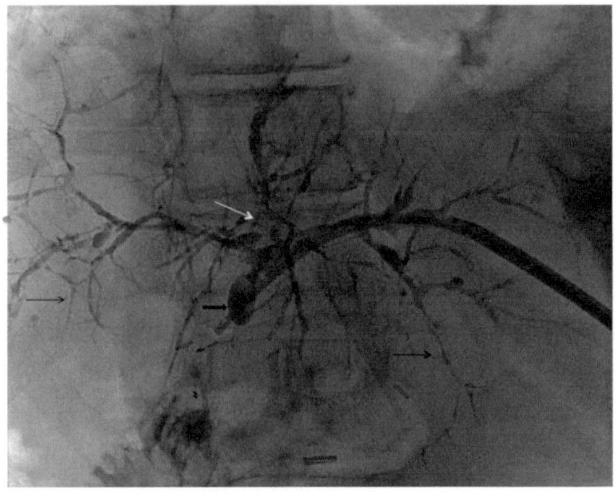

Fig. 15.2 A catheter placed into the left duct (segment 2) has been injected in a patient who has undergone prior hepatico-jejunostomy. Cholangiography demonstrates a typical appearance of severe PSC with multiple short strictures of the intrahepatic bile ducts that result in a "beaded" appearance (*thin black arrows*). Some strictures appear confluent (*white arrow*). Despite severe disease there is not significant biliary ductal dilation. All liver segments can be identified although abnormal, except for segment 8. The anastomosis is not well visualized on this image, but an extrahepatic diverticulum is suggested (*thick arrow*)

There are no definitive cholangiographic features of malignancy, although perihilar location for CCA is most common. The suspicion of cancer is increased with discovery on MRI/MRC of a new dominant stricture, focal bile duct thickening or irregularity, and venous phase enhancement of an associated mass [6]. Clinical signs include new evidence of biliary obstruction, worsening enzymes, and elevation of CA19-9 greater than 100 U/mL in the absence of cholangitis [6]. Early stricture recurrence after dilation is also a suggestive feature.

Percutaneous Transhepatic Drainage and Stricture Dilation

One of the first descriptions of PTD and stricture dilation in PSC patients by May et al. described an experience at the Mayo Clinic in 14 PSC patients with dominant strictures presenting with intractable pruritus and jaundice or recurrent episodes of bacterial cholangitis [10]. Access was transhepatic ($n=9$) or via T-tube ($n=5$). PTD was completed and followed, after 24–48 h, with stricture dilation utilizing short inflation times of less than one minute of 10 atm PTA balloons ranging in size from 5 to 8 mm for intrahepatic and 6–10 mm for extrahepatic strictures. Internal-external drainage catheters of 10–14 Fr. were placed. Strictures were dilated in all 14 patients. Treatment resulted in a decrease in the number of cholangitic episodes. In nine patients (64 %) with recent onset of jaundice (<6 months), a decrease in bilirubin was seen. PTD was complicated by bacteremia or cholangitis in 5 (36 %) patients. One-third of patients with symptomatic resolution initially had symptom and stricture recurrence at 6–18 months.

Skolkin et al. described attempted PTD and stricture dilation in 15 PSC patients, utilizing transhepatic access ($n=13$) or indwelling T-tubes ($n=2$) [11]. In all patients, alkaline phosphatase was three times normal, and ten of these patients had bilirubin elevation. Clinical indications included jaundice, pruritus, or a progressive rise in alkaline phosphatase and/or bilirubin. All patients had multifocal, intrahepatic strictures, and a majority also had confluence or extrahepatic strictures. Stricture dilation was performed serially with 4–10 mm PTA balloons with inflation pressures of 6–10 atm for 5 min. Five 14 Fr. internal-external drainage catheters were placed with exchange at 6–8 weeks for an average of 4.5 months. PTD was successful in 14 patients, 13 of which improved symptomatically. An average of 9 h in 3.7 sessions was required to accomplish these results. Five of 13 patients developed recurrence, four were retreated, and one underwent liver transplantation. A majority of patients demonstrated biochemical improvement or no change, after drain removal compared with before drain placement, with recurrent enzyme elevation after 10 months on average. Fever complicated all procedures. One patient experienced arterial bleeding secondary to a pseudoaneurysm. Escalation of care from complications occurred in 7 (47 %) patients. There were no deaths.

Following these early studies in PSC patients, endoscopic experience and technology improved elevating this approach over percutaneous intervention due to a better complication profile and improved tolerance without external drains. The infrequent presentation of PSC patients for percutaneous intervention has limited further reports, with most authors' experience combined in reports of benign strictures of all cause. Successful drain placement is thought to be lower for non-dilated ducts (70 % in non-dilated ducts compared to 95 % in dilated ducts) [12]. This gap in results appears to narrow with center experience.

Endoscopic interventions in multiple small series of PSC patients have been reported. Three series published since 2004 have included greater than 100 patients describing experiences collected over 20 years [2–4]. The endoscopic approach has evolved to include dilation of symptomatic extrahepatic and central right and left intrahepatic strictures with short if any course of internal drainage to follow, usually only in patients with cholangitis. All these reports are non-randomized and most retrospective. Symptomatic and biochemical improvement has been demonstrated [2, 4, 13], as well as improved survival and survival free of transplantation, when compared to predictive models [3, 9, 13, 14].

The series by Chapman et al. is the only report to describe a group of patients who failed endoscopy and required percutaneous therapy, despite the fact that endoscopic failures are likely part of most experiences [4]. In this retrospective series of 128 PSC patients followed for a mean period of 9.8 years, 20 % underwent transhepatic access procedures (a total of 37 cases). In the group of patients undergoing PTD, dominant strictures were present in 81 % and CCA with complex strictures in 43 %, compared to an overall incidence in their report of dominant strictures in 63 % and CCA in 16 %. Fifteen percent of patients in the percutaneous intervention group had stone disease approached by combined procedures utilizing lithotripsy. This data suggest that patients requiring transhepatic therapy are a selected population with advanced disease and particularly poor survival as a result of a high incidence of dominant strictures related to CCA. So although symptomatic and biochemical improvement following transhepatic intervention is thought to mirror endoscopic results, the severity of disease in patients referred for percutaneous intervention likely confounds outcome comparison between methods.

Our experience includes a subset of patients referred for PTD in their last months before transplantation. We reviewed a small series of ten patients listed for transplantation and referred for transhepatic drainage after failed endoscopy for acute cholangitis ($n=6$) or worsening jaundice ($n=4$), with a mean bilirubin at presentation of 20 mg/dL (5.5–38.7 mg dL) [15]. Seven of ten patients free of CCA had biopsy-proven cirrhosis. This represented 12 % of the PSC patients evaluated for orthotropic liver transplantation at the University of Colorado between July 1991 and June 1998. Intrahepatic disease was severe in most patients and extrahepatic or hilar disease was present in all. Two patients presented with stone disease.

Internal-external drainage was successful in nine patients, one with endoscopic assistance. External drainage only was purposely completed in one patient with fungal cholangitis. Drains were left in place until transplantation (mean 186 days; range 13 to 385 days), with multiple subsequent procedures for anticipated and unanticipated drain exchange. Eight patients demonstrated modest biochemical improvement. Two patients were hospitalized with fungal sepsis until transplant, eight were discharged of which six were transplanted during follow-up, and two remained listed. Complications occurred in four patients (40 %) including severe pancreatitis requiring a 6-day hospitalization, fever and mild pancreatitis, a portobiliary fistula treated conservatively with drain manipulation, and a small biloma that did not require drainage. There were no complications that affected liver transplant status. These data support an infrequent role for PTD in end-stage PSC patients with cirrhosis to control symptoms and infection, while awaiting transplantation.

Complications and Management

Complications of percutaneous intervention vary with indication, and as yet there is very little PSC-specific literature for PTD. Major complications (8–10 %) described following biliary drainage for all indications include sepsis (2.5 %), hemorrhage (2.5 %), inflammatory/infections (abscess, peritonitis, cholecystitis, pancreatitis) (1.2 %), pleural including pneumothorax or bile leak (.5 %), and death (1.7 %) [12]. Minor complications include tube-related pain and drain migration or occlusion.

Postprocedural pain related to intercostal drain placement can last for several weeks despite nerve blocks and oral narcotics. If the percutaneous tract is too near the undersurface of a rib, pain may not resolve without tube reposition or intercostal nerve blocks. Rarely a drain requires replacement to a more favorable position. Biliary drains require exchange at 6–8 week intervals to preserve patency. Once the drain tract matures, this is a relatively painless procedure, often done without sedation. Despite routine administration of antibiotics for all procedures, periprocedural cholangitis is frequent. Although bile cultures are often positive in PSC patient who have had no prior biliary intervention, colonization of the biliary tree from obstructed indwelling internal stents or internal-external drains has decreased enthusiasm for long-term drain placement. So as not to compromise transplant, the duration of drain placement should be minimized and if possible the drains removed prior to transplantation. Choledochojejunocutaneous fistula creation (Hutson loop) to permit repeat percutaneous dilation without need for drain placement had some initial appeal but has become unpopular with the increasing role of transplantation and the increased complexity introduced by prior surgery. Hutson loops are still sometimes performed in the management of recurrent pyogenic cholangitis [16, 17].

Transgression of an arterial branch can lead to hemobilia that most often is treated with percutaneous embolization. Transgression of a venous branch generally is self-limited and managed with tube repositioning to tamponade bleeding. In PSC populations, intrahepatic duct rupture following dilation (a complication rarely described) may be seen after balloon dilation and may cause bleeding. Planned placement of a drain across the stricture is usually sufficient for control of bile leak and for tamponade of bleeding.

Bile leak most commonly is the result of placement of a "too high" (cephalad) right-sided intercostal drain that crosses the pleural space. A second percutaneous drain to divert bile may be required before the offending drain can be removed. Tract embolization with bile diversion permits healing, while pleural collections are controlled with drainage.

Although not studied in matched populations, ERCP appears to have a lower complication rate than percutaneous therapy [18]. Complication rates in retrospective reports of endoscopic interventions have varied from 1 to 20 %, improving with experience [2, 4, 9, 14]. Serial procedures are better tolerated without the need for indwelling external drains. Hospitalization following PTD is also avoided. While endoscopy does require deep sedation or general anesthesia at every procedure, after initial drainage, percutaneous intervention requires either no or mild sedation.

Conclusion

Although increasingly infrequent, percutaneous intervention in patients with PSC may be required when patients are unsuitable for endoscopic intervention. PTC, although more technically difficult than in malignant obstruction with a dilated biliary tree, has similar results in providing diagnostic cholangiographic detail to diagnosis PSC and define dominant strictures. PTD generally follows all intervention aside from the rare instance when the procedure is limited to PTC. Stricture brushing and biopsy may be used to confirm cancer. Dilation and drainage improve biochemical patterns, symptoms, and cholangitis similarly to an endoscopic approach with a higher complication profile, including drain-related pain. Patient referral after failed endoscopy selects a population of end-stage patients with dominant strictures and frequent CCA impacting survival.

References

1. Aljiffry M, Renfrew PD, Walsh MJ, et al. Analytical review of diagnosis and treatment strategies for dominant bile duct strictures in patients with primary sclerosing cholangitis. HPB (Oxford). 2011;13(2):79–90.
2. Gotthardt DN, Rudolph G, Klöters-Plachky P, et al. Endoscopic dilation of dominant stenoses in primary sclerosing cholangitis: outcome after long-term treatment. Gastrointest Endosc. 2010;71(3):527–34.
3. Gluck M, Cantone NR, Brandabur JJ, et al. A twenty-year experience with endoscopic therapy for symptomatic primary sclerosing cholangitis. J Clin Gastroenterol. 2008;42(9):1032–9.
4. Chapman MH, Webster GJ, Bannoo S, et al. Cholangiocarcinoma and dominant strictures in patients with primary sclerosing cholangitis: a 25-year single-center experience. Eur J Gastroenterol Hepatol. 2012;24(9):1051–8.
5. Björnsson E, Lindqvist-Ottosson J, Asztely M, et al. Dominant strictures in patients with primary sclerosing cholangitis. Am J Gastroenterol. 2004;99(3):502–8.
6. Rizvi S, Eaton JE, Gores GJ. Primary sclerosing cholangitis as a premalignant biliary tract disease: surveillance and management. Clin Gastroenterol Hepatol. 2015;13(12):2152–65.
7. Darwish Murad S, Kim WR, Therneau T, et al. Predictors of pretransplant dropout and posttransplant recurrence in patients with perihilar cholangiocarcinoma. Hepatology. 2012;56(3):972–81.
8. MacCarty RL, LaRusso NF, Wiesner RH, et al. Primary sclerosing cholangitis: findings on cholangiography and pancreatography. Radiology. 1983;149(1):39–44.
9. Stiehl A, Rudolph G, Klöters-Plachky P, et al. Development of dominant bile duct stenoses in patients with primary sclerosing cholangitis treated with ursodeoxycholic acid: outcome after endoscopic treatment. J Hepatol. 2002;36(2):151–6.
10. May GR, Bender CE, LaRusso NF, et al. Nonoperative dilatation of dominant strictures in primary sclerosing cholangitis. AJR Am J Roentgenol. 1985;145(5):1061–4.
11. Skolkin MD, Alspaugh JP, Casarella WJ, et al. Sclerosing cholangitis: palliation with percutaneous cholangioplasty. Radiology. 1989;170:199–206.
12. Saad WE, Wallace MJ, Wojak JC, et al. Quality improvement guidelines for percutaneous transhepatic cholangiography, biliary drainage, and percutaneous cholecystostomy. J Vasc Interv Radiol. 2010;21:789–95.
13. Ponsioen CY, Lam K, van Milligen de Wit AW, et al. Four years experience with short term stenting in primary sclerosing cholangitis. Am J Gastroenterol. 1999;94(9):2403–7.
14. Baluyut AR, Sherman S, Lehman GA, et al. Impact of endoscopic therapy on the survival of patients with primary sclerosing cholangitis. Gastrointest Endosc. 2001;53(3):308–12.
15. Cahalan D, Shrestha R, Kumpe D, et al. Results of percutaneous biliary drainage in patients with severe primary sclerosing cholangitis. Paper presented at the Society of Cardiovascular and Interventional Radiology Annual Meeting, Orlando, March 1999.
16. Wigdan A, Gallinger S, Pratzer A, et al. Recurrent pyogenic cholangitis with hepatolithiasis – the role of surgical therapy in North America. J Gastro Surg. 2008;12(3):496–503.

17. Fontein DB, Gibson RN, Collier NA, et al. Two decades of percutaneous transjejunal biliary intervention for benign biliary disease: a review of the intervention nature and complications. Insights Imaging. 2011;2(5):557–65.
18. Alkhatib AA, Hilden K, Adler DG. Comorbidities, sphincterotomy, and balloon dilation predict post-ERCP adverse events in PSC patients: operator experience is protective. Dig Dis Sci. 2011;56(12):3685–8.

Liver Transplantation for PSC

16

Kendra Conzen and Trevor L. Nydam

Liver transplantation is widely accepted as the definitive treatment for patients with end-stage liver disease secondary to cirrhosis. Primary sclerosing cholangitis (PSC) is a chronic immune-mediated inflammatory disease of the intrahepatic and extrahepatic bile ducts which leads to cholestasis, fibrotic strictures, and duct obliteration. PSC eventually results in cirrhosis in more than half of affected individuals. Therapeutic options are limited. Medical management, endoscopic interventions, and surgical resection of biliary strictures are not curative and have little impact on disease progression. A majority of persons who do not undergo liver transplantation ultimately die from liver failure due to biliary cirrhosis or from hepatobiliary cancer [1–5]. Cholestatic liver disease is the primary etiology of ESLD in 8.2 % of liver transplant recipients [6]. Median survival of patients with PSC ranges from 10 to 21 years from time of diagnosis until liver transplant or death [1, 3, 4, 7–10]. This chapter will discuss indications for liver transplant in PSC, pretransplant evaluation, intraoperative technique, and postoperative outcomes.

K. Conzen, MD • T.L. Nydam, MD (✉)
Division of Transplant Surgery, Department of Surgery, University of Colorado School of Medicine, Aurora, CO, USA
e-mail: trevor.nydam@ucdenver.edu

Indications

Indications for liver transplantation in the setting of PSC include decompensated cirrhosis, recurrent cholangitis, refractory pruritus, and early-stage malignancy not amenable to resection (intrahepatic hepatocellular carcinoma or hilar cholangiocarcinoma) [11]. In many cases, ongoing biliary inflammation, fibrosis, and developing strictures progress to cirrhosis. One-quarter of PSC patients have cirrhosis at time of diagnosis, though less than 4 % present with clinical symptoms of portal hypertension [1, 3]. Presence of ascites or varices at diagnosis is associated with a higher rate of disease progression in the first 5 years [1]. Similar to other forms of chronic liver disease, the presence of complicated cirrhosis warrants evaluation for transplantation.

Recurrent cholangitis is an all too common complication of ongoing PSC and represents an indication for transplantation not found in other chronic liver disease. Again, ongoing biliary inflammation and fibrosis lead to strictures and relative biliary obstruction resulting in recurrent bacterial cholangitis. Frequent hospital admissions and endoscopic interventions lead to a state of chronic illness and poor quality of life. While this morbidity associated with recurrent cholangitis is significant, it does not appear to lead to increased mortality on the waitlist and does not contribute to the patients' MELD score [12]. This and the scarcity of standard-criteria cadaveric grafts make the practice of petitioning for MELD

L.M. Forman (ed.), *Primary Sclerosing Cholangitis*, DOI 10.1007/978-3-319-40908-5_16

exception points a continued debate. For this reason, live donor liver transplantation (LDLT) has proven to be a reliable and attractive option for these patients.

Severe, refractory pruritus can be profoundly morbid condition that can cause suicidal ideation and chronic cutaneous excoriations. With these associated conditions, liver transplantation should be considered albeit with the same waitlist and allocation limitations.

The lifetime risk of cholangiocarcinoma (CCA) is 10–15 % in PSC patients, more than one-quarter of which present within 1 year of the initial PSC diagnosis [1–5, 8, 10, 13]. In a select group of patients, CCA is an accepted indication for transplantation with good outcomes. A patient with small, localized, hilar CCA can be transplanted within a rigorous protocol of neoadjuvant chemoradiation and aggressive staging. Tumors that do not fit within this strict protocol are considered contraindications to transplantation with cadaveric grafts.

Recipient Evaluation

General criteria for evaluating PSC patients for liver transplantation are similar to criteria for non-PSC patients. This should include a thorough history and physical examination to identify any comorbid medical conditions that are contraindications to transplantation. Although surgical management of extrahepatic bile duct strictures is rare in the setting of PSC, prior biliary surgery for any indication can complicate the liver transplant operation [14]. Cholangiography is the preferred diagnostic intervention for PSC with characteristic findings of segmental bile duct strictures with focal dilations (beading) and mural irregularities of intra- and extrahepatic bile ducts. Liver biopsy may be useful in identifying individuals with small-duct variant of PSC but is not recommended for routine evaluation because PSC does not uniformly affect the liver and a high probability for sampling error exists [15]. Ancillary testing includes laboratory testing, abdominal imaging to evaluate for hepatobiliary masses and assess patency of hepatic vessels, cardiopulmonary testing, bone density assessment, and age-appropriate routine cancer screening (colonoscopy, mammography, Pap smear, PSA level), including tumor markers (CA 19–9 and CEA). Inflammatory bowel disease (IBD) is present in 60–80 % of PSC patients, and PSC patients have a tenfold increased risk of colorectal adenocarcinoma, underscoring the importance of surveillance colonoscopy and IBD management in patients being considered for transplantation [2, 4, 11, 16–19]. A significant subset of PSC patients (approximately 14 %) has other immune-mediated inflammatory or autoimmune disease, which is associated with lower rates of transplant-free survival [20].

Graft Allocation

Priority on the waitlist for liver transplantation is currently determined by the Model for End-Stage Liver Disease (MELD) score. The MELD score, implemented in 2002 and revised in January 2016, is a formula used to predict 90-day mortality. It is calculated from serum bilirubin, creatinine, INR, and sodium values. As mentioned previously, for PSC patients the MELD system has several limitations. Patients with severe, intractable pruritus or recurrent cholangitis commonly have low INR and creatinine levels, thereby limiting the ability of the MELD score to accurately reflect the severity of disease symptoms and ongoing morbidity [21]. Quality of life can be disproportionately poor in patients with low MELD [22]. MELD also fails to predict the progression of PSC.

Additional MELD points (MELD "exception" points) may be granted to patients with conditions that are not accurately reflected in the MELD calculation, such as a documented history of recurrent cholangitis. It was previously believed that patients with recurrent cholangitis were at increased risk for severe complications, including increased mortality. However, recent analysis of UNOS data suggests that PSC patients with recurrent cholangitis do not suffer higher rates of death and actually have lower waitlist mortality compared to non-PSC patients [12, 21].

Additionally, removal for deterioration in condition is equivalent between PSC and non-PSC groups [21]. In 2006, a consensus conference attempted to narrow upgrade criteria to recurrent bacteremia or sepsis secondary to PSC [23]. Yet, in most regions the petitions continue to be reviewed in a nonstandardized fashion, and a majority of patients are approved with limited symptoms or complications of bacterial cholangitis. Due to minimal comorbid conditions, these patients continue to be transplanted at a high rate [24].

Development of an early-stage primary liver cancer warrants a request for a standardized MELD exception. Liver transplantation offers more than 80 % cure rate for early-stage hepatocellular carcinoma (HCC). Patients with HCC tumors who meet Milan criteria (1 tumor <5 cm or 2–3 tumors each less than 3 cm in diameter) are eligible and have maximal anticipated benefit [25]. As mentioned prior, CCA disproportionately affects patients with PSC, and transplantation for CCA has not yet achieved the high cure rates seen with HCC. Yet, highly specialized treatment protocols such as that published by the Mayo Clinic have improved survival in patients with localized, early-stage, hilar CCA [26]. Pretransplant management includes neoadjuvant chemoradiation, assessment of disease progression (tumor size and vascular invasion) with cross-sectional imaging, lymph node sampling with endoscopic ultrasound, and surgical exploration prior to proceeding with transplantation. The attrition rate is significant, leading to a very selective group of patients, but overall survival is good in multiple high-volume centers [27]. Recurrence of CCA post-liver transplant is high, and only select patients with isolated, hilar CCA, <3 cm, who have completed the protocol with neoadjuvant chemoradiation and aggressive staging should be considered [11, 26].

Donor Selection

The waitlist for a graft from a standard donor after brain death (DBD) has become increasingly competitive, with an average MELD score above 30 at time of transplant and wait times greater than 2 years in some regions in the United States [6]. As described above, disease and symptom severity is poorly reflected in the MELD score, and wait times for PSC patients are long. To reduce time to transplantation, PSC patients and transplant surgeons must consider nonstandard donor livers, specifically allografts from donors after cardiac death (DCD), public health service (PHS)-increased risk donors, extended criteria donors (e.g., older donor age), and living donors. The advantages of reducing wait time for transplant in an attempt to reduce waitlist mortality are not without consequence. A retrospective analysis of UNOS data comparing use of DCD vs. DBD livers in PSC patients revealed a significantly increased risk of graft loss in the DCD allograft recipients (hazard ratio 2.4) [28]. The use of DCD livers may disproportionately affect outcomes in PSC patients compared to non-PSC recipients. Specifically, a higher rate of graft loss due to biliary complications has been reported [28]. New protocols for administration of intraoperative hepatic artery thrombolytics with improvement in biliary outcomes in DCD allografts have recently been published, but it remains to be seen if these benefits are realized in the PSC recipient subgroup [29].

PSC patients are more likely to be transplanted with allografts from living donors than are non-PSC patients [30]. Outcomes in LDLT for PSC are better than LDLT done for other chronic liver diseases [31]. When considering live donor options, one must be aware of the potential presence of undiagnosed PSC in family members of recipients. A genetic predisposition exists, with a 100-fold increased risk in first-degree relatives. PSC prevalence is 0.7 % among all first-degree relatives of patients with PSC and 1.5 % among siblings [32]. Certain HLA alleles (B8, DRB1*03, DRB1*13) and other genes have been implicated in the pathogenesis of PSC, but no diagnostic assay exists for which to screen potential donors [33]. Therefore, any family members undergoing donor evaluation should have laboratory testing (including serum bilirubin, AST, ALT, alkaline phosphatase, GGT), cross-sectional imaging (CT or MRI), cholangiography (MR or endoscopic), and possible liver biopsy. A history of inflammatory bowel disease in a potential donor, while not an absolute contraindication, should encourage one to proceed cautiously.

The Operation

Preparation of the patient in the operating room is similar to that of patients being transplanted for other indications. General anesthesia is administered by an experienced liver transplant anesthesiologist. Adequate venous access for large-volume resuscitation is established, and hemodynamic monitors are placed (e.g., intra-arterial blood pressure catheters, transesophageal echocardiography probe or Swan-Ganz catheter, continuous pulse oximetry). Antibiotic selection and duration in the perioperative period should take into consideration a history of cholangitis in the recipient.

Intraoperatively, many of the technical considerations for the native hepatectomy and vascular reconstruction of the donor liver are the same as for other recipient subgroups. The technical aspect of greatest contention is that of restoration of biliary continuity to the allograft. For most non-PSC recipients, the preferred method is creation of an end-to-end choledochocholedochostomy, or duct-to-duct, anastomosis. Historically, this was not used in PSC patients due to concerns about the risk of residual disease in the extrahepatic bile duct. Reconstruction to the recipient duct was believed to increase the risk of anastomotic stricture and disease recurrence in the allograft. Therefore, Roux-en-Y choledochojejunostomy (RYCJ) was the preferred method for biliary reconstruction in PSC patients, even if there was no gross evidence of disease in the extrahepatic duct at time of surgery. However, RYCJ is not without morbidity. RYCJ configuration can lead to bacterial overgrowth of the biliary system and is significantly associated with an increased risk of ascending cholangitis, 25 % vs. 9 % in duct-to-duct patients within the first year after transplant [34–36]. In some studies, the risk of late development of non-anastomotic strictures is higher in the Roux-en-Y group, which may be related to recurrent inflammation from higher rates of cholangitis [35]. Diagnosis and management of biliary obstruction is more challenging with RYCJ because only the most skilled endoscopists can navigate the Roux limb, thus necessitating percutaneous transhepatic interventions. Anastomotic strictures in RYCJ are more likely to require surgical intervention to correct than strictures with duct-to-duct anatomy [37]. This may be due to difficulty with endoscopic access to Roux limbs. There is also a small, but known, risk of gastrointestinal bleeding from the jejunojejunostomy.

In light of these disadvantages, there has been a trend toward duct-to-duct biliary drainage in PSC patients without gross disease of the extrahepatic bile duct. Retrospective analyses of outcomes in recipients with duct to duct are promising. A recent meta-analysis found no difference in rates of biliary strictures (anastomotic or non-anastomotic), biliary leaks, PSC recurrence, 1-year graft survival, or risk of cholangiocarcinoma [36]. Duct-to-duct anastomosis is associated with reduced risk of late non-anastomotic strictures and reduced risk of cholangitis [35]. Al-Judaibi and Sutton found no difference in biliary stricture or leak rates when duct to duct was performed in patients with grossly normal extrahepatic bile ducts, but did report that postoperative cholangiography is used more frequently in duct to duct [35, 38, 39]. It should be realized that, unless a pancreaticoduodenectomy is performed at time of transplant, the most distal aspect of the common bile duct remains in situ, regardless of the method selected for biliary reconstruction. Posttransplant occurrence of de novo cholangiocarcinoma in the extrahepatic duct remnant is rare, ranging from 0 % in some series to a few isolated case reports [35, 40, 41]. Type of biliary duct reconstruction is not associated with development of de novo cancer in the remnant duct [41]. Long-term overall survival and graft survival between types of biliary reconstruction are comparable at 5 and 10 years [35, 37].

When considering duct-to-duct reconstruction in PSC patients, the surgeon should carefully evaluate preoperative imaging and intraoperative appearance of the recipient's extrahepatic duct. Normal radiographic appearance; negative cytologic bile duct brushings preoperatively; the absence of periductal inflammation, edema, or wall thickening in the operating room; and confirmed patency of distal duct with passage of a probe may be conducive to duct-to-duct reconstruction [35, 41]. If the recipient duct is not amenable to reconstruction, either due to concerns about disease involvement or size discrepancy, choledochoduodenostomy presents another option for biliary drainage of the allograft. It excludes the recipient's remnant duct, but maintains normal anatomic configuration of the GI tract, allowing for future endoscopic access. Early results are promising and do not demonstrate increased risk of leak, cholangitis, or strictures compared to standard RYCJ or duct-to-duct reconstruction [42, 43]. The success of this approach in the PSC subgroup of recipients is yet to be determined.

Posttransplant Outcomes

Overall posttransplant survival is higher for recipients with PSC than for those with alcohol- or viral hepatitis-related cirrhosis. Graft and overall patient survival exceeds 80 % at 5 years, and earlier reports indicated no significant difference between recipients of living or deceased donor allografts [44, 45]. Analysis of UNOS data reveals a 95.4 % 5-year patient survival for LDLT in PSC patients (vs. 87.5 % for DDLT, ns) [45]. Five-year graft survival for LDLT is 87.1 % vs. 79.2 % for DDLT, not significantly different [45]. However, a multivariate analysis controlling for MELD score suggests that risk of graft or life loss with LDLT for PSC patients is significantly less compared to DDLT for low MELD patients (mean MELD <20) [31]. The rate of re-transplant is the same in PSC for LDLT versus DDLT [45].

Patients transplanted for PSC are at risk for all the posttransplant complications associated with other indications including hepatic artery thrombosis, venous inflow and outflow obstruction, anastomotic stricture, viral infection, acute and chronic rejection, and ischemic cholangiopathy. These posttransplant complications need to be ruled out prior to assigning the diagnosis of recurrent PSC to the patient with posttransplant cholangitis, bile duct changes, or graft dysfunction. However, PSC does recur following transplant in an estimated 10–35 % of patients and is amenable to medical and endoscopic treatments previously described for primary disease including re-transplantation [46].

It is believed that patients transplanted for PSC are at higher risks for acute cellular rejection (ACR) than patients transplanted for other indications [47]. Yet, these early studies were mostly done when the immunosuppression regimen consisted of cyclosporine and azathioprine. The current immunosuppression regimen typically consists of a perioperative steroid taper with a calcineurin inhibitor and mycophenolate mofetil combination for long-term maintenance. While it remains unclear if ACR rates are significantly different, this combination is associated with higher rates of posttransplant IBD. Therefore, in a patient with recurrent flares, a combination that again includes azathioprine should be considered [48].

Incidental or undiagnosed CCA occurs with high frequency. It is estimated that up to 29 % of pathology specimens from PSC patients who die or undergo liver transplant contain CCA [1]. Recurrence after transplant is relatively uncommon in these patients where incidental tumors are found on explant pathology. As described previously, patients with known hilar CCA who undergo neoadjuvant chemoradiation with aggressive staging at a high-volume center can expect a 65 % recurrence-free survival at 5-year posttransplant [27]. Again, this is a highly selective group of patients, but these outcomes are good relative to those expected with resection of CCA.

Posttransplant Quality of Life

Liver transplant successfully cures most PSC patients of their preoperative symptoms. Pruritus, jaundice, and fatigue resolve and overall subjective health status improves [49, 50]. Health-related quality of life questionnaires demonstrate good posttransplant functional status, equivalent to or better than recipients of liver transplant for other etiologies [51, 52]. Additionally, PSC patients have a higher rate of return to work than other groups [52].

Conclusion

Liver transplantation is currently the only curative therapy for primary sclerosing cholangitis and is associated with excellent overall survival and improved quality of life. Living donor and nonstandard deceased donor allografts may reduce waitlist time for PSC patients with severe disease symptoms and low MELD scores. Biliary reconstruction of the allograft with the recipient's native bile duct should be considered. Transplantation as treatment for hilar cholangiocarcinoma may offer a significant survival benefit in a select group of patients with good response to neoadjuvant chemoradiation. Thorough evaluation of posttransplant complications is necessary to distinguish recurrent PSC or acute cellular rejection from other causes of allograft dysfunction.

References

1. Broome U et al. Natural history and prognostic factors in 305 Swedish patients with primary sclerosing cholangitis. Gut. 1996;38(4):610–5.
2. Bergquist A et al. Hepatic and extrahepatic malignancies in primary sclerosing cholangitis. J Hepatol. 2002;36(3):321–7.
3. Tischendorf JJ et al. Characterization, outcome, and prognosis in 273 patients with primary sclerosing cholangitis: a single center study. Am J Gastroenterol. 2007;102(1):107–14.
4. Boonstra K et al. Population-based epidemiology, malignancy risk, and outcome of primary sclerosing cholangitis. Hepatology. 2013;58(6):2045–55.
5. Folseraas T, Boberg KM. Cancer risk and surveillance in primary sclerosing cholangitis. Clin Liver Dis. 2016;20(1):79–98.
6. Kim WR et al. Liver. Am J Transplant. 2016;16 Suppl 2:69–98.
7. Wiesner RH et al. Primary sclerosing cholangitis: natural history, prognostic factors and survival analysis. Hepatology. 1989;10(4):430–6.
8. Ponsioen CY et al. Natural history of primary sclerosing cholangitis and prognostic value of cholangiography in a Dutch population. Gut. 2002;51(4):562–6.
9. Bambha K et al. Incidence, clinical spectrum, and outcomes of primary sclerosing cholangitis in a United States community. Gastroenterology. 2003;125(5):1364–9.
10. Kingham JG et al. Incidence, clinical patterns, and outcomes of primary sclerosing cholangitis in South Wales, United Kingdom. Gastroenterology. 2004;126(7):1929–30.
11. Chapman R et al. Diagnosis and management of primary sclerosing cholangitis. Hepatology. 2010;51(2):660–78.
12. Goldberg DS et al. Risk of waitlist mortality in patients with primary sclerosing cholangitis and bacterial cholangitis. Liver Transpl. 2013;19(3):250–8.
13. Khaderi SA, Sussman NL. Screening for malignancy in primary sclerosing cholangitis (PSC). Curr Gastroenterol Rep. 2015;17(4):17.
14. Tsai S, Pawlik TM. Primary sclerosing cholangitis: the role of extrahepatic biliary resection. Adv Surg. 2009;43:175–88.
15. Karlsen TH et al. Primary sclerosing cholangitis. Best Pract Res Clin Gastroenterol. 2010;24(5):655–66.
16. Soetikno RM et al. Increased risk of colorectal neoplasia in patients with primary sclerosing cholangitis and ulcerative colitis: a meta-analysis. Gastrointest Endosc. 2002;56(1):48–54.
17. European Association for the Study of the Liver. EASL Clinical Practice Guidelines: management of cholestatic liver diseases. J Hepatol. 2009;51(2):237–67.
18. Singh S et al. Incidence of colorectal cancer after liver transplantation for primary sclerosing cholangitis: a systematic review and meta-analysis. Liver Transpl. 2013;19(12):1361–9.
19. Singh S et al. Inflammatory bowel disease after liver transplantation for primary sclerosing cholangitis. Am J Gastroenterol. 2013;108(9):1417–25.
20. Rupp C et al. Non-IBD immunological diseases are a risk factor for reduced survival in PSC. Liver Int. 2013;33(1):86–93.
21. Goldberg D et al. Waitlist survival of patients with primary sclerosing cholangitis in the model for end-stage liver disease era. Liver Transpl. 2011;17(11):1355–63.
22. de Vries EM et al. Biomarkers for disease progression of primary sclerosing cholangitis. Curr Opin Gastroenterol. 2015;31(3):239–46.
23. Freeman RB et al. Waiting list removal rates among patients with chronic and malignant liver diseases. Am J Transplant. 2006;6(6):1416–21.
24. Goldberg D et al. Lack of standardization in exception points for patients with primary sclerosing cholangitis and bacterial cholangitis. Am J Transplant. 2012;12(6):1603–9.
25. Mazzaferro V et al. Liver transplantation for the treatment of small hepatocellular carcinomas in patients with cirrhosis. N Engl J Med. 1996;334(11):693–9.

26. Rea DJ et al. Liver transplantation with neoadjuvant chemoradiation is more effective than resection for hilar cholangiocarcinoma. Ann Surg. 2005;242(3):451–8; discussion 458–61.
27. Darwish Murad S, et al Efficacy of neoadjuvant chemoradiation, followed by liver transplantation, for perihilar cholangiocarcinoma at 12 US centers. Gastroenterology. 2012a;143(1):88–98.e83; quiz e14.
28. Sundaram V et al. Donation after cardiac death liver transplantation in primary sclerosing cholangitis: proceed with caution. Transplantation. 2015;99(5):973–8.
29. Seal JB et al. Thrombolytic protocol minimizes ischemic-type biliary complications in liver transplantation from donation after circulatory death donors. Liver Transpl. 2015;21(3):321–8.
30. Goldberg DS et al. Current trends in living donor liver transplantation for primary sclerosing cholangitis. Transplantation. 2011;91(10):1148–52.
31. Goldberg DS et al. Superior survival using living donors and donor-recipient matching using a novel living donor risk index. Hepatology. 2014;60(5):1717–26.
32. Bergquist A et al. Increased prevalence of primary sclerosing cholangitis among first-degree relatives. J Hepatol. 2005;42(2):252–6.
33. Karlsen TH et al. Genome-wide association analysis in primary sclerosing cholangitis. Gastroenterology. 2010;138(3):1102–11.
34. Aberg F et al. Infectious complications more than 1 year after liver transplantation: a 3-decade nationwide experience. Am J Transplant. 2011;11(2):287–95.
35. Sutton ME et al. Duct-to-duct reconstruction in liver transplantation for primary sclerosing cholangitis is associated with fewer biliary complications in comparison with hepaticojejunostomy. Liver Transpl. 2014;20(4):457–63.
36. Pandanaboyana S et al. Meta-analysis of Duct-to-duct versus Roux-en-Y biliary reconstruction following liver transplantation for primary sclerosing cholangitis. Transpl Int. 2015;28(4):485–91.
37. Damrah O et al. Duct-to-duct biliary reconstruction in orthotopic liver transplantation for primary sclerosing cholangitis: a viable and safe alternative. Transpl Int. 2012;25(1):64–8.
38. Wells MM et al. Roux-en-Y choledochojejunostomy versus duct-to-duct biliary anastomosis in liver transplantation for primary sclerosing cholangitis: a meta-analysis. Transplant Proc. 2013;45(6):2263–71.
39. Al-Judaibi B et al. Duct-to-Duct Biliary Anastomosis Yields Similar Outcomes to Roux-en-Y Hepaticojejunostomy in Liver Transplantation for Primary Sclerosing Cholangitis. Hepat Mon. 2015;15(5):e18811.
40. Landaverde C et al. De-novo cholangiocarcinoma in native common bile duct remnant following OLT for primary sclerosing cholangitis. Ann Hepatol. 2009;8(4):379–83.
41. Esfeh JM et al. Duct-to-duct biliary reconstruction in patients with primary sclerosing cholangitis undergoing liver transplantation. HPB (Oxford). 2011;13(9):651–5.
42. Bennet W et al. Choledochoduodenostomy is a safe alternative to Roux-en-Y choledochojejunostomy for biliary reconstruction in liver transplantation. World J Surg. 2009;33(5):1022–5.
43. Campsen J et al. Choledochoduodenostomy in pediatric liver transplantation. Pediatr Transplant. 2011;15(3):237–9.
44. Kashyap R et al. Comparative analysis of outcomes in living and deceased donor liver transplants for primary sclerosing cholangitis. J Gastrointest Surg. 2009;13(8):1480–6.
45. Kashyap R et al. Living donor and deceased donor liver transplantation for autoimmune and cholestatic liver diseases–an analysis of the UNOS database. J Gastrointest Surg. 2010;14(9):1362–9.
46. Graziadei IW et al. Recurrence of primary sclerosing cholangitis following liver transplantation. Hepatology. 1999;29(4):1050–6.
47. Kugelmas M et al. Different immunosuppressive regimens and recurrence of primary sclerosing cholangitis after liver transplantation. Liver Transpl. 2003;9(7):727–32.
48. Jorgensen KK et al. Immunosuppression after liver transplantation for primary sclerosing cholangitis influences activity of inflammatory bowel disease. Clin Gastroenterol Hepatol. 2013;11(5):517–23.
49. Gross CR et al. Quality of life before and after liver transplantation for cholestatic liver disease. Hepatology. 1999;29(2):356–64.
50. Saldeen K et al. Follow-up after liver transplantation for primary sclerosing cholangitis: effects on survival, quality of life, and colitis. Scand J Gastroenterol. 1999;34(5):535–40.
51. Ruppert K, et al. In a 12-year study, sustainability of quality of life benefits after liver transplantation varies with pretransplantation diagnosis. Gastroenterology. 2010;139(5):1619–29, 1629.e1611–1614.
52. Aberg F et al. Influence of liver-disease etiology on long-term quality of life and employment after liver transplantation. Clin Transplant. 2012;26(5):729–35.

Recurrent Primary Sclerosing Cholangitis After Liver Transplantation

17

James F. Trotter and Mark G. Swain

Primary sclerosing cholangitis (PSC) is a chronic liver disease that accounts for a relatively small fraction of liver transplant recipients. At our center, Baylor University Medical Center, 5 % of liver recipients have PSC, while at other centers the fraction may be as high as 15 % [17]. Nationally, the Scientific Registry of Transplant Recipients (SRTR) reported that 4 % of deceased-donor liver transplant (DDLT) patients were performed for PSC in 2014 [23]. Identical numbers are seen in Europe where 4 % of liver transplant recipients have PSC according to the European Liver Transplant Registry [1]. Although relatively small in number, PSC patients have some of the best outcomes after liver transplant. A relatively large fraction survives into the second decade after transplant for several reasons. First, advances in surgical techniques and immunosuppressive therapy have led to significant increases in long-term patient and graft survival over the past two decades. In fact, graft half-life has increased from 5.8 years in 1989 to 10.5 years in 1998, most of which has been realized by improved outcomes within the first year of transplant [32]. Another important factor is that PSC transplant recipients are typically younger than patients with other types of liver disease. Therefore, they have fewer comorbidities which could jeopardize the success of the transplant and a longer potential posttransplant lifespan compared to other recipients. Finally, as will be discussed, recurrent disease occurs in some patients, but graft failure after recurrence is relatively uncommon. This review will focus on the diagnosis, risk factors, and management of recurrent disease after liver transplant in PSC patients.

Recurrent Disease After Transplant

There are variable reported rates for recurrent PSC after liver transplantation, ranging from 2 to 40 %. This variation can be explained, in part, by four important general considerations regarding any type of recurrent disease in liver transplant recipients [36]. First, the diagnostic accuracy of recurrent disease in liver recipients can be problematic, because common posttransplant complications may appear clinically, histologically, or radiologically similar to recurrent disease. For example, the differentiation between mild acute cellular rejection and recurrent hepatitis C or early recurrent AIH may be difficult. For recurrent PSC, the cholangiographic findings of ischemic injury or chronic rejection or an anastomotic stricture may be

J.F. Trotter, MD (✉)
Director, Hepatology, Baylor University Medical Center, 3410 Worth Street #860, Dallas, TX 75246, USA
e-mail: james.trotter@baylorhealth.edu

M.G. Swain, MD, MSc, FRCPC, FAASLD
Cal Wenzel Family Foundation Chair in Hepatology, Professor of Medicine, Head, Division of Gastroenterology and Hepatology, University of Calgary, Section Head, Section of Gastroenterology and Hepatology, Calgary Zone, Alberta Health Services, TRW Building, 3280 Hospital Dr., NW, Calgary, Alberta, Canada T2N 4N1

L.M. Forman (ed.), *Primary Sclerosing Cholangitis*, DOI 10.1007/978-3-319-40908-5_17

indistinguishable from recurrent PSC. One proposed set of criteria for PSC disease recurrence includes a. cholangiogram showing non-anastomotic biliary strictures occurring >3 months after transplantation; b. exclusion of other conditions associated with biliary strictures (including hepatic artery thrombosis, cytomegalovirus, chronic rejection); and/or c. liver biopsy showing fibrous cholangitis and/or fibro-obliterative lesions [19]. Second, the discovery of recurrent disease is a function of time as well as ascertainment bias. In the case of PSC, recurrent disease may not be evident for years and a relatively small fraction of patients actually develop recurrence (approximately 1/5) at a rate of approximately 3–5 % per year. Therefore, the longer a cohort is followed, the greater the likelihood of recurrence, and the larger the size of each reported cohort, the lower the variation in recurrence between the cohorts. These three factors (small number of PSC recipients, relatively low rate of recurrence, and increasing rate of recurrence over time) contribute to the wide variation in reported rates of PSC recurrence which are largely drawn from single-center reports. The rate of recurrence is also directly related to the vigor with which recurrent disease is sought. Some centers perform protocol liver biopsy and imaging, thereby potentially reporting recurrence of subclinical recurrent disease. However, most centers perform liver biopsy only reflexively (i.e., on the basis of biochemical or clinical abnormalities), and, therefore, recurrent disease is discovered in its later stages. In the case of PSC, the definitive diagnostic test, endoscopic retrograde cholangiopancreatography (ERCP) or magnetic resonance cholangiopancreatography (MRCP), may be too invasive or expensive, respectively, to warrant disease surveillance. The third important general consideration about recurrent disease is that immunosuppression may have a positive or negative impact on recurrence. The ill effects of immunosuppression are most evident in patients with viral hepatitis (hepatitis B and C). For patients with an autoimmune liver disease, including PSC, immunosuppression may have a protective effect against these disorders. Therefore, variations in immunosuppressive regimens between transplant centers and transplant eras could impact the incidence of recurrent disease. Finally, current data on recurrent disease may not reflect outcomes of future long-term survivors. By all accounts, current liver recipients are sicker at the time of transplant and their donor organs are older than those in previous years. In addition, the level of immunosuppression is also much lower than the early era of transplant. To the extent that these factors alter recurrent disease, graft loss, and patient survival, they could alter the outcomes for current recipients compared to earlier transplant cohorts.

Diagnosis of Recurrent PSC

As noted above, the diagnosis of recurrent PSC depends to some extent on the vigor of posttransplant surveillance. Since there is no effective therapy to prevent recurrent PSC or alter its natural history, protocol biopsies or imaging in asymptomatic patients are not recommended. Therefore, most patients with recurrent disease are usually identified by lab test abnormalities or clinical symptoms. The most common liver function test abnormality associated with recurrent PSC is an elevation in the alkaline phosphatase followed by an elevated bilirubin. Elevation in the alkaline phosphatase may be related to the type of biliary anastomosis performed at the time of transplant. Traditionally, PSC patients undergo complete resection of their biliary tree and therefore require a Roux-en-Y anastomosis (choledochojejunostomy), a biliary anastomosis fashioned from the small bowel and the donor common hepatic duct. Elevations in the alkaline phosphatase up to 200 IU/l are common in patients with a Roux anastomosis, although higher levels may signal the development of recurrent biliary strictures thereby warranting further evaluation. Resection of the entire recipient biliary tree (with subsequent Roux-en-Y anastomosis) has historically been preferred to remove the possibility of strictures and cholangiocarcinoma developing in the recipient's remnant duct. However, there have been a number of studies evaluating duct-to-duct anastomosis (choledochocholedochostomy) compared to a Roux-en-Y in PSC patients. Some of these studies have reported fewer biliary strictures with a DD anastomosis [3, 43] or no difference [10, 11, 16, 20, 22], and two have found higher rates [41, 46]. A recent meta-analysis of ten studies of nearly 1000 patients found no difference in the overall incidence of biliary or anastomotic strictures between the two types (duct-to-duct vs. Roux) of anastomosis in PSC patients [39]. In fact, cholangitis was more common in the Roux-en-Y group (OR 2.9, $p=0.02$). Up to 69 % of PSC patients in these studies had a DD anastomosis with the average being 48 %. There are advantages of a duct-to-duct anastomosis over a Roux-en-Y. Most important is the ease of access to the biliary tree for diagnostic or therapeutic studies via an ERCP (duct-to-duct) compared to percutaneous transhepatic cholangiography (PTC) (Roux-en-Y). Intraoperatively, the duct-to-duct anastomosis is faster and an easier to perform, especially in PSC patients with inflammatory bowel disease who may have undergone previous bowel surgery. Such patients may have a complicated operation due to adhesions, and isolation of sufficient jejunum for the Roux limb can be difficult. Aside from liver function test abnormalities, the most common symptoms of recurrent disease are similar to patients with PSC before transplantation. Jaundice, fever, or abdominal pain should alert the clinician to the possibility of recurrent disease. In patients, with either asymptomatic LFT elevations or clinical symptoms, hepatic imaging with ultrasound is the first step in the evaluation. However, the definitive diagnosis of recurrent PSC requires cholangiography either noninvasively with MRCP or invasively with ERCP or PTC. The choice of diagnostic technique depends on the clinical setting and center preference. For patients with asymptomatic, mild elevations in alkaline phosphatase, noninvasive imaging may be sufficient. However, in patients with clinical symptoms or marked liver test abnormalities, invasive imaging with cholangiography is indicated so that therapeutic treatments (biliary drainage procedures) can be applied if necessary. Because most PSC have had a Roux-en-Y biliary anastomosis, the most common approach for cholangiography is percutaneous transhepatic cholangiography. However, depending on the operator and patient, cholangiography may be successfully performed via an endoscopic approach in up to 90 % of cases [5, 12, 27, 33]. For patients undergoing invasive cholangiography, pre-procedural antibiotics may be helpful in preventing post-procedural clinical symptoms of cholangitis. However, one study evaluating ERCP complications in PSC patients (including non-transplant patients) reported a significantly higher rate of post-procedural cholangitis in the PSC group (4 %) compared to non-PSC patients (0.2 %, $p<0.0002$) despite routine use of antibiotics before the procedure in PSC patients [6].

Similar to the diagnosis of PSC before transplantation, the role of liver biopsy in the diagnosis of recurrent PSC is limited. The typical histologic findings of recurrent PSC include cholangitis, cholestasis, and "onionskin" fibrosis of the bile ducts. In some cases, recurrent PSC may be discovered by liver biopsy in patients with elevated AST/ALT and suspected acute cellular rejection. In patients with a cholestatic pattern of liver function tests, the biopsy could reveal chronic rejection which typically presents in this fashion. While the biopsy may be sufficient for the diagnosis of recurrent PSC by some criteria (see above), patients with histologic evidence of recurrent PSC should undergo biliary imaging with either MRCP, ERCP, or PTC to confirm the diagnosis and measure its extent and severity.

Once biliary strictures have been identified by either noninvasive or invasive cholangiography, the diagnosis of recurrent PSC requires elimination of other potential causes of this finding. The most common postoperative complication associated with biliary strictures is hepatic artery thrombosis or stenosis. Therefore, the patency of the hepatic artery should be evaluated in all patients with biliary strictures with either hepatic arterial Doppler ultrasound (DUS) or hepatic angiography depending on the clinical setting. At most centers, hepatic arterial DUS is sufficient to rule out hepatic arterial problems. If the DUS is sufficiently abnormal, then arteriography is indicated to confirm the diagnosis and perform hepatic arterial stenting, if indicated. Surgical revascularization is rarely helpful for the treatment of recurrent strictures except in special circumstances. Other causes of biliary strictures should be considered including chronic rejection, cytomegalovirus disease, ABO incompatibility between donor-recipient, prolonged donor cold ischemia time, retained biliary stent, recurrent cholangiocarcinoma, and donor after cardiac death (DCD). In some PSC patients, the precise cause of biliary strictures (recurrent PSC vs. another cause) may be difficult to ascertain. However, the treatment of the strictures is largely the same regardless of their etiology.

Treatment of Recurrent PSC

Once identified, the treatment of recurrent PSC is no different than before transplantation. For mild cases, some clinicians will prescribe ursodiol if the patient is not already receiving it. Theoretically, ursodiol may prevent the development of biliary sludge and stones which could lead to recurrent bouts of cholangitis and long-term graft damage. However, as noted below, there is no evidence that this treatment prevents recurrent PSC or improves the natural history of recurrent disease. In pretransplant PSC patients, neither regular dose ursodiol (13–15 mg/kg/day) nor high dose ursodiol (17–23 mg/kg/day or 28–30 mg/kg/day) has demonstrated efficacy [30, 31, 38]. In fact, high-dose ursodiol in pretransplant PSC has been linked to a higher rate of colonic neoplasia [13, 24]. Therefore, ursodiol is not recommended for PSC patients with or without recurrent disease, although some clinicians may prescribe it. In some mild cases, recurrent cholangitis or suspected recurrent cholangitis may be treated with either oral or intravenous antibiotics without biliary drainage procedures. In addition, patients with recurrent cholangitis may benefit from continuous low-dose oral antibiotic therapy to prevent recurrent symptoms. Aside from preventing recurrent cholangitis, there is limited data in pretransplant PSC patients that short-term antibiotics (12 weeks, vancomycin, metronidazole, or minocycline) are associated with a significant reduction in alkaline phosphatase by about 50 % with some short-term improvement of symptoms [42, 44]. While antibiotics are a helpful component in the treatment of acute cholangitis, biliary drainage is the most effective means of symptomatic improvement. The most common means of biliary drainage is through the placement of percutaneous biliary drainage tubes. However, as noted above, in selected cases endoscopic placement of biliary stents may be used. Typically, biliary drainage tubes or stents must be changed ever 8–12 weeks. In general, the size of the drainage tubes is increased at each session until a maximally tolerated drainage tube or stent is in place. Percutaneous biliary tubes are most effective for patients with isolated strictures in the large ducts (common hepatic or right or left hepatic ducts). Patients with more diffuse disease in the smaller ducts typically have less benefit from percutaneous drains. The total duration of biliary drainage is a decision made based on the judgment and experience of the treating physician with some input for the patient. In most instances, biliary drains should stay in for at least 3–6 months but in many instances for much longer. Their presence in the bile duct over a long period of time may help in reestablishing patency of the biliary duct by increasing the diameter of the stricture, especially if continuous "upsizing" of the drainage tubes is possible. The decision to remove the biliary drain depends on the clinical situation and assessment of the patient's response to the drains over time. In patients with favorable characteristics, the duration of the biliary drains could be as short as 3–6 months. These characteristics include localized disease, significant improvement in liver tests, absence of recurrent cholangitis, and patency of the biliary system on cholangiography. However, patients without these features may require chronic indwelling biliary drains. In some cases, the input of the patient is helpful in making this decision. The advantages of removal of the drains (absence of external biliary drain appendage, absence of ongoing biliary drain exchanges) must be balanced with the potential risks (recurrent clinical cholangitis, replacement of the biliary drains requiring percutaneous procedure with attendant risk and pain).

Over time numerous studies have identified potential risk factors for PSC recurrence. Unfortunately, the list of risk factors is very long and diverse. Collectively, these risk factors are not particularly informative in terms of how to effectively avoid recurrence through specific management recommendations. These risk factors include younger recipient age [45], older donor age [21], male sex [34, 45], sex mismatch [28], acute cellular rejection [4, 25, 35], steroid-resistant rejection [7, 29], CMV infection or mismatch [14, 25, 35], related donor [15], use of extended-donor criteria graft [2], presence of inflammatory bowel disease [21], INR [21], and presence of CCA before transplantation [8]. In summary, there is no specific modifiable or non-modifiable risk factor which would change the selection of patients for liver transplant or their management afterward.

Similar to pretransplant disease, patients who develop severe (recurrent) PSC may be considered for (re)transplantation. However, in the current era of high-MELD liver transplantation, many of these patients are very ill and debilitated at the time of retransplantation. The addition of advancing age and the ill effects of years of immunosuppression further adds to this problem. Consequently, some patients may not be considered eligible for retransplantation or once re-listed may sufficiently deteriorate leading to removal from the list. Finally, while biliary drains help greatly in the symptomatic treatment of recurrent PSC, some patients become what may be termed as "biliary cripples." Such patients have enough biliary drainage to prevent MELD score sufficient for transplantation with inadequate drainage to prevent chronic debility from ongoing cholangitis.

Natural History of PSC After Liver Transplant

As noted above, patients with PSC have among the best prognosis of any group of liver transplant recipients. Recent data from the Scientific Registry of Transplant Recipients show that patients with cholestatic liver disease (about ½ of whom have PSC) have the highest posttransplant survival rate of any patient disease cohort with 5-year graft survival rates of 78 % [23]. Data from the European Liver Transplant Registry reports 72 % 5-year graft survival rates [1]. The Nordic Liver Transplant Registry included 796 PSC patients with a 5-year graft survival rate of 75 % which was only exceeded by PBC [17]. PSC recurrence occurs in some patients as reported in numerous studies. Data from a meta-analysis evaluated 14 studies of 940 patients undergoing liver transplant for PSC with a median follow-up of 58 months [18]. They reported a recurrence rate of 17 %. Because some of the smaller studies reported the highest recurrence rates, the weighted recurrence risk is only 11 %. They also reported insufficient data to determine any effect of immunosuppression (tacrolimus vs. cyclosporine) on outcomes. Large studies subsequent to this meta-analysis have reported similar results. Data from the University of Colorado reported 22/130 (17 %) with recurrent disease with a median follow-up of 66 months [8] See Fig. 17.1. Fifteen of 22 patients with recurrent PSC were successfully treated

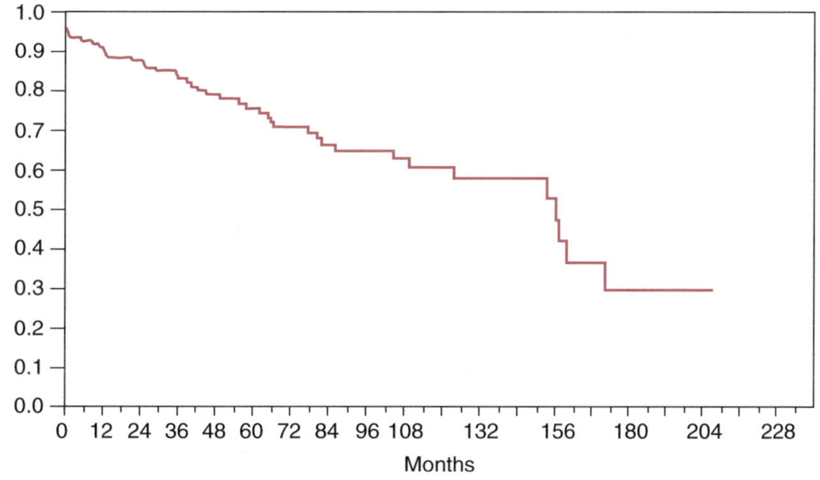

Fig. 17.1 PSC recurrence-free survival after transplant (From: Campsen et al. [8])

medically with ursodiol or biliary drainage, but 7/22 progressed to retransplantation. A multicenter report from the United Kingdom of 679 PSC patients found 81 (14.3 %) patients developed recurrent PSC and 37 (48.7 %) of whom developed graft failure [40]. Another large single-center trial from the United Kingdom of 200 PSC patients followed for a median time of 1957 (approximately 65 months) reported 37 % recurrent disease and 8 % graft loss rate from recurrence [9]. A German multicenter report of 335 PSC patients followed for a mean of 99 months found 20.3 % with recurrent disease and 5-year graft survival rates slightly lower than other reports at 69 % [21].

Living Donor Liver Transplantation

In terms of recurrent PSC after LDLT, there is limited information of about posttransplant outcomes. Data from the A2ALL Study reported that PSC patients had a significantly higher survival rate compared to other disease etiologies [37]. Data from a Japanese survey study on 114 PSC patients all undergoing LDLT at 29 institutions reported a recurrence rate of 27 % and graft loss rates of 69 % in patients with recurrent disease. They reported the following as risk factors for recurrent disease in multivariate analysis: high MELD scores, first-degree-relative donors, postoperative CMV infection, and early biliary anastomotic complications [15]. However, since there is no DDLT comparator group, these data are difficult to place in context. An analysis of the SRTR registry compared patient and graft survival rates for autoimmune and cholestatic disease (including PSC) for LDLT vs. DDLT recipients. There was no difference in patient or graft survival rates for LDLT vs. DDLT in this cohort [26].

Summary Paragraph

An uncommon indication for liver transplantation, PSC is associated with excellent long-term survival rates largely due to the relatively young age of recipients and their absence of comorbid medical conditions which could jeopardize the success of the operation. However, disease recurrence occurs in about one in six patients. The diagnosis may be suspected by elevated liver function tests, typically the alkaline phosphatase or bilirubin, and requires confirmation with either liver biopsy or cholangiography with ERCP or cross-sectional imaging. While numerous risk factors for recurrence have been reported, none have practical implications. There is no known therapy for recurrent disease that predictably changes its natural history. Most patients are administered ursodiol, and symptomatic cholangitis is treated with antibiotics and biliary drainage procedures, as indicated. Recurrent disease can be managed effectively, and graft loss requiring retransplantation does not occur in most cases.

References

1. Adam R. Evolution of indications and results of liver transplantation in Europe. A report from the European Liver Transplant Registry (ELTR). J Hepatol. 2012;57:675–88.
2. Alabraba E, Nightingale P, Gunson B, Hubscher S, Olliff S, Mirza D, Neuberger J. A re-evaluation of the risk factors for the recurrence of primary sclerosing cholangitis in liver allografts. Liver Transpl. 2009;15:330–40.
3. Al-Judaibi B, Hernandez Alejandro R, Uhanova J, Marotta P, Mosli M, Chandok N. Duct-to-duct biliary anastomosis yields similar outcomes to Roux-en-Y hepaticojejunostomy in liver transplantation for primary sclerosing cholangitis. Hepat Mon. 2015;15:e18811.
4. Alexander J, Lord JD, Yeh MM, Cuevas C, Bakthavatsalam R, Kowdley KV. Risk factors for recurrence of primary sclerosing cholangitis after liver transplantation. Liver Transpl. 2008;14:245–51.
5. Azeem N, Tabibian JH, Baron TH, Orhurhu V, Rosen CB, Petersen BT, et al. Use of a single-balloon enteroscope compared with variable-stiffness colonoscopes for endoscopic retrograde cholangiography in liver transplant patients with Roux-en Y biliary anastomosis. Gastrointest Endosco. 2013;77:568–77.
6. Bangarulingam SY, Gossard AA, Petersen BT, Ott BJ, Lindor KD. Complications of endoscopic retrograde cholangiopancreatography in primary sclerosing cholangitis. Am J Gastroenterol. 2009;104:855–60.
7. Brandsaeter B, Schrumpf E, Bentdal O, Brabrand K, Smith HJ, Abildgaard A, et al. Recurrent primary sclerosing cholangitis after liver transplantation: a magnetic resonance cholangiography study with analyses of predictive factors. Liver Transpl. 2005;11:1361–9.

8. Campsen J, Zimmerman MA, Trotter JF, Wachs M, Bak T, Steinberg T, Kam I. Clinically recurrent primary sclerosing cholangitis following liver transplantation: a time course. Liver Transpl. 2008;14:181–5.
9. Cholongitas E, Shusang V, Papatheodoridis GV, Marelli L, Manousou P, Rolando N, et al. Risk factors for recurrence of primary sclerosing cholangitis after liver transplantation. Liver Transpl. 2008;14:138–43.
10. Damrah O, Sharma D, Burroughs A, Rolando N, Fernando B, Davidson B, Rolles K. Duct-to-duct biliary reconstruction in orthotopic liver transplantation for primary sclerosing cholangitis: a viable and safe alternative. Transpl Int. 2012;25:64–8.
11. Distante V, Farouk M, Kurzawinski TR, Ahmed SW, Burroughs AK, Davidson BR, Rolles K. Duct-to-duct biliary reconstruction following liver transplantation for primary sclerosing cholangitis. Transpl Int. 1996;9:126–30.
12. Dellon ES, Kohn GP, Morgan DR, Grimm IS. Endoscopic retrograde cholangiopancreatography with single-balloon enteroscopy is feasible in patients with a prior Roux-en-Y anastomosis. Dig Endoscopy. 2014;26 Suppl 2:109–15.
13. Eaton JE, Silveira MG, Pardi DS, Sinakos E, Kowdley KV, Luketic VA, et al. High-dose ursodeoxycholic acid is associated with the development of colorectal neoplasia in patients with ulcerative colitis and primary sclerosing cholangitis. Am J Gastroenterol. 2011;106(9):1638–45.
14. Egawa H, Taira K, Teramukai S, Haga H, Ueda Y, Yonezawa A, et al. Risk factors for recurrence of primary sclerosing cholangitis after living donor liver transplantation: a single center experience. Dig Dis Sci. 2009;54:1347–54.
15. Egawa H, Ueda Y, Ichida T, Teramukai S, Nakanuma Y, Onishi S, Tsubouchi H. Risk factors for recurrence of primary sclerosing cholangitis after living donor liver transplantation in Japanese registry. Am J Transpl. 2011;11:518–27.
16. Esfeh JM, Eghtesad B, Hodgkinson P, Diago T, Fujiki M, Hashimoto K, et al. Duct-to-duct biliary reconstruction in patients with primary sclerosing cholangitis undergoing liver transplantation. HPB (Oxford). 2011;13:651–5.
17. Fosby B, Melum E, Bjøro K, Bennet W, Rasmussen A, Andersen IM, et al. Liver transplantation in the Nordic countries – an intention to treat and post-transplant analysis from The Nordic Liver Transplant Registry 1982–2013. Scan J Gastroenterol. 2015;50:797–808.
18. Gautam M, Cheruvattath R, Balan V. Recurrence of autoimmune liver disease after liver transplantation: a systematic review. Liver Transpl. 2006;12:1813–24.
19. Graziadei IW, Wiesner RH, Batts KP, Marotta PJ, LaRusso NF, Porayko MA, et al. Recurrence of primary sclerosing cholangitis following liver transplantation. Hepatology. 1999;29:1050–6.
20. Heffron TG, Smallwood GA, Ramcharan T, Davis L, Connor K, Martinez E, Stieber AC. Duct-to-duct biliary anastomosis for patients with sclerosing cholangitis undergoing liver transplantation. Transplant Proc. 2003;35:3006–7.
21. Hildebrand T, Pannicke N, Dechene A, Gotthardt DN, Kirchner G, Reiter FP, et al. Biliary strictures and recurrence after liver transplantation for primary sclerosing cholangitis: a retrospective multicenter analysis. Liver Transpl. 2016;22:42–52.
22. Hoekstra H, Buis CI, Verdonk RC, van der Hilst CS, van der Jagt EJ, Haagsma EB, Porte RJ. Is Roux-en-Y choledochojejunostomy an independent risk factor for nonanastomotic biliary strictures after liver transplantation? Liver Transpl. 2009;15:924–30.
23. http://srtr.transplant.hrsa.gov/annual_reports/2012/pdf/03_liver_13.pdf.
24. Imam MH, Sinakos E, Gossard AA, Kowdley KV, Luketic VA, Harrison EM, et al. High-dose ursodeoxycholic acid increases risk of adverse outcomes in patients with early stage primary sclerosing cholangitis. Aliment Pharmacol Ther. 2011;34:1185–92.
25. Jeyarajah DR, Netto GJ, Lee SP, Testa G, Abbasoglu O, Husberg BS, et al. Recurrent primary sclerosing cholangitis after orthotopic liver transplantation: is chronic rejection part of the disease process? Transplantation. 1998;66:1300–6.
26. Kashyap R, Safadjou S, Chen R, Mantry P, Sharma R, Patil V, et al. Living donor and deceased donor liver transplantation for autoimmune and cholestatic liver diseases – an analysis of the UNOS database. J Gastrointest Surg. 2010;14:1362–9.
27. Katanuma A, Isayama H. Current status of endoscopic retrograde cholangiopancreatography in patients with surgically altered anatomy in Japan: questionnaire survey and important discussion points at Endoscopic Forum Japan 2013. Gastrointestin Endosc. 2013;77:568–77.
28. Khettry U, Keaveny A, Goldar-Najafi A, Lewis WD, Pomfret EA, Pomposelli JJ, et al. Liver transplantation for primary sclerosing cholangitis: a long term clinicopathologic study. Hum Pathol. 2003;34:1127–36.
29. Kugelmas M, Spiegelman P, Osgood MJ, Young DA, Trotter JF, Steinberg T, et al. Different immunosuppressive regimens and recurrence of primary sclerosing cholangitis after liver transplantation. Liver Transpl. 2003;9:727–32.
30. Lindor KD. Ursodiol for primary sclerosing cholangitis. Mayo Primary Sclerosing Cholangitis-Ursodeoxycholic Acid Study Group. N Engl J Med. 1997;336:691–5.
31. Lindor KD, Kowdley KV, Luketic VA, Harrison ME, McCashland T, Befeler AS, et al. High-dose ursodeoxycholic acid for the treatment of primary sclerosing cholangitis. Hepatology. 2009;50:808–14.
32. Lodhi SA, Lamb KE, Meier-Kriesche HU. Solid organ allograft survival improvement in the United States: the long-term does not mirror the dramatic short-term success. Am J Transplant. 2011;11:1226–35.
33. Lopes TL, Baron TH. Endoscopic retrograde cholangiopancreatography in patients with Roux-en-Y anatomy. J Hepatobiliary Pancreat Sci. 2011;18:332–8.

34. Mogl MT, Albert K, Pascher A, Sauer I, Puhl G, Gül S, et al. Survival without biliary complications after liver transplant for primary sclerosing cholangitis. Exp Clin Transplant. 2013;11:510–21.
35. Moncrief KJ, Savu A, Ma MM, Bain VG, Wong WW, Tandon P. The natural history of inflammatory bowel disease and primary sclerosing cholangitis after liver transplantation – a single-centre experience. Can J Gastroenterol. 2010;24:40–6.
36. O'Grady JG. Phenotypic expression of recurrent disease after liver transplantation. Am J Transplant. 2010;10:1149–54.
37. Olthoff KM, Smith AR, Abecassis M, Baker T, Emond JC, Berg CL, et al. Defining long-term outcomes with living donor liver transplantation in North America. Ann Surg. 2015;262:465–755.
38. Olsson R, Boberg KM, de Muckadell OS, Lindgren S, Hultcrantz R, Folvik G, et al. High-dose ursodeoxycholic acid in primary sclerosing cholangitis: a 5-year multicenter, randomized, controlled study. Gastroenterology. 2005;129:1464–72.
39. Pandanaboyana S, Bell R, Bartlett AJ, McCall J, Hidalgo E. Meta-analysis of duct-to-duct versus Roux-en-Y biliary reconstruction following liver transplantation for primary sclerosing cholangitis. Transpl Int. 2015;28:485–91.
40. Ravikumar R, Tsochatzis E, Jose S, Allison M, Athale A, Creamer F, et al. Risk factors for recurrent primary sclerosing cholangitis after liver transplantation. J Hepatol. 2015;63:1139–46.
41. Schmitz V, Neumann UP, Puhl G, Tran ZV, Neuhaus P, Langrehr JM. Surgical complications and long-term outcome of different biliary reconstructions in liver transplantation for primary sclerosing cholangitis-choledochoduodenostomy versus choledochojejunostomy. Am J Transpl. 2006;6:379–85.
42. Silveira MG, Torok NJ, Gossard AA, Keach JC, Jorgensen RA, Petz JL, Lindor KD. Minocycline in the treatment of patients with primary sclerosing cholangitis: results of a pilot study. Am J Gastroenterol. 2009;104:83–8.
43. Sutton ME, Bense RD, Lisman T, van der Jagt EJ, van den Berg AP, Porte RJ. Duct-to-duct reconstruction in liver transplantation for primary sclerosing cholangitis is associated with fewer biliary complications in comparison with hepaticojejunostomy. Liver Transpl. 2014;20:457–63.
44. Tabibian JH, Weeding E, Jorgensen RA, Petz JL, Keach JC, Talwalkar JA, Lindor KD. Randomised clinical trial: vancomycin or metronidazole in patients with primary sclerosing cholangitis – a pilot study. Aliment Pharmacol Ther. 2013;37:604–12.
45. Vera A, Moledina S, Gunson B, Hubscher S, Mirza D, Olliff S, Neuberger J. Risk factors for recurrence of primary sclerosing cholangitis of liver allograft. Lancet. 2002;360:1943–4.
46. Welsh FK, Wigmore SJ. Roux-en-Y Choledochojejunostomy is the method of choice for biliary reconstruction in liver transplantation for primary sclerosing cholangitis. Transplantation. 2004;77:602–4.

Index

L.M. Forman (ed.), *Primary Sclerosing Cholangitis*, DOI 10.1007/978-3-319-40908-5

D

E

MIX
Papier aus verantwortungsvollen Quellen
Paper from responsible sources
FSC® C105338
FSC
www.fsc.org

If you have any concerns about our products,
you can contact us on
ProductSafety@springernature.com

In case Publisher is established outside the EU,
the EU authorized representative is:
Springer Nature Customer Service Center GmbH
Europaplatz 3, 69115 Heidelberg, Germany

Printed by Libri Plureos GmbH
in Hamburg, Germany